Susan La Flesche Picotte, M.D.

Susan La Flesche Picotte, M.D.

Omaha Indian Leader and Reformer

By Benson Tong
Foreword by Dennis Hastings

UNIVERSITY OF OKLAHOMA PRESS : NORMAN

Also by Benson Tong

Unsubmissive Women: Chinese Prostitutes in Nineteenth-Century San Francisco (Norman, 1994)

Portions of chapter 6, "This Curse of Drink," were previously published as "Allotment, Alcohol, and the Omahas" in the *Great Plains Quarterly* 17, no. 1 (Winter 1997).

Published with the assistance of the National Endowment for the Humanities, a federal agency which supports the study of such fields as history, philosophy, literature, and language.

ISBN: 0–8061–3140–3

1 2 3 4 5 6 7 8 9 10

In memory of my mentor, teacher, and friend,
Gerald Thompson (1947–98),
who shared my reverence for the native peoples of
North America

Contents

Illustrations

Foreword

Susan La Flesche Picotte was born into the Omaha Nation in a tepee in 1865. She went on to become the first Indian woman doctor, graduating from the Woman's Medical College of Pennsylvania on March 14, 1889. After a year as intern in the Woman's Hospital of Philadephia, she obtained a government appointment and went back home to serve as physician to the Omaha reservation boarding school.

Soon Indians from all over the reservation began coming to Susan for help. The reservation was thirty miles long by fifteen miles wide, and she made house calls by walking or driving a buggy, most often alone, across the rugged land. In the homes of the sick, she often served as nurse and cook and, in many cases, as funeral director and member of the clergy.

Susan La Flesche Picotte's accomplishments, her generosity, intelligence, and her humanitarian achievements deserve our attention and admiration. There has been a need for a full-length biography of Susan La Flesche Picotte, and that need is met in this very good book. Through this biography, Dr. Susan emerges as a notable hero in American history. I am tremendously impressed by Benson Tong's comprehensive research into both published and oral records and by his dedication to honoring the past and seeing Susan's story preserved for all—especially for the Omaha Nation, an almost forgotten people.

Before we can set out on the road to success, we have to know where we are going; before we can know that, we must determine where we have been. It seems that a basic requirement is to study the history of our past civilizations. The changes that have been made in recent years regarding recorded versions of American history, or Omaha history in particular, are still continuing today. The extent of this change is governed not so much by a voluntary reappraisal among historians as by the pressure of once-forgotten peoples, who have only recently attained the awareness, cohesiveness, and political power which have motivated them to demand these changes.

The new voices that we are witnessing in recorded history today reflect a recognition of the demands of the dispossessed and over-looked *peoples* who have had a role in history to receive, finally, the attention to which they are entitled. By including the stories of Indians, women, and others, we expand our history in a solid positive direction which addresses the uniqueness of their contributions. Such a new course can help provide Omahas and other neglected peoples with a sense of identity and belonging—a means of overcoming a collective inferiority complex. These stories can provide inspiration for us, motivate us, and help improve scholastic interest among our young people.

The correction of past injustice is not simply a service to those who have been wronged, it is a service to everyone. For we cannot correctly understand the present, if we have a distorted interpretation of the past.

DENNIS HASTINGS

Walthill, Nebraska

Acknowledgments

Unlike my first book, *Unsubmissive Women: Chinese Prostitutes in Nineteenth-Century San Francisco*, this work posed almost no logistical problems and required few favors from far-flung friends. Still, it was a challenge to cover the thousands of miles traveled by Susan La Flesche Picotte during the course of her lifetime. From Lincoln, Nebraska, to Hartford, Connecticut, I searched and collected the fragmented evidence. In this endeavor, I received the able assistance of my dearest friend, William John Bigelow, who accompanied me on several of these exacting trips. I am deeply grateful to him for the company and encouragement.

The late Gerald Thompson, who passed away suddenly in 1998, was a source of inspiration to me since the early days of my graduate work. His guidance enabled me to transform a master's thesis into a published work, and his paternal support kept me on course during the years. He guided me even though the rewards of mentoring are meager at best. For all the gifts he freely offered, I will remember him always with profound gratitude.

Diane Britton and Ronald Lora read the original version of this manuscript. Over the years, I have learned much from them; both introduced me to the complex sociopolitical milieu of the turn of the century. From that introduction, I developed a fascination with Progressive-Era reforms—a subject covered in this biography. I must also thank Glenda Riley of Ball State University, Muncie, Indiana, who graciously agreed, despite a hectic schedule, to read this work. I appreciate her insightful comments and suggestions, which led me to reconceptualize my image of Susan La Flesche Picotte.

Almost all academics depend on a circle of colleagues to help them survive the brunt of professional demands. I am no exception. An unexpected incident in the fall of 1994, however, turned some colleagues into close friends. During a period of my work when few listened and many turned away, Leslie Heaphy, Regan A. Lutz, and David Brown drew near and offered me much needed mental and emotional support. They reaffirmed my faith in friendship and its value. Exemplifying the virtue of "speaking kindly to each other," to quote Omaha chief Big Elk, they provided eloquent testimony of goodwill and tolerance, values I hold dearly. We have gone our separate ways as we have answered our respective professional callings, but those common bonds will never be severed.

I would also like to acknowledge the indispensable, professional aid of the staffs of the Nebraska State Historical Society; National Archives; Connecticut State Library; Hampton University Archives; Presbyterian Historical Society; National Anthropological Archives, Smithsonian Institution; and the Archives and Special Collections on Women in Medicine, The Medical College of Pennsylvania and Hospital.

I end these acknowledgments by returning to John. Since 1990 he has been a selfless friend. His support was crucial in producing the first book, and years later he is still around, despite the many twists and turns in my personal life. Though not a historian, John was more than happy to be carried away to different spaces and times, and in return he generously shared what he learned with me. For his steadfastness, I owe him an unmeasurable debt and my deepest affection.

Introduction

While choosing materials to use in teaching my first Native American history class, I came across Valerie Sherer Mathes's biographical article on Susan La Flesche Picotte, M.D. (1865–1915). Intrigued, I read the essay and soon decided that her remarkable and inspiring life deserved a book-length biography. Throughout this book, Susan La Flesche Picotte and the rest of her family members are often identified by their first names. My intent is to avoid confusion created by multiple use of the family name. In doing so, I mean no disrespect to Dr. Picotte's or her family's legacy.

Born into the fairly acculturated, pragmatically oriented Omaha tribe, young Susan, a mixed blood, grew up in a time of tumultuous change. By the mid-nineteenth century, the growing dominance of American capitalism, operating in the name of expansive nationalism, and an ethnocentric understanding of republican citizenry, had forced the Omahas to give up most of their traditional economy. Since 1854 the tribe had accepted life on the reservation, although a traditionalist faction continued to look to the Indian past for mental and emotional guidance. Faced with the pressures of attempting to integrate the warrior tribal culture with the realities of reservation life, many Omahas, her father Chief Joseph La Flesche included, chose to journey toward acculturation and the selective adoption of Euro-American culture. But they made the transition without losing their ties to their former lifeway.

Susan's life clearly exemplified that journey as she struggled to keep her place in two worlds—the world of the Omahas and that of the Euro-Americans. Along the way, she assumed the challenging role of the cultural mediator, or broker—one who promoted certain elements of the larger white society, but was ever-mindful of the value of her Indian roots. As a mediator, she became the embodiment of two lifeways. She lived in a cultural borderland, which she employed as a bridge between peoples. Though undoubtedly influenced by the cross-cultural tensions that enveloped her, Susan chose to move into the role of culture broker following several personal experiences within cross-cultural environments.[1]

The Americanization policy, with its emphasis on education, opened the door for the young Omaha woman to step into the world of Western knowledge. She became the first American Indian woman to graduate from a medical college—a unique achievement for Native Americans of any gender during that period. Though she practiced Euro-American medicine, she never belittled traditional remedies. In fact, Susan attributed her interest in curing people to her childhood curiosity about the medicine men and their work. Thus, like many other cultural intermediaries of the past, she traced the trajectory of her life from early tribal influences.

As an OIA (Office of Indian Affairs) physician, she served her people with compassion and selflessness. In her capacity as medicial missionary for the Women's National Indian Association and later for the Board of Home Missions of the U.S. Presbyterian Church, Susan offered succor, both physical and spiritual, to Omahas deprived of adequate medical attention and distanced from many traditional beliefs.

As a promoter of various causes, ranging from prohibition to the anti-tuberculosis campaign, Susan came to the forefront of public attention. In her crusade for temperance and preventive health measures, Susan became the quintessential Progressive-Era reformer. Her work—ranging from medical care to evangelism—positioned her, in a time of fluid socioeconomic conditions, as a link between local communities and regional and national structures.[2]

Motivated by her strong Presbyterian faith and the legacy of her family's activism, Susan threw herself into the role of cultural intermediary, even at the cost of tribal factionalism. She was probably also propelled by the intangible sense of self-satisfaction and, to some extent, the sense of personal power that she derived from her labors. However, at times her indomitable strong will and the projected brokerage placed her at cross purposes with the interests of some tribal members.

But Susan, like the rest of her family, never severed her ties to the Indian community. Her efforts to establish a hospital on the reservation, despite her own poor health, bear witness to her dogged determination. In middle-age she fought, following in the footsteps of her father, for the Omahas' sovereignty in land management. Though fully aware that she could jeopardize her good standing with the Indian Office, she spoke openly and bluntly, attacking the creaky bureaucracy that had denied the Indians their claims and land titles. Like most cultural mediators, Susan frequently sought to convince Euro-Americans of the rights and racial potential of Indians. In the struggle for land autonomy, she argued time and again that her people, given their success in attaining "civilization," deserved to be shorn of the shackles of OIA paternalism.

However, Susan was not a very systematic thinker when it came to reform of Indian policy. She argued for freedom, while all the time she pleaded for government protection against the "evils" of white society. Susan largely agreed with white reformers that she herself was living proof of what Indians could accomplish under the sway of "civilization." It may have been this belief that led her to conclude that other Indians could also survive and prosper in the white-dominated world, but this was a facile conclusion. Many Native Americans were simply unprepared to answer the call of progress, a fact of which she was well aware. Susan never resolved the conflict between her calls for protection and for autonomy. The problems of the day were too complex, and so a clear-cut answer proved to be elusive.

In failing to arrive at a satisfactory solution for the Indian predicament, Susan suffered an identity crisis to some degree. Earlier in life Susan had expounded the virtues of Euro-American values, but later, uncertainty colored her sense of self. This is not surprising since she lived in a complex world of multiple, often conflicting, loyalties. Further, cultural exchange is a dynamic process that rarely allows a person to retain equilibrium. Susan began to question some of the outcomes of the "de-Indianization" process, particularly land allotment in severalty and citizenship. In so doing, she reevaluated her self-perception and her perception of others. This indecisive, fluid element in Susan's image of selfhood supports the argument that identity, being in part a relationship of the "Other" to oneself, "is always a structure that is split, it always has ambivalence within it."[3] Certainly Susan is proof that even the most educated Indians, in redefining their sense of self, did not always fit into the linear, assimilationist model of change. The process of transformation from a traditional to an acculturated Indian was ongoing, persistent, and multifaceted, and it was not necessarily irreversible.

Until the end of her life, Susan took pride in her Indianness as well as pride in her accomplishments within the dominant white society. She had moved successfully between the two worlds that encompassed her life. Though early in her public career she may have given some Euro-American contemporaries the impression that she accepted Victorian gender sensibilities, she actually adhered little to that prescriptive, white middle-class ideal. Like so many other American women of all backgrounds, she resisted the metaphor of separate spheres and its attendant unequal power relations.[4]

Susan, in fact, projected a syncretic Indian feminine identity, one rooted in shifting native gender roles that merged traditional beliefs with cultural innovation. She took on some accoutrements of Western civilization but her "Indianness" remained intact. An examination of her life may reflect a typical life study in what anthropologists label "permissive diversity," or biculturalism. The latter, however, is somewhat misleading, because biculturalism suggests a phenomenon of restriction of or detraction from Indianness. But becoming bicultural is not a matter of accepting all change—of becoming 100 percent

American. In fact biculturalism, or cross-cultural mixing, can be seen as a form of recovering and reconstructing identity, a form of decolonization. James A. Clifton argues that those who undergo this transformation become cognitively and "culturally enlarged."[5] Further, if an Indian is quintessentially "a moral idea," as N. Scott Momaday believes, and the criteria for adjudging Indianness is a lived identity, then Susan certainly qualifies as an Indian.[6] And she achieved that personal success in spite of poor health and family problems.

As with other biographies of women, this biography of Susan La Flesche Picotte is also a vehicle for exhibiting a particular time period from a feminine perspective.[7] Though Susan's public career spanned less than a quarter of a century, she earned a place in the hearts and minds of her contemporaries for her attempts to reduce the chasm between two seemingly irreconcilable cultures. Like many other cultural brokers, she had "breached language barriers, clarified diplomatic misunderstandings, softened potential conflict, and awakened that commonality shared by the human race."[8] She became, in essence, the model cultural mediator—one who tried to improve the quality of human life while fostering mutual understanding across the racial divide.

Susan La Flesche Picotte, M.D.

CHAPTER ONE

"I Never Saw a Battle"

"My mother has seen many battles. The younger Indians, of course, have never seen a battle and only know of them from the stories of the old warriors," recalled Dr. Susan La Flesche. The year was 1908; the place, Walthill, Nebraska. An Omaha tribal leader and a campaigner for Indian policy reform, La Flesche was the subject of an interview by the *Omaha World Herald*. Asked to recollect the colorful, "bloody" past, she replied: "When we used to go on buffalo hunts, we always had signals in case the enemy appeared. The Sioux were our enemies at that time and often used to steal upon hunting parties and scalp them." However, in the next moment she admitted that "as a child I was accustomed to keep a sharp lookout, but I never saw a battle."[1] Susan La Flesche had grown up and had become the first female Native American physician, but by the time the infant Susan entered the world of the Omahas, or "Upstream People," in 1865, tumultuous upheavals had already transformed the sacred native landscape in Nebraska.

The original environment of the Omahas was not Nebraska but most probably the Great Lakes region. According to the Sacred Legend, or tribal creation story, the Great Spirit, or *Wakon'da*, brought the Omahas out of the water to live "near a large body of water in wooded country."[2] The forebears of the Omahas were originally members of a single Dhe'giha division of Siouian speakers that also included the Kansa, Quapaw, Osage, and Ponca Indians. Over the course of centuries they migrated down the Ohio River to the Mississippi, where a separation occurred among the cognate tribes. The Omahas and the Poncas went up the Mississippi, and by the late seventeenth century they had reached the eastern side of the Missouri River in western Iowa.[3]

During the next century, following several pitched battles with the Yankton Sioux, the Upstream People journeyed west and eventually crossed the Missouri. The Omahas and the Poncas moved steadily southward until they finally arrived in Nebraska sometime in the early 1720s.[4] Following a separation from the Poncas and a failed settlement attempt, the tribe established its primary village—the "Big Village"—at Omaha Creek, on the west side of the Missouri.[5]

Guided by a practical, self-reliant ethos—one encapsulated by their creation legend's refrain, "and the people thought"—the Omahas creatively harnessed the natural resources of their ecosystems.[6] The tallgrass prairies, river valleys, and mixed-grass plains served as the boundaries of their world. Within this world, the Omahas created a subsistence economy based on agriculture and hunting—an economy that offered security and sustenance. In so doing, they engaged in a traditional way of life that transcended the limits of their environment.[7] This pragmatic, worldly mind-set became a part of young Susan's sense of self.

Before the late-nineteenth century the Omahas' traditional cycle of economic life began in the chilly, damp month of April with ceremonies to consecrate corn seeds, the product of Mother Earth. According to an article Susan wrote in 1912, after the chanting of the maize ritual song the women received the sacred red corn grains and mixed them with seeds from the previous harvest.[8] In early May the Indian women, whose economic roles complemented those of the men, cleared and burned the vegetation. Then, the blessed corn seeds were planted, followed by beans, watermelons, squash, pumpkins, and some tobacco. By late June or early July, the cultivated fields and the village of earth-covered lodges were abandoned for the buffalo hunt, while the crops matured in the simmering heat of the Midwest summer.[9]

Before each seasonal hunt could proceed the Omahas performed the ritual of the white buffalo robe, which called upon spiritual powers to aid in the chase. Then the whole tribe moved out to help with the hunt. These were "nice times" for Susan and her sisters, but the hunt was also a crucial economic activity. The summer and winter hunts provided about half of the Indians' food. In addition, the bison served as raw material for clothing, shelter, tools, utensils, and weapons. As in most tribes, the Omaha women were responsible for processing the gains of the hunt, which included drying and jerking the meat and dressing and tanning the skins.[10]

By early September the women, saddled with the burden of meat and hides, and the rest of the hunting party would return to the village to be greeted by the sight of the blooming prairie goldenrod. The backbreaking harvest season had arrived. After the joyful feasting and celebration, and after the corn had been safely harvested and stored away, the tribe broke up into small hunting parties. The arduous winter hunt often stretched into spring when the early buds of flora were emerging, and then the whole cycle or "annual round" would begin anew.[11]

Women played a pivotal role in completing this annual cycle. As in other indigenous societies, Omaha women inhabited a specific realm, separate and apart from that of the men. However, their world coexisted in balanced reciprocity with that of the men. The labors of both men and women were acknowledged as necessary for the well-being of the tribe. Thus there was no gender-based status distinction. Furthermore, the division of labor by gender did not preclude men from assisting women in female-specific tasks, or vice-versa.

Similarly absent was the European and American division between domestic and public domains, a division that created a hierarchy. For example, though Omaha men dominated religious life, women were not necessarily on the periphery; many rituals, from those associated with birth to those surrounding death, offered opportunities for women to forge social ties with male members of the tribe. As in most native cultures, the status of Omaha women hinged on wealth, kinship ties, and work performance.[12]

Following the arrival of European colonization, women suffered less decline in status and influence than their male peers. In Susan's time Indian women, living under the aegis of western patriarchal assumptions, held highly limited or no formal authority within tribal government, but they continued to exert influence through internal tribal networks and their roles in reproduction and production. In adult life, Susan would benefit from this gender parity.[13]

In prereservation days the Upstream People traded with neighboring tribes, particularly with the Poncas, to supplement their subsistence economy. Much of the trading was actually reciprocal gift giving and was carried out through the Omahas' Wa'wan or calumet ceremony, which was used to establish fictive relationships between trading parties.[14] The Omahas' trading network expanded in the early 1700s to include Europeans and reached its peak by century's end.[15]

By the late 1790s contact with whites had made life easier, particularly for the Omaha women. Indians secured horses for hauling and relied more on finished household items. Firearms were especially useful, because they facilitated hunting and warfare. To secure valuable guns and horses, the Omahas planted less and hunted more. Their traditional appreciation for practical innovations or ideas probably allowed the permeation of white ways into the *uki'te*, or tribe, without severe factionalization. Not until Susan's lifetime did fragmentation become obvious. Even then, the bond of uki'te (also meaning "to fight") encompassed concepts of community and a sense of unity and continued to facilitate adaptation. Growing up in that milieu, Susan could not help but be affected by the strength of uki'te.[16]

For Omahas the absorption of new influences did not signal the decay or diminution of their culture. Instead, by incorporating European technology and ideas, the Omahas kept their culture viable, and new innovations became as much a part of their traditions as the old ways. But European influence also left an indisputable negative impact on the tribe. Contact brought diseases, particularly smallpox. During their famous journey up the Missouri River in 1804,

Meriwether Lewis and William Clark reported that the Omaha population, estimated at two thousand people in the mid-1790s, had been reduced by one-half after smallpox struck in the winter of 1800–1801. This tragedy was not the first or the last epidemic that struck the tribe.[17] Such biological devastation had long-term repercussions; in Susan's lifetime the population of the Omaha tribe was estimated at less than 1,200 members.

Less fatal, but no less unfortunate, were the intertribal hostilities spurred on by the keen competition for guns and trade goods. An endless cycle of defense and retaliation ensued when raiding parties of nearby enemies such as the Otos and Missouris, Pawnees, and Poncas swooped down on the *hu'thuga*, or camp. Complicating the picture further were the pressures of powerful nomadic hunters such as the Teton and Yanktonai Sioux peoples from the north, who also staked a claim on the limited bison range. As a young girl, Susan heard many stories of these attacks from her elders. The Sioux depredations continued into the mid-nineteenth century and were exacerbated by those of the Sauks from the east.[18]

These pressures on the tribe eventually led to population loss and destroyed villages. Later, when Indians became primary producers in the European-dominated trading network, the emphasis of the Omaha economy shifted from subsistence to production-for-exchange. As a result, the time women spent in processing furs inflated, and the tribal economy became reliant on the Euro-American market—a dependence that persisted as a hallmark of reservation life into the early twentieth century. As an adult Susan, along with her fellow Omahas, would suffer the consequences of this dependency.[19]

Still, at least before the advent of allotment in severalty in the 1880s, the Upstream People preserved much of their traditional way of life. Much of this success could be attributed in part to workable political institutions and cohesive religious beliefs. The Omahas' Council of Seven Chiefs, with its system of hereditary clan leaders, preserved order and unified the various clans. The existence of a chiefly lineage within each clan minimized competition, accommodated family and individual achievement, and maintained tribal cohesion. Even at the height of Euro-American paternalism, this level of unity never entirely disappeared, and that in turn facilitated Susan's rise to tribal leadership.[20]

The Omahas also drew their strong sense of determination from their religion. The Omahas conceived the world as being animated by Wakon'da—so Susan wrote in a 1912 article. Susan's people believed that they came into contact with Wakon'da through rituals and that this ensured success in future endeavors. Religion gave the Omahas their identity, their purpose in life, binding them with the sense of uki'te.[21]

"Holding the people together," to quote the Sacred Legend, was also what historian Michael C. Coleman would later call the Omahas' "non-violent rearguard action"—a successful mechanism that involved avoiding physical conflict with white nations and simultaneous selective adoption of European ways. Susan's generation would continue that strategy of survival. Certainly, the Omahas were never compelled to defend their territory through the use of physical violence. In fact, during much of the last quarter of the eighteenth century these Indians, led by Chief Blackbird, used the strategic location of their Big Village on the middle Missouri to dictate the terms of trade with the Europeans, playing Spanish, English, and later, American traders off against each other. They also reduced the threat from upstream tribes by denying them access to white traders and guns.[22]

That period marked the apogee of Omaha power. But the smallpox outbreak of 1800–1801 and the subsequent demise of the "feared and respected" Chief Blackbird robbed them of centralized authority and capable warriorship. Another decade would pass before the next strong leader, Big Elk, emerged.[23] By then the United States, following the purchase of Louisiana in 1803, had become the arbiter of Indian fortunes and would soon shape Susan's pathway of life.

With the penetration of American traders into the Missouri Valley, the Omahas were drawn closer into the fur trade. Earlier, when the French and Spanish controlled the region, it had been a seller's market, and the Omahas had benefitted from that advantageous position. The wealth accumulated through trading often was offered to tribal leaders as a way to enhance personal and familial prestige. But when the American Fur Company monopolized the trade after the mid-1820s, the Omahas became caught in a buyer's market and, consequently, received less for their labor. Slowly, the Indians surrendered their economic autonomy and became dependent on white traders for goods and services.[24]

The Omaha tribe was rapidly being co-opted into the burgeoning market revolution that grew out of early American industrialism. Dependency, however, also resulted in close cultural encounters. This was evident at the major trading post of Bellevue, not far from the Big Village. At Bellevue, the dominant cohort was the mixed-blood offspring of company employees and their Omaha wives.

Susan's father, Joseph La Flesche (E-sta-ma-za, or Iron Eye), was one such offspring of these "country" marriages. La Flesche's father was a French Canadian fur trader. Joseph La Flesche, Sr., in the tradition of the *coureur de bois*, lived among the Indians. He met Joseph's mother and lived with her, but sometime later he left the tribe and remarried a Ponca woman. Joseph La Flesche, Sr., eventually made his way to Bellevue where, until he died at an unknown age, he was employed by the resident trader, Peter A. Sarpy.[25]

While the background of Joseph's father is indisputable, the same cannot be said about that of his mother. Wa-tun-na, Susan's paternal grandmother, was either Omaha or Ponca. Her tribal affiliation remains an issue today and, consequently, has cast a shadow over Susan's and her natal family's claim to Omaha membership. The nineteenth-century ethnologist James Owen Dorsey claimed that Wa-tun-na was a Ponca. Years later, after Joseph's death, the anthropologist Alice C. Fletcher interviewed a cousin of the family who attested that Wa-tun-na was an Omaha. Francis La Flesche (1857–1932), Joseph's son, who collaborated with Fletcher on *The Omaha Tribe* (1911), offered a genealogy in that landmark work showing that his grandmother was indeed an Omaha. A few friends and descendants of the La Flesche family, however, insisted that she was a Ponca. R. H. Barnes, a modern anthropologist, concluded that Wa-tun-na was a Ponca and that she married an Omaha man after abandoning her frequently absent white spouse. Barnes attributes the confusion about her tribal affiliation to the immediate family's need to identify Wa-tun-na as Omaha so that Joseph's claim to head chieftainship was indisputable.[26]

Equally unclear is Joseph's year of birth. At the time of his death, obituaries reported that he was born in 1822. But later his son Francis (the product of another marriage and so Susan's stepbrother) placed the date as 1818.[27]

Young Joseph joined the tribal community in a time of turmoil. Though the Omahas "never stained their hands with the blood of a white man," to quote Joseph's adopted grandfather, Chief Big Elk, they had to defend themselves against the aggressive onslaughts of the Dakota Sioux.[28]

The arrival of dispossessed tribes exacerbated the situation. Eastern Indians—removed beginning in the mid-1820s to the Missouri Valley so as to make way for Euro-American westward expansion—were resettled on the lands of the Osage, Kansa, and Sioux. This in turn forced the latter tribes, in search of new bison range, to encroach upon the territories of the Pawnees, Otos and Missouris, and Omahas.[29] Those aggressive thrusts into the Omahas' homeland eventually drove the Upstream People away. Deprived of their resource base, they were forced "to prowl over the country like so many hungry wolves" in a desperate search for the bison herds that were retreating westward.[30]

By the time Joseph entered adolescence, the incessant demands of the fur trade and concomitant indiscriminate hunting had resulted in an obvious depletion of beaver and bison. By 1830 periods of Indian starvation were increasing. The Omahas, according to Indian agent John Dougherty, "starv[ed] almost half the year, and [were] very badly clad." Dougherty warned that the Omahas "must cultivate the soil or perish by hunger." Of course the Omahas cultivated crops, but their agricultural efforts reaped insufficient food for the long winters.[31] This period of prolonged poverty demoralized the Omahas and set the stage for their further dispossession in the late nineteenth century, as Susan later witnessed.

Joseph probably suffered little of this privation as a child. Transferred at the age of five to the care of two aunts when his mother left to remarry, the young Omaha came under the guidance of his own father, who returned after a long absence, in the early 1830s. Young Joseph grew up exposed to the cross-cultural trading his father engaged in with Indians and non-Indians. Also, the occasional trips to

St. Louis provided another window to the Euro-American world. He picked up French as well as a few other Indian languages.[32] Thus, early in life, Joseph's world view expanded, as would Susan's under his guidance, beyond the boundaries of the native landscape and into dynamic cultural borders.

When Joseph was still an infant, the United States Army, with the bitter lesson of the War of 1812 still intact, envisioned a cordon of forts from Green Bay on the Great Lakes westward to Montana as a means of preventing future British infiltration into the rugged northern regions. To carry out the monumental task of establishing the forts, three army expeditions were mustered. The Missouri Expedition received the assignment to cover the Upper Missouri region.[33]

Accompanying the Missouri Expedition troops was an army physician, John Gale, Susan's maternal grandfather. Born in 1795, Gale hailed from New Hampshire. He joined the army during the War of 1812 and apparently obtained his medical knowledge on the job during the war. When peace arrived, the army transferred him to the New Hampshire Rifle Regiment to participate in the Missouri Expedition. Late in the summer of 1818 Gale and the troops traveled up the Missouri River to Council Bluffs at present-day Fort Calhoun, Nebraska. When a shortfall in appropriations halted their farther ascent of the river, the troops stayed at Council Bluffs and built Fort Atkinson.[34]

Meanwhile, Dr. Gale had fallen in love with a young woman of Omaha-Oto-Iowa descent called Nicomi, Susan's maternal grandmother. Though the army's social policies opposed soldier-Indian miscegenation, many high-ranking officers on the frontier often openly expressed admiration and affection for frontiersmen who took Indian women as wives and mistresses. Military personnel could relate to Indian women on a human level because, unlike Indian men, they were not seen as a threat to whites. Nineteenth-century Euro-Americans saw all women, regardless of racial background, as less inscrutable and more approachable than men. Further, unlike white women who were bound by Victorian constraints, Indian women exhibited qualities of independence and power that some army personnel admired. Though Gale's romantic liaison with Nicomi never attained the respectability of a proper western marriage, it probably represented genuine human involvement.[35]

The conjugal union between the Yankee man and Omaha woman resulted in two children, one of whom died in infancy. The other child, born in 1822, was Mary, Susan's mother. Mary was separated early in life from her father when Nicomi refused to let him take the child with him when his garrison was ordered back to St. Louis. But before he left Nebraska, Gale persuaded his friend Peter Sarpy to take care of his Indian family. Not long after, in 1830, Dr. Gale died at Fort Armstrong on the upper Mississippi at the age of thirty-five. There is little evidence to show that Gale's Euro-American roots ever shaped Susan's sense of self.[36]

A few years after Gale's departure from Nebraska, Sarpy, also of French descent, asked for Nicomi's hand. This amalgamation suited Sarpy's self-interests; through his marriage to Nicomi, Sarpy gained the Omahas' trade and their protection against hostile tribes.[37]

Nicomi, for her part, apparently manipulated Sarpy in order to gain material goods and affection. Nicomi clearly was a strong, outspoken woman. She always used the Omaha language, refusing to speak French or English. She saw herself (and her child) in terms of her ranking within Indian society. Her awareness of her "Indianness" and of white society's possible threat to her only child prompted Nicomi's decision to keep Mary under her care. She probably wanted Mary to maintain her bonds of Indian kinship. However, it was Nicomi who persuaded Sarpy, most likely because she recognized the value of education, to send Mary to St. Louis to attend school. But Nicomi herself did not like living in hustle-bustle St. Louis and soon chose to return to the reservation.[38]

Mary Gale grew up as determined as her mother and just as proud of her Indian heritage. At least in Mary's case, her parents' cross-cultural marriage had not produced a next generation that reflected a Europeanized family. Refusing to use the French she had picked up at school, Mary, like Nicomi, spoke only the Omaha language. Mary understood English, but, as the adult Susan once explained, "she will not speak it unless she has to." It is probable that Susan, like her mother Mary, inherited some of Nicomi's pride and strong willpower.

Mary Gale (Waoo-Winchatcha), in spite of her half-English descent, acquired a firm social identity as an Indian. She was known as "The One Woman," a position of honor, and also as the "Dream Woman," because of a vision she revealed to her native people.[39]

When Mary became part of Sarpy's life she also became acquainted with other members of the mixed-blood community, including the man she would marry, Joseph La Flesche. By then, the young man had chosen to cast his lot with his mother's people. Unlike the métis people of Canada, who underwent a process of ethnogenesis, American mixed bloods were bereft of a unique and identifiable identity. Like most American mixed bloods, Joseph identified more closely with full-blood members of his tribe than he did with mixed bloods of other tribes or with his European heritage. His matrilocal residency pattern confirmed his social identity as an Omaha. Joseph, or Iron Eye, immersed himself in Omaha lore and customs; he performed the *wathin'ethe*, the "count" or traditional gift-giving, in order to enter an exclusive Omaha society. The fact that he later aspired to the chieftainship revealed that he sought status within the Omaha value system.[40] By remaining within the orbit of traditionalism, Iron Eye preserved his claim to Indianness and ensured that Susan stood a chance of doing so as well.

It is estimated that Susan's parents, Joseph and Mary, entered into wedlock sometime in 1845 or 1846. Less than ten years later and just before his death in 1853, Chief Young Elk (the son of the deceased Chief Big Elk) adopted Joseph in a public ceremony and announced that Joseph would inherit the chieftainship of the Elk clan. Most probably Joseph was also accepted into Big Elk's clan, We'zhinshte of the Earth (Hongashenu) moiety. Since chieftainship within each clan was hereditary, this adoption and entry into the Elk clan was necessary. But La Flesche did not become first principal chief of the Omaha tribe until approximately 1855, after principal chief Logan Fontenelle (from another clan) had been killed by the Sioux.[41]

Well before La Flesche assumed the chieftainship position, non-Indian speculative pressure on his homeland had forced the tribe, through the Treaty of Prairie de Chien (1830), to surrender their claims to lands east of the Missouri River. A subsequent treaty in

1836 resulted in the cession of land between the western boundary of the state of Missouri and the Missouri River. But the most significant, and perhaps most painful, loss came in 1854. In that year, the Omahas ceded their tribal largess in northeastern Nebraska, retreating subsequently to a tract of 300,000 acres adjacent to the Missouri, which became the federally supervised reservation where Susan was born. In return for selling their land, along "with the ashes of their ancestors," the Omahas were promised a tribal annuity of $40,000 for the next thirty years.[42]

Often the Omahas were left to fend for themselves. Although the 1854 treaty and earlier agreements provided annuities, the process of issuing payments was fraught with loopholes that traders and agents exploited to their advantage. Since 1840 the swelling stream of westward-bound emigrants along the Platte, heeding the call of Manifest Destiny, had further threatened the survival of the tribe. These tired, weary, but excited travelers "fouled the water, used up the wood, ruined pastures, and drove off game animals," according to historian Robert A. Trennert, Jr. Trailing not too far behind the emigrant trains were non-Indian hunters who "wantonly killed the buffalo," sometimes keeping only the tongues. Latter-Day Saints (Mormons), in search of their new Zion, squatted for two years on the Omahas' ancestral land and depleted all remaining game. Daily life was abysmal. "Scouring the country in every direction," many Indians struggled to survive on roots and little else, one missionary recounted. The Omaha population plunged from fourteen hundred in the late 1830s to eight hundred in 1855.[43]

But lines of fracture did not run through the Upstream People, because strong leadership held the tribe together despite the incessant stress. Chief Big Elk, leader from 1811 to 1849, maintained sufficient control over his people. Big Elk, after a visit to Washington, D.C., in 1837–38, advised his people to adapt to the changing world. The next chief, Young Elk, similarly warned his people of the "coming flood." Accommodation with the United States was touted as the only option left. When Joseph La Flesche assumed one of the two head chieftainships in mid-century, the Omahas had already gained a reputation as the "friends of the whites," and thus their offspring, like Susan, would soon be viewed as ideal cohorts for the "civilization" process.[44]

Joseph La Flesche implicitly supported the process of "civiliza-tion" by continuing the policy of nonviolent rearguard action. Employed at one point by the American Fur Company and later as the proprietor of a trading store and ferry service, Susan's father was familiar with Euro-American ways. Under the guidance of Young Elk, Joseph imbued his adopted father's call for accommodation and adaptation. Looking back, Joseph observed: "After a while the white men came, just as the blackbirds do, and spread over the country . . . it matters not where one looks now one sees white people . . . his [the Indian's] only chance is to become as the white man."[45] Joseph clearly knew that his people had few other recourses, and from her father, Susan would learn likewise.

The whites' inundation of the Nebraska landscape intensified in the 1850s. The creation of the territory of Nebraska in 1854 after the passage of the Kansas-Nebraska Act drew swarms of settlers who fanned across the country. No longer tainted with the "Great American Desert" image, the plains bustled with change and movement. Emigrants and travellers were joined by speculators in the clamor for unhindered access to the region. The federal government responded with the policy of "concentration," or the relocation of tribes and the compression of tribal estates to create right-of-ways through native lands. The Office of Indian Affairs (OIA) wanted the Omahas and other tribes to relocate away from main migratory routes of white settlers so that their traffic through the plains would be unhindered. During the 1850s over fifty treaties, including the one that the Omahas signed in 1854, had been negotiated with a wide cross section of tribes. In all, Indian title to 174 million acres of land was extinguished. Manifest Destiny had triumphed, but at the expense of the Indians.[46]

For Joseph La Flesche, the advancement and superiority of whites seemed unquestionable following his visit to Washington, D.C., as part of the Omaha delegation that signed the 1854 treaty. While in the capital, he stood in awe of the wide cobblestone streets, imposing brick buildings, horse-drawn metal trolley cars, and the teeming crowds of non-Indian people. When he returned to the reduced tribal estate, he addressed his people about the future: "Look ahead, and you will see nothing but the white man."[47]

Following the 1854 treaty, the Omahas exchanged their expansive homeland for a relatively small reservation. Located in the Blackbird Hills of northeastern Nebraska, the landscape that Susan became familiar with featured rich soil and bountiful natural resources. The advantages, coupled with unusually strong government support, resulted in the Omahas' showing dramatic "signs of improvement in their condition" within a few years, as reported by an Indian agent.[48]

For some Omahas, "improvement" entailed breaking some time-honored traditions. One segment of the tribe, the "young men's party" or "Progressives," led by Susan's father, established their own village of frame and log houses. Traditionalists, scattered on two earth-lodge and tipi settlements, derisively called it the "Village of Make-Believe White Men."[49]

Joseph, the leader of the village, reportedly was the first Omaha to build a plastered, frame house west of the Missouri. He and his family moved to the two-story home that Susan grew up in sometime in late 1857. The La Flesche family then cleared and broke forty-five acres for cultivation in the rich, flat bottomland beside the Missouri Valley. They planted corn, wheat, potatoes, fruits, apples, grapevines, and a vegetable garden.[50]

Joseph realized that modern homes and commercial farming did not provide sufficient defense against white encroachment and that only Euro-American education could help young Omahas accommo-date change in the late-nineteenth century. Equipped with education, extolled La Flesche, Indians could then labor in positions akin to those of Euro-Americans. Consequently, he asked the Presbyterians, who had established a school for the Omahas in Bellevue, Nebraska, to accompany them to their new reservation. There Presbyterian officials erected a new mission. Its centerpiece was a three-story limestone building that served as a residence for missionaries and as dormitories and schoolrooms for the pupils. The mission sat on a bluff overlooking the steamboat landing and agency buildings. A three-mile-long road connected the complex with the La Flesche village. With nineteen wooden dwellings by 1861, the village lasted nearly twenty years. Apparently with some help from the mission school, it produced tribal leaders, Susan included, for years.[51]

On the reservation, Chief La Flesche wielded his power effectively in the enforcement of social order. In his fight against heavy drinking, Susan's father showed his mettle, and this crusade left an impression on young Susan. Alcohol made its appearance in the Missouri Valley in the early 1800s as a result of the expansion of the fur trade. The stories of the baneful impact of alcohol on Indians, of cultural deprivation and destitution, abound in contemporary accounts.[52]

Like other tribes of the central plains, the Omahas did not escape the influence of *pede'ni*, "firewater" or alcohol. By the mid-1850s heavy drinking afflicted a significant number of Omahas, enough to prompt the tribal council to support Chief Joseph La Flesche's proposal to break the drinking habits of some of his people. Some twenty years earlier young La Flesche had witnessed the senseless murder of an innocent Indian by a drunken Indian—an incident that had shaped his commitment to temperance.[53] At the start of the campaign against drinking, Chief La Flesche thundered: "My children, drink is bad for the red man. We need to know what we are doing, and whiskey makes us fools. We will have no more drink while Joseph lives."[54]

Under La Flesche's leadership, a police force of thirty men—an updated version of the tribes' military or soldiers' society—was organized and uniformed. Besides maintaining order, they were to inflict corporal punishment on any drunken Omaha, regardless of the offender's rank. One well-known tribal anecdote told the story of Two Crows, a member of the police force, who summoned his comrades to inflict the prescribed punishment on him after one drinking bout. The punishment, according to the Presbyterian missionary R. J. Burtt, was "severe enough to lay 'em up for a week."[55]

Iron Eye was conscious of the need to move the Omahas toward "civilization," but he never espoused total assimilation into the dominant society. Although Iron Eye adopted Euro-American clothing, he never denigrated those who retained the "blanket," or "robe," as their form of dress. He did not speak out against the pipe dances or the traditional exchange of gifts. Even though he practiced commercial farming, he continued to participate in the biannual bison hunts, bringing Susan and her siblings along. Joseph was also present for the last buffalo hunt in 1876. During such hunts, he and his family lived in a tipi. To enforce his ban against drinking, he resorted to a traditional punishment, namely flogging. Later in life the Indian chief embraced Christianity, but he never gave up polygamy. He sent away his third wife as a gesture of compromise, but kept his second wife, Ta-in-ne. La Flesche endorsed white farming, allotment, education, and later citizenship for the Indian, but he felt that all this had to be carried out "through accommodation to Omaha traditions, not through assimilation to white ways."[56] To that end, Joseph argued that the protection of the Omaha treaty rights must be paramount; otherwise, the traditional way of life, based on economic and political independence, would fade away. That mind-set would also come to infuse Susan's world view.

Iron Eye spoke out often about the wrongs that had been done to the Indians and about their right to be treated fairly and justly. Suspicious of the Indian agents' conduct, Iron Eye drew up a code of ethics in 1860 to regulate the agents' dealings with the tribe. With the help of local Presbyterian missionaries, he kept close tabs on the issuance of annuity payments. He demanded payments in coin, not paper money or material goods, and pushed for the expenditure of tribal funds on agricultural tools, medicine, and other necessities.[57]

By the early 1860s, La Flesche's leadership had born fruit. The fields of the "Make-Believe White Men" village flourished, yielding enough surplus for commercial sale in Sioux City. The reservation as a whole produced a bounteous harvest in 1861; there was so much food that they gave away some to their starving neighbors, the Poncas.[58]

On the social front, success was no less resounding. Conservative Omahas rebuffed the evangelization of the Presbyterian missionaries and their schooling program but unanimously backed the progressive-led tribal council in its efforts to stamp out alcoholism on the reservation. In 1864 the whole tribe demonstrated their commitment to temperance. In that year, the Omahas agreed to accommodate a segment of the Winnebago tribe, then on the brink of starvation, on their reservation. To maintain intertribal harmony and order, the Omaha Tribal Council drew up a set of by-laws for the Winnebagos to live by. The first by-law read: "Any member of said tribe of Winnebagos who may be found intoxicated or in whose possession any spirituous liquors may be discovered, shall be severely punished whether chief, or otherwise."[59]

On the whole, such close social control succeeded in checking the spread of this social disease. In his 1881 annual report, Arthur Edwards, the field official of the consolidated Omaha and Winnebago agency, lavished praise on his charges; they were, he wrote, "strictly temperate."[60] This situation persisted at least until La Flesche's death in 1888. A year later, annual reports of Indian agents and inspectors indicated that there was still little drunkenness among the Omahas.[61]

Iron Eye's efforts on behalf of his tribe were those of a cultural intermediary or broker. Living in the cultural frontier—a "place where peoples with different . . . identities meet and deal with each other"—he learned to assume, accommodate, and coordinate different roles.[62] A successful merchant trader, he also sought recognition as an Indian chief. Making full use of his linguistic skills and connections with non-Indians, Joseph La Flesche sought to bridge the gap between his tribe and the dominant society. He also served as the link between the native political structure and regional and national sources of white power.

La Flesche acknowledged that the Euro-American world offered something of value. Moving within the pattern of accommodation, he adapted selectively from other cultures and became a teacher of his own people. But he never cast aspersions on the traditional way of life; in fact, he chose to maintain some elements of it. La Flesche attempted to straddle the cultural divide, and though successful in a number of instances, he often found himself in precarious positions. He ran the risk of losing the friendship of local OIA officials when he stood up for Omaha treaty rights. However, to have done otherwise would have caused the Omahas to lose confidence in him as their leader. Later, living in the cultural middle ground, La Flesche would face more such challenges. His children, Susan included, would also encounter such dilemmas.

When La Flesche's daughter Susan was born in 1865, the Omahas were at a pivotal crossroad in their tribal history. Susan's words "I never saw a battle" revealed how much had changed since the dawn of the nineteenth century. No longer brave warriors and skillful hunters, the Omahas now lived within well-defined boundaries surrounded by land-hungry settlers and military garrisons. Like their former enemies—the Sioux, Sacs and Foxes, and Pawnees—the Omahas were mired in a cycle of treaties, land sale, and broken promises. The glorious battles of the past were over, gone forever. But though the Omahas' history had included adaptation and change up to this point, it had also been filled with a sense of persistence and continuity. Beyond the 1860s, the Omahas' story was one of discovering new beginnings.

The new challenge that the Omahas faced in the post–Civil War years came in the form of the federal government's aggressive pursuit of assimilation set against the backdrop of the country's relentless Social Darwinistic drive for economic development and rigid nationalism. To that end, education for Indian children was conceived as a central tenet of the "civilization" plan. Susan La Flesche, like thousands of Indian children at the turn of the century, would find herself at the receiving end of this effort.

CHAPTER TWO

"For the Delight of Those Days"

"I am a little Indian girl twelve years old. I go to school at the Omaha agency," wrote Susan La Flesche in a brief but informative 1877 letter to the *St. Nicholas Magazine*, a well-known juvenile periodical. In that year Susan and three other sisters, Susette or "Bright Eyes" (1854–1903), Rosalie (1861–1900), and Marguerite (1862–1945), each wrote to the periodical.[1] These unique writings provide a glimpse into the state of mind of young Omahas growing up in a time of convulsive changes.

Focusing on her white education, Susan reported the following in a matter-of-fact tone: "I study geography, history, grammar, arithmetic, and spelling. I read in the Fifth Reader. I have three older sisters and two brothers. Sometimes father, mother, and grandmother come to see us."[2] The content of her letter revealed some of the dynamics of the shifting power relationship between American Indians and Euro-Americans of the late-nineteenth century. More pointedly, it outlined the contours of the Euro-American educational system on the Omaha reservation. The system was designed to transform seemingly wild, roaming Indians into self-sustaining, self-respecting citizens of the republic.[3]

Undoubtedly, the underlying Euro-American assumption was that Indians grew up in an environment devoid of values, culture, and emotional ties. In truth, Indians "lavish[ed] all attention on their children," according to an article that Susan wrote as an adult in defense of her people. She also indicated, perhaps with some exaggeration, that Omahas were unreserved in "show[ing] their affection" for the young ones.[4] However, it is clear that the upbringing of the younger generations remained paramount in the minds of the Omaha elders; no other task consumed so much time.[5] While she was growing up, Susan received constant emotional and cognitive nourishment not only from her mother but also from a concentric circle of people, including her father, grandmother, siblings, and distant relatives. These extended kinship ties bound Susan to her homeland and tribal heritage and later gave some legitimacy to her claim to mediate on behalf of her people.

Mary Gale gave birth to her daughter Susan in a buckskin tipi, most probably during the height of a summer bison hunt. The exact year of Susan's birth, like that of her father, remains a mystery. According to a questionnaire she filled out in November 1888, she was born in Oakland, Nebraska, in June 1866. But her tombstone at the Bancroft, Nebraska, cemetery reads June 17, 1865. Her marriage certificate, dated June 30, 1894, noted that she was twenty-nine years old at the time of betrothal; thus, supposedly she was born in 1865.[6]

Susan's arrival coincided with the rapid disappearance of the Omahas' traditional way of life. The future looked uncertain, even bleak. Though her family prospered—Chief La Flesche owned fifty head of cattle, harvested on the average two thousand bushels of corn, and made a lot of money as the reservation's trader and moneylender—this wealth did not trickle down to the common Omaha. Most Omahas suffered from tuberculosis, measles, or pneumonia, wore threadbare moccasins, and went without meat, surviving instead on birds and roots. Throughout the 1860s, the population of the tribe increased only marginally. Summer swarms of grasshoppers and prolonged periods of drought decimated crops. Deprived of their essential foodways, the Omahas suffered malnutrition. When malnourishment was coupled with disease, a steady toll ensued.[7] The debilitating reservation era had arrived.

The Omahas' customs came under attack during those years from zealous OIA (Office of Indian Affairs) agents who deliberately undermined the powers of the hereditary chiefs. Eventually agents replaced those so-called "uncooperative" chiefs with compliant, hand-picked leaders, also known as "paper chiefs." Aside from the splinter within the leadership echelon, the tribe was also divided on the question of acculturation—La Flesche's "young men's party," or Progressives, versus the "chiefs' party," or traditionalists. There was also a small group of nonaligned chiefs.[8] Tribal dissension had set in, and it would later dog Susan's claim to cultural brokerage and tribal leadership.

Predictably, the Omahas were buffeted from all sides by the government, hostile white settlers, and rapacious opportunists all out to make a quick dollar at the Indians' expense. By the 1860s the rubric of Manifest Destiny had radically undercut the concentration policy of the late antebellum period. Following the end of the Civil War, the mid-America was seething with activity. Miners, driven by the dream of striking gold or silver, continued to cross the plains on their way to far western rivers and mountains. Construction crews crisscrossed the plains as they pushed to extend railroad lines. Settlers, many part of the great European immigration of the late-nineteenth century, had poured into Nebraska and surrounded the Omaha reservation as they staked out the free land that had been offered under the Homestead Act of 1862. Ranchers, in particular, staked out land to raise herds of longhorns, thus launching great cattle empires. Ranchers, farmers, and other settlers could also purchase more fertile lands from railroad companies, which helped, through their interconnecting lines, to open up the country west of the Mississippi River. Speculators took advantage of the Morrill Act of 1863, which allowed states to sell public-domain land to build endowments for colleges.[9] In March of 1865 the Omahas sold almost one hundred thousand acres in the northern portion of their reservation to the United States. On this northern section, the federal government carved out a reservation for the destitute Winnebagos.[10] The following year, the Nebraska territorial legislature voted to ask the federal government to expel all Indians from the state. The vote was almost inevitable.

The thrust of continental domination was gathering momentum as the stoic and agrarian age of Washington and Jefferson gave way to the pell-mell mentality of the Gilded Age. Consequently, during their early reservation years the Omahas saw land losses, tribal fragmentation, patterns of forced and voluntary acculturation, the gradual demise of the buffalo hunt, and usurpation of their traditional sources of power. Perhaps most tragic was the loss of the traditional hunt, because without it the Omahas could not perform the renewal ceremony for the Sacred Pole, which represented the unity of the tribe.[11] Even as the rest of the country began to take on the concept of a unified nation—symbolized by the successful completion of the transcontinental railroad in 1869—the Omaha tribe stood on the verge of disintegration.

Chief Joseph La Flesche understood that the end of the Omahas' traditional way of life was near, but less than a year after Susan's birth, he lost his position as chief of the Omahas. The events leading up to this turning point had much to do with a struggle for power between the Omaha agent Robert W. Furnas (1864–66) and Chief La Flesche, or Iron Eye. Furnas accused La Flesche of insubordination and obstructionism, but the most serious charge was that La Flesche cheated his people of their share of the wealth by lending money at usurious rates and barring his people from dealing with licensed traders. La Flesche's mysterious opposition to an 1865 treaty amendment providing for universal education on the reservation also incensed Furnas.[12]

The fragile relationship fell apart when Furnas removed La Flesche from his position as reservation trader. This move was defensible, since only American citizens could assume such positions.[13] By the spring of 1866 Furnas had persuaded his superiors that La Flesche should be deposed as chief. Apparently this did not elicit much opposition from the Omahas, which only augmented Furnas's case against La Flesche. Bereft of the support of his tribe and perhaps tired of the political bickering, Chief Iron Eye and his family hastily fled the reservation on the night of April 17, 1866. After a few months the family returned home, but Joseph La Flesche would never again hold a seat on the tribal council. Henceforth, his only recognition came as the leader of the "young men's party."[14] Susan never recounted this series of events herself, but the incident must have further weakened the La Flesche family's tentative claim to tribal leadership and probably pushed the family even more toward the cultural borderland.

The loss of his highly esteemed position certainly jolted La Flesche and may have played a part in his decision not to give Susan an Indian name. Perhaps Joseph La Flesche realized that the precarious balance between accommodation and tradition might prove unworkable for future generations of Omahas. Joseph thought that his children should be exposed to Omaha ways in order to claim an Indian identity but should not embrace all traditions, at least not to the extent that they would suffer the stigma of being a traditional Indian living in a white-dominated world. No doubt Joseph's affiliation with local Presbyterian missionaries—he converted sometime in the 1860s—had much to do with his decision to place his children on the periphery of the traditional cultural matrix.[15] Consequently Susan, unlike her older sister Susette, or Inshtatheamba, did not at the age of three or four go through the turning of the child ceremony, during which she would have been given an Indian name. The turning of the child ceremony was one of the many rituals central to Omaha religious life. Like rituals surrounding birth, marriage, and death, the naming ceremony was performed to launch a person on the next stage of life's journey. This ceremony, which took place in springtime "after the first thunders had been heard, when grass was well up, and the birds were singing," also symbolized the child's formal admission into the tribe and spiritual oneness with Wakon'da.[16]

Nor did Susan receive the "mark of honor," which would indicate that she was one of the most distinguished women of the tribe, being the daughter of Iron Eye, a leader and member of the "Night Dance Society," who had contributed one hundred acts or gifts. According to her father, the tattoos on the forehead and upper chest would "be detrimental in . . . future [white] surroundings." Since the recipient of the mark, or tattoo, receives the power of Wakon'da and then radiates it out into the hu'thuga, or camp circle, Joseph's decision may have also been a symbolic attempt to distance his faction from the rest of the tribe.[17] This distancing also left an impression on Susan: it allowed her to be receptive to the other side of the cultural divide and to acknowledge its inherent value.

But Susan was not isolated from the cultural practices of the tribe. She later recalled being fascinated by the sacred bundles, packs of buffalo skins that often contained pieces of bones, feathers, and bird skins. The bundles constituted the centers of power and were often drawn upon for help during battles and other crises. Susan was also highly curious about the medicine men and their work, particularly their use of a walnut bowl to compound herbs and roots from which healing drinks were concocted. In a 1908 interview, she hinted that her interest in curing people began in those early childhood years.[18]

Like other Indians, young Susan learned mostly by application and imitation, rather than rote memorization of principles. Joseph La Flesche may have forsaken his ancient faith, but philosophically he remained an Omaha, always basing his beliefs and actions on careful thought and serious thinking. His children, including Susan, shared that stance. Knowledge and understanding came not from intuition but through training, and such training was considered pivotal before one could be accepted as a mature member of the tribe. The instruction took the form of play that imitated adult life and offered the children recreation and reinforcement of their education in Omaha lifeways.[19]

Over time Susan came to appreciate the centrality of work to female Indian identity and status, and this would mold her sense of responsibility for herself and others. The desire to labor on behalf of the community was gradually and almost imperceptibly forged in the crucible of her formative years. Put to work at the tender age of four or five, young Susan learned from her mother to forage for wood, carry water, and run other light errands. Susan detested carrying water, as evidenced in a speech she made later in life: "It was a weary, toilsome walk, clear down to the spring and back again under the hot sun, through the stubble, barefooted and we were happy little mortals when our dreaded work was finished." Like other young girls, she helped unpack horses returning from a hunt; the animals would later be led by young boys to water and "tether in the grass." In her early adolescent years Susan learned how to erect a tipi and how to dress skins and dry bison meat.[20]

Because the La Flesche family engaged in farming, Susan also became conversant with the cycle of planting and harvesting crops. She and her family sowed corn, hoed potatoes, and weeded vegetables. With her other sisters, Susan helped with the grueling chores of harvest time. As an adult, Susan would recall that yearly ritual: "Oh! For the delight of those days, as the reaper cut down the golden grain and we went eagerly forward striving to see who could keep nearest the machine." Susan remembered how after each harvest, she and other children would stand on "top of a high hill, looking down on a field of harvesting wheat . . . watch[ing] the moon rise, flooding the valley with silvery light and casting clear shadows around the trees."[21]

It was deemed necessary that Susan possess full knowledge of the practical skills of existence since the Omahas depended upon their women for the processing of daily necessities and supplies. Both sexes held each other in high esteem, because their survival depended on mutual effort. The different aspects of female and male roles combined in a symmetry that was essential to the tribe's continuity. Omaha women, operating in the absence of a power hierarchy, were the equals of men and were highly valued in traditional society. Susan's childhood training prepared her to assume a position in Omaha society.[22]

Dressed in a calico dress and with her hair in braids, Susan also received instruction in proper social etiquette and good manners. All Omaha children were inculcated with the values of industry, politeness, and consideration for others. But unlike the boys, young girls came under special scrutiny. Discipline for the girls was more stringent, while the boys enjoyed greater liberty. Young girls like Susan tried to master the demeanor of well-bred Omaha women. They practiced sitting on their left hip, and rising from a sitting posture noiselessly, without drawing too much attention. According to Omaha custom, young members of the tribe were not allowed to interrupt an elder who was speaking. Other social taboos included passing between a person and the fire, staring at a stranger, or asking for the stranger's name.[23]

From her father, Susan and her sisters came to appreciate the value of compassion and charity. Her elder sister Susette remembered that he once taught her a poignant lesson. As a little girl Susette received a small bird that she enjoyed playing with. Her father called Susette and asked her to put it carefully on the ground, away from tents and the people, and to utter: "God, I give you back your little bird. Have pity on your bird." Susan once heard her father admonishing a transgressor: "He who is present at a wrongdoing and lifts not a hand to prevent it is as guilty as the wrongdoers." Iron Eye also said: "When you see a boy barefooted and lame, take off your moccasins and give them to him. When you see a boy hungry, bring him to your house and give him food." Joseph implied that as a member of a privileged family, young Susan had a responsibility to the poor and the weak. This lesson in fellowship became embedded in Susan's mind and would serve as a central tenet of her personal philosophy.[24]

Susan and other young girls were trained separately from the boys, but both sexes did spend time playing together. Since they had no factory-made toys, they depended on nature to amuse themselves. The children made toys out of clay, modeling men and animals. Susan and her siblings shaped dishes out of clay and built houses made of mud.[25] Sometimes, according to Susan, young Omaha girls, according to Susan, would "go off and play camp life . . . playing to perfection the part of the mothers." They would set up a little tent for the purpose of playing house,and quite often Susan took her meals in the tent with other little girls and siblings.[26]

Not all games imitated real life. Some were simply fun, even silly. *Ke-tum-bae-ah-ke-ke-tha* (contending with the eyes by looking) was a group game in which the object was to see whose sober face would smile first; when that happened, water was poured over the offender or the loser's head was snapped at with fingers. *Ou-hae-ba-shun-shun* (crooked path) involved the children following a leader and committing acts of mischief as they wound around trees, bushes, and tufts of grass.[27]

Many amusements followed the rhythm of the seasons. After the springtime thaw of the frozen land, when all life-forms had stirred from the winter slumber, the Omaha youngsters played a game in which they imitated animals such as the turkey, whose antics Susan recounted as an adult in an unpublished essay entitled "The Dance of the Turkey." Flapping their hands and fingers in imitation of the turkey's tail, the children hopped and jumped, singing the song of "Wa-han-the-shu-gae," or the "dance of the turkeys."[28] During the parched Nebraskan summers, Omaha children went on their "hunt." When they went on a hunt, Susan and the girls would harness up some of the boys as ponies and would pack upon them the play-tent poles, tent cover, and all sorts of bundles. Other boys acted as warriors who rode "imaginary horses, [and] shot imaginary buffaloes" with their long spears of grass. Indeed, the children played many games that mimicked the occupations of mature Omaha life. Going on the hunt, taking down and putting up tents—with the tall stalks of sunflowers serving as poles—and attacks on enemies all furnished incidents for play.[29]

Then the air turned cooler as the northern winds swept through the pliant grasses and swaying sunflower stalks, and autumn had arrived. The young girls would collect the dried corncobs and fashion them into dolls, dressing them in worn-out pieces of calico. They housed their dolls in miniature tipis made from sunflower stalks and old blankets. In an article published in 1892, Susan recounted how she used to make stick horses from sunflower stalks, and on these she would ride barefooted in and out of the earth lodges.[30]

The first snowflakes marked the onset of winter activities. To make a sled, Indian children cut great slabs of ice from the river and trimmed them into the proper shape. Then a layer of grass was pressed down on the slabs and frozen into place. Soon Susan and the rest of the playful group, shrieking and screaming, were away at a furious speed.[31] It is probable that such traditional play activities impressed upon Susan the value of the old ways and helped her to avoid assuming, as she crossed over to the other side of the cultural divide during later years, a manner of white-like superiority or cultural paternalism.

During the long, bitterly cold winter months, the four La Flesche sisters sat on the hard ground around a warm, crackling fire and pressed their grandparents to share yarns of yesteryear with them. At some point, Susan and her sisters learned about the Sacred Legend, the tribal creation story. Their elders taught them about the creatures who shared the sky and earth with them and about the ancient origins of the Omaha people. Through this instruction, the La Flesche children probably came to understand the Omahas' belief that their people belonged to the land the lived on. That awareness most likely shaped young Susan's appreciation for the sacred nature of the native landscape and the Omahas' claim to their land.

Writing later in life, Susan recalled how she and her sisters used to also listen to ghost stories and to tales of buffalo hunts and battles with the dreaded Sioux. In particular, ghost stories drew a reaction from Susan; she often looked up at the opening of the roof of the lodge and feared that she might see a dog looking down. According to an Omaha belief, if a dog looked down through the opening into the lodge then someone in the company would die soon. A sense of relief descended on her when she saw only dark skies and twinkling stars above her.[32]

One of the stories Susan listened to was told by her grandmother Nicomi, and years later Susan would relate the tale to the ethnologist James Owen Dorsey. This was the story of Ichtinike (Orphan) and the turkeys. Ichtinike is an Omaha trickster—a cultural figure who represents the perversity, ambiguity, and contradiction of life. Trickster tales convey life lessons by exposing human flaws. Through such myths Susan's grandmother and other Omaha adults taught tribal values to their young charges without the tedium of direct instruction; learning, in fact, became a joyful process.[33] In this particular tale, Ichtinike, looking for food, spotted some turkeys feeding on an elevated ground among the arrowhead plants. Ichtinike asked himself: "How [what] shall I do in order to eat them?" Shortly, he figured a strategy. Carrying a raccoon-skin robe on his back, he ran close by the turkeys. The turkeys stopped him, and he agreed to sing some songs for them. In return, Ichtinike asked them to dance for him. He asked the turkeys to close their eyes; otherwise, their eyes would turn red. Then, he nabbed the turkeys as they pranced around him. The story clearly underscores the Omahas' reliance on pragmatic thought, always asking themselves how they could better their situation. In a period of Euro-American colonization such a line of questioning became even more urgent. The appreciation for a practical, self-reliant thought process would later shape Susan's approach to life.[34]

However, Susan's parents' support for white education meant that she would certainly be exposed to it. Mary Gale apparently could accept the childrens' prolonged absences from home while they were away at school because she knew they could reap benefits from the whites' instruction. There was no doubt where Joseph stood on this matter. He went so far as to demand that his children converse in Omaha and French only with their parents; with one another they had to use English. Because Susan was the youngest, she probably enjoyed an early exposure to English via her sisters, and that knowledge gave her an early edge in cultural brokership. In a speech delivered in 1886 before a white audience, Susan commented that "they [her parents] cannot speak English, but they felt the need of education, and did not want us to go through what they had experienced."[35] Despite the threat of a severance of the parent-child bond, Mary and Joseph aggressively pushed their offspring into the embrace of the missionaries' educational system.

On the other hand, it is entirely possible that Susan was packed off to school for part of the year, probably at the age of three, because she was too young to work productively and required too much attention. A mission teacher in 1868 reported that many of the parents, motivated by those reasons, had enrolled their female toddlers. Susan recalled that when she began school she was so small that "when [she] went to sleep the big boys used to put [her] in the high old-fashioned desks they used in those days."[36]

Susan's white education, which eventually took her to far-flung places, began in a limestone building only a few miles away from home. This was the Presbyterians' mission school. Completed in 1857, the imposing three-story boarding school was funded through the sale of four quarter sections of land, surrendered by the Omahas under the 1854 treaty that Joseph had signed. Under contract with the federal government, the Presbyterians accepted the responsibility of using the school as the primary agency for the "moral improvement and education" of the tribe.[37]

Like other nineteenth-century evangelical Americans, the well-meaning but ethnocentric mission officials toiled to transform the Indians into self-supporting, productive Christians. They demanded that the Indians reject their "heathen" past and embrace the Jeffersonian, pietistic, rural-American way of life. This attitude was very much in line with the government's Indian policy, which grew out of the replacement model of cultural change. Cultural identity was conceived as a zero-sum phenomenon: one was either Indian or non-Indian. To make a Native American lose his or her "Indianness," the process of "civilization" had to be invoked. According to the Presbyterians, "civilization" was linked inextricably to the successful propagation of Christianity and to finding a new economic life within the competitive system of private property. The missionaries felt that without these new values, Indians would backslide and all efforts would be wasted. This all-encompassing religious and social vision drove the missionaries' agenda for most of the nineteenth century.[38]

The Presbyterian missionaries directed most of their energies at the children, believing that white ways learned at an early age would become permanent and irreversible. Susan and her fellow students received what historian Michael C. Coleman later described as a "three-pronged education—religious, vocational, and academic" designed to "lift Indians into the privileges and responsibilities of citizenship in the Christian civilization and in the United States."[39]

Laboring to save souls, the missionaries sincerely believed that circumstances, not race, held the Indians back. Reverend William H. Hamilton, who served the Omaha people for nearly half a century, once wrote: "The improvement of the children is about what might be expected of persons in their situation, not rapid, but still learning something." The length of time that would be needed for "civilization" concerned mission officials, but they never doubted the malleability of the native people. This viewpoint was very much in step with the legacy of the eighteenth-century Enlightenment—faith in the unity of mankind and belief in environmental explanations of human diversity.[40]

These expectations were applied to both sexes; the missionaries believed that Indian girls as well as boys possessed the potential to become Christian citizens. In 1857 missionary I. R. Rolph, then serving on the Omaha reservation, wrote to the Board of Foreign Missions of the Presbyterian Church that it made his "courage wane to think of educating boys here . . . if they have only the prospect before them of taking up . . . with a partner for life whose ambition would be only for hunters [sic] fare and satisfied with the habits of the wigwam."[41] It was believed that education for the Indian woman would not only ensure her personal happiness and eternal salvation, but would also support the perpetuation of the Anglo-American family through her influence on her young ones.[42]

The missionaries' viewpoint fell in line with the nineteenth-century prescriptive, middle-class European and American ideology of womanliness. This ideal stemmed in part from a larger effort to halt the blurring of the line between the public and private spheres, a process set in motion by the aggressive forces of industrialization and modernization. As the patriarchal family unit threatened to come apart, society tried to impose a gendered, hierarchical binary in an attempt to re-create order. Women, in the ideal form, occupied a separate "sphere" of domesticity. At home, women were expected to parlay their intuitive morality into a source of power, which they were to draw upon to nurture their children and temper their husbands' unbridled passions. Supposedly pure, pious, and domesticated, middle-class American women were proscribed from entering the public realm, the exclusive domain of men. This so-called "cult of true womanhood," or domestic ideology, relegated women to the home, the center of their orbit. Within that private realm, women were expected to exercise their spirit of self-sacrifice and self-abnegation, thus balancing men's self-assertive and competitive natures in the public sphere.[43] In reality, few American women could afford or wanted to live up to those expectations; working-class, black, and immigrant women sidestepped those boundaries of womanhood and forged different life-styles.[44]

The Presbyterian missionaries on the Omaha reservation tried to echo that separate-sphere ideology. The education of Indian girls emphasized the honing of vocational skills. Susan learned the Euro-American version of household arts—the preparation and serving of food, sewing, knitting, and laundry. Male students, however, spent their time mastering husbandry and taking care of the mission farm. Such separate vocational training reflected prescribed, unequal gender roles in the Euro-American society: men at work, women at home. This ideal was in somewhat stark contrast to traditional Omaha role expectations for the sexes. While each sex did, as in Euro-American culture, inhabit a particular realm, gender parity and fluidity in gender roles marked the traditional Omaha lifeway.[45]

In the classroom, Susan had the opportunity, in theory, to improve her English speaking, reading, and writing skills. Like white children, Susan and other Omaha students used the McGuffey readers and primers. She also received limited instruction in certain academic subjects such as arithmetic, geography, and music. The student body, which numbered on the average forty, also memorized biblical lessons. Particular attention was paid to the testaments. Religious instruction must have struck a chord with Susan; later in life, she would assume the role of a native missionary, attempting to convert her people to Christianity.[46]

Seemingly, Susan did not gain a lot of academic knowledge from the missionary teachers. The teachers simply did not apply well the prescribed curriculum. As an adult, Susan recalled those days with a tinge of humor: "I can't say as I learned very much, for sometimes the teacher used to put a newspaper over his head, calmly lean back in his seat and repose in placid slumber." There is little evidence that she was ever exposed to literature, science, or history. Her world view probably expanded little beyond the immediate surroundings.[47]

In fact, some of the missionaries' writings seemed to suggest that the students, both boys and girls, were more valued for their labor than their minds. In one letter, for example, the Reverend Hamilton concluded that the girls, though "quite small," were "better workers" than the boys. Such an attitude, if pervasive, probably tempered any enthusiasm for a more comprehensive curriculum for Indian girls. However, to the credit of the teachers, the school was praised by visitors as "well-organized" and "doing a great deal of good"; evidently, the teachers did the best they could given the limited resources.[48]

Throughout Susan's stay at the boarding school, the enrollment fluctuated between twenty and fifty students. The instability in class size stemmed from factionalism within the tribe; many parents kept their children away from the school because they feared the wrath of the leaders of the "paper chiefs' party." In fact, the majority of the students' parents were affiliated with the "young men's party." Poor enrollment may have kept the academic program at a modest level.[49]

Susan probably did not suffer unduly in the boarding school. Familiar with the notion of discipline, she adjusted to the demanding daily regimen. The fact that her parents could visit her as often as they desired, and that she could do likewise, cushioned the pangs of loneliness.[50] Because of her early exposure to the English language, Susan had fewer problems grappling with a foreign curriculum than some of the other children. Being the product of a culture that had been incorporating white traits for a long time, Susan was open to new ideas, and the adaptive life-style of her family and tribe eased her adjustment to a white-controlled environment. Unlike most children who spent time in a government or missionary boarding school, Susan probably did not perceive the curricula as an invasion of her personal and cultural being or feel that her acquiescence was a form of racial betrayal. Finally, her family's conversion to Christianity and her parents' close association with the missionaries—both Joseph and Mary acted as interpreters for them—probably eased any misapprehensions Susan had about spending time away from home. To some extent, this formative experience must have laid the foundation for Susan's receptiveness to the ways of the "Other."

But Susan did not remain in the Presbyterian school for long, because the implementation of Indian reform—the "Peace" or "Quaker Policy"—in 1869 led to the eventual termination of the mission school and its program. Quaker day schools were substituted in its place. The day schools were part of the agenda of education and civilization—touted as the panacea for Indian-white conflicts.

The federal government, tired of the Plains Indian Wars of the 1860s and under strong pressure from eastern reformers to find a nonviolent solution to the "Indian Question," chose the route of "conquering by kindness." Bloody army action, including the Sand

Creek Massacre of 1864 and the rout of Cheyennes and Sioux in Kansas three years later, had evoked the reformers' bitter denouncement. In 1867, in response to the charges of military blunders and miscarriages of justice, Congress created a commission, made up of mostly humanitarian reformers, to find alternatives to warfare with the Indians. This Indian Peace Commission placed the blame squarely on whites and called for the "civilizing" of Indians so that Native Americans and non–Native Americans could "mingle together," stating that then "war would have been impossible."[51]

In 1867–68 the peace commission was charged with the responsibility of securing new treaties with northern and southern plains tribes. President Andrew Johnson also instructed the commission to consolidate western Indians on one of three designated larger reservations. While the peace secured for the northern plains lasted for nearly a decade, comity on the southern plains was short-lived. Southern plains tribes, frustrated by the delay of promised provisions, struck out in anger and hunger against nearby settlers and their properties. Soon warfare broke out again.[52]

When the U.S. Army responded with the infamous rout at the so-called Battle of the Washita on November 27, 1868, and the subsequent relentless campaign of that winter, some American reformers became revolted by the grisly reports of violence. They agreed that the army should continue to move Indians onto reservations, but now the process of "civilization" would be realized under the supervision of morally upright concerned citizens who would serve as the new Indian agents, replacing those who were deemed to be unscrupulous or inefficient.[53]

President Ulysses S. Grant, who oversaw this policy shift, envisioned using army officers as Indian agents, but unwilling to give up an important source of patronage, Congress opposed him. In retaliation, Grant accepted civilian nominees that had been chosen by the country's Protestant leaders. Thus, the Peace Policy employed religion as a way to assimilate and acculturate Indians. It was, indeed, a "mission policy," one focused on social reform and good ethical behavior, leading, at least in theory, to absorption of the Indians into white society.[54]

One particular Protestant denomination not only answered the call, but to some extent led the way. The Society of Friends, or Quakers, in a memorial submitted to Grant in early 1869 urged him to "promote their [the Indians'] education, their industry, their morality."[55] Following Grant's positive response, the Hicksite Friends, one of the two branches of the Society of Friends, were assigned the Northern Superintendency, which included the Omaha Agency. Samuel Janney, the new superintendent, placed his faith in the redemptive power of education, allotment, and farming—three fundamental tenets largely echoing mainstream thought on Indian reform. In addition, the Quakers, like the Presbyterians, adhered to social norms for female and male occupations. Like their predecessors, the Quakers saw themselves as models of the prescriptive, Victorian gender ideology. From them, Susan would continue to hear about white social attitudes on the "proper," ideal roles of men and women.[56]

For almost a decade, until the age of fourteen or fifteen, Susan came under the sway of the Friends. She spent years attending a Quaker day school. The Presbyterians were forced to close their school shortly after the first Quaker agent arrived on the reservation in June 1869. Interdenominational strife—not at all uncommon on reservations—was one catalyst for the chain of events that led to the school's eventual closure. Reverend William Hamilton, the superintendent of the mission school, never got along with the first Friends agent, Edward Painter. The small white community on the reservation suspected Painter of cheating the Omahas on their wheat transactions. Painter, in turn, accused Hamilton of school mismanagement; supposedly, his negligence led to poor attendance.[57]

Factionalism among the Omahas further fanned the flames of heated discord. Painter sided with "paper chiefs," who resented the La Flesche party, which was allied with the missionaries. The paper chiefs had succeeded in persuading Painter to transfer the $3,750, drawn annually from the Omahas' annuity to support the mission school, to fund the establishment of new day schools. This move on the part of the paper chiefs clearly was rooted in their resentment of Hamilton and the mission school, because many of the children of the "make-believe white men" attended the school. Of course, the change would also strike a blow against La Flesche's party, which had rallied around the Presbyterian authorities.[58] This rupture within the tribe reverberated into the late-nineteenth century and later implicated Susan for her association with the La Flesche party.

The government contract for the mission school was withdrawn, after a summer of accusations and counter-accusations, in September 1869, and by the end of the month the students had been sent away.[59] Quaker officials then established their day schools, which, they argued, would show better attendance since the students could return to their families on a daily basis. But, as it turned out, attendance remained small and irregular, and the schools drew mainly the children of "progressive parents."[60] Susan continued to mingle almost exclusively with semiacculturated youngsters. Her world was becoming more "white" than "red."

Ironically, the school that Susan now attended had been used as a blockhouse, which stored ammunition and military supplies during the height of the plains wars. Susan later remembered how she and other children had walked to the school, located three miles from home. She wrote: "The neighbor's children used to wait for us, so 15 or 20 of us, with our bright tin pails, trooped off, arriving in time for school at 9 o'clock." When school was out at "4 o'clock [we] had a gay time rushing home over the prairies, feeling free to loiter, and sometimes reaching home at sunset."[61]

Susan's day school, like the former mission school, taught her the rudiments—reading, writing, spelling, arithmetic—and, in addition, a few academic subjects like history and geography, in preparation for further education at an industrial boarding school. The Quaker school, unlike the Presbyterian institution, did not give students specific instruction in farm work and household training. Perhaps the Friends' divergence here was related to their separation of conversion from "civilization." Seemingly, Susan enjoyed the focus on book learning and did well. A shorter, and less regimented, schedule probably resulted in more "conscientious children," to borrow Susan's words. In one 1871 report, their teachers wrote that the Omaha childrens' "progress in learning . . . will compare favorably with any school of white children." Edwin C. Kemble, an Indian inspector, visited the day schools in 1874 and found that the students were making excellent strides in their education.[62] For Susan, this early exposure to Euro-American knowledge forged her sensitivity to the chasm dividing Indian and white cultures and, possibly, attuned her to the choices that confronted late-nineteenth-century Native Americans.

Susan's success at school had much to do with changes at home. Sometime in 1876 or 1877, after her older sister Susette had secured a teaching position on the reservation, the four sisters moved out of their parents' home and into a "little brown house" adjacent to Susette's school. Being the youngest, Susan took care of the odd, but light, errands. According to Susan, Susette insisted that the sisters converse with one another only in English. While living with her sisters for at least a couple of years, Susan made rapid improvement in her command of the language, which put her in good stead for higher education.[63]

Susan apparently relished the years she spent with the Quaker teachers. The Friends were convinced of the inherent spirituality of the Indians and felt that Native Americans could, like themselves, access the Inner Light or spiritual revelation. Their teachers, consequently, offered a generalized Christian education but avoided direct, active proselytism. They did set up Sabbath or Sunday schools, but they allowed educated Omahas some rein on the instruction. In fact, Susette led some of the meetings. Susan and her other sisters also attended these gatherings. This indirect approach, an affirmation of the egalitarianism of the Inner Light, was a stark contrast to the Presbyterians' didactic method of conversion. The Omahas, including the La Flesche sisters, were drawn to the Friends' sense of tolerance, which meshed well with the Omahas' traditional reverence for openness to new ideas.[64]

On the other hand, the Friends' downplaying of rituals diverged from the general admiration Plains tribes had for church ceremonies that paralleled their own religious teachings. This might explain why the La Flesche sisters, particularly Susan, did not adhere to Quakerism for the long run. Susan eventually returned to the fold of Presbyterianism.[65]

Despite the relative success of the Quaker schools, they did not escape the pressure of tribal factionalism and interdenominational tensions. With the support of the Presbyterians, members of the "young men's party" pleaded with the government as early as 1877 to reinstate support for the mission school. In an 1879 letter, Joseph La Flesche claimed that "the Quaker teachers had accomplished little in educating the Omaha youth." He emphatically stated that they did not want the day schools and "wish[ed] for the boarding school back." The lack of progress in "English learning" was cited as the main cause for the agitation.[66] Perhaps there was some truth in it; according to Hamilton, "even the Quakers feel and acknowledge the day schools a failure." Strapped for funds, most Indian schools across the country during the Peace Policy floundered and then failed.[67]

In 1879, not impressed with the Friends' educational efforts, Joseph must have encouraged Susan to follow the footsteps of Susette, who some years earlier had left the prairies and headed for Elizabeth, New Jersey. Through a connection with the relative of a local Presbyterian missionary, Susette had enrolled at the Elizabeth Institute for Young Ladies in 1869. At the end of her three-year stay, the principal of the institute placed her at the "head of her classes." Despite graduating with honors, Susette could not secure a teaching position on the Omaha reservation, because she was not white, until she threatened to bring the issue to the attention of the American public.[68]

By the time Susan was ready to embark on her own journey to the East, Susette had already made a mark in the consciousness of white Americans. Susette came to national attention as an advocate for the destitute Poncas. Following the Poncas' tragic removal to Indian Territory in 1877, Standing Bear and thirty other Poncas fled back to their homeland in northeastern Nebraska in the winter of 1879. But the U.S. Army caught up with the fugitives, and not long after, the group of Poncas were placed on trial. The Poncas successfully defended themselves and returned to their former land along the Niobrara River. Susette not only testified at the trial, but also led a fact-finding visit to the Ponca reservation. Then she began a long lecture tour of eastern cities—a tour designed to bring the plight of the Poncas to the attention of reformers and humanitarians.[69]

During Susette's tour the newspapers billed her as an "Indian Princess," thus identifying her with a popular, romanticized image of Native American women—a legacy of Pocahontas that bore no relation to reality. Indian women who were presumed to exemplify this image were admired because they were helpful to Euro-Americans and had accepted white culture. Considered "exceptional" Indians, these women were believed to possess superior qualities of intellect and morality, which enabled them to understand and embrace white, Christian civilization. In the perception of white Americans, Susette fit this image, because of her level of education, command of English, blood ties to the upper strata of the tribal society, and refined Victorian mannerisms.[70] This distorted understanding of Susette would later be repeated in the case of Susan. Euro-Americans remained oblivious to the fact that such women had to make difficult choices when engaging in cross-cultural contact; they were forced to confront the possibility of weakening their traditional identity even as they considered the potential gain that accommodation of white ways provided them.

Susette's role as an advocate for Native American rights and citizenship thrust forward the La Flesche family as exemplary Indians, and that attention facilitated Susan's entrance into white-dominated, social-benevolence networks. Susette's national prominence also paved the way for Susan's entry into the Elizabeth Institute. Accompanied by Marguerite, Susan spent nearly two and a half years at the institute, but little is known about this period in her life. Records related to the school are nonexistent, but published histories of the city of Elizabeth reveal that the school was established in 1861. Run by Nettie C. Read and Susan H. Higgins, the school offered English, elocution, Latin, and French. Additional subjects included German, philosophy, physiology, literature, drawing, and music. Students could pursue either the regular or the college preparatory courses. Susan probably chose the former, since she later had to return to the East for more education before beginning medical school. Her lessons in physiology class must have nurtured her interest in medicine.[71] This period away from reservation life further contoured Susan's cross-cultural agility; living in a predominantly

Euro-American environment must have impressed upon her the cultural advantages of the dominant society.

In 1882 Susan and Marguerite returned to the reservation. By then, Susan had grown into a slender, dark-complected seventeen-year-old woman with well-defined facial features that became, with age, increasingly angular. As Susan had changed, so had the Omahas. The Omahas had taken another significant step on the road to acculturation by agreeing to division of the reservation. Allotment of land, which would end the holding of land in common and move American Indians into private ownership of the land, was the challenge of the decade and beyond, and Susan's personal life would become inextricably linked to this route of "de-Indianization."

The parceling of land into quarter sections of 160 acres for each family was nothing new, because during the 1870s Quaker agents had carried out the Omahas' request for allotment in severalty as outlined in the 1865 treaty. Unwilling to leave Nebraska and share the fate of other removed tribes, the Omahas chose accommodation to white ways, including land titles and individual farms. Not that the Omahas had much choice; the last bison hunt in the winter of 1876–1877 ended with the Omahas scouring the plains and begging for food. Too poor to engage in commercial husbandry, they had to turn to the model of the white farm. With oxen and plows, the Omahas began to break up the black soil of the prairie and farm their tracts of land. Like white farmers, they now took their chances of bearing the brunt of grasshopper plagues and prolonged droughts.[72]

But the removal of the Poncas to Indian Territory worried the Omahas, because it had revealed that the Great Father's promise to safeguard their reservation was meaningless. Unfortunately, their fears were not unfounded. Because Congress never officially approved the allotment schedule, the Omahas did not own the land they had tilled.[73] After the panic over the possibility of losing their land had subsided somewhat, "progressive" Omahas, led by Joseph La Flesche, called upon the ethnologist Alice C. Fletcher, then working on the reservation, to help them secure proper titles to their land. Already convinced that Indians could move up the ladder of social evolution, Fletcher agreed. She had little problem persuading policy-makers in the nation's capital; by then, several bills providing for allotment in severalty had already been submitted. All that was needed was someone to push for the vote, and this she did with considerable success.[74]

For their part, "progressive" Omaha Indians accepted the Omaha Allotment Act of 1882, the forerunner of the Dawes, or General Allotment, Act of 1887, to avoid the possibility of losing all their land and being removed to Indian Territory. Some traditionalists, however, were less optimistic; they harbored some trepidations about the proposed legislation. Still, members of the Omaha Council considered division of the land a way to escape the supervision of the Indian Office. A tribal petition to Congress expressed their desire to preserve cultural and political independence: "This great country, that we called our own . . . is fast filling up with white people . . . we want to stay here as long as we live . . . . We ask that Congress. . . secure to us and our children what belongs to us."[75] Perhaps more than anything else, this defense of what remained of the ancestral homeland drew most of the wrangling tribal members together and, at least temporarily, papered over the cracks within the leadership ranks.

The Omahas had accepted the allotment legislation in hopes of halting the process of dispossession, but that would not prove the case. In fact, though aimed at creating individuality and "a desire to accumulate property," the allotment of land led to tribal destitution and dissipation by the turn of the century. This attempt to bring "civilization" to the Omahas, in essence to Americanize the Indians, did little to bring them closer to the rights and privileges of citizenship.[76]

But in the euphoria of having secured their titles via the 1882 legislation, the Omaha Indians celebrated their triumph. They welcomed Fletcher's return, this time to carry out the land allotment program among the Omahas. Fletcher wrote that during the early summer of 1883, she surveyed and registered the assigned land "amid torrid heats and torrid storms." It was during this time that Fletcher's path crossed Susan's.[77]

At this juncture, Susan assisted at the mission school. Reopened in December 1879, the mission school enrolled only female students by the time Susan joined the staff. In a questionnaire she later filled out for the Hampton Institute, Susan revealed that she taught for about six months at the school. An 1883 report by an OIA inspector identified Susan as the assistant to Mrs. Margaret C. Wade, the missionary teacher. This was probably a pleasant experience for Susan; the school was small and manageable. Inspectors, who looked for regimentation, lavished praise on the school; it was "comfortable," "in good order," and the students "looked well" and were "orderly."[78]

One wet day in July 1883, Susan's brother Francis—interpreter for the allotment work—brought Fletcher to the mission school. Fletcher, suffering from a severe chill, was very ill, with what was later diagnosed as inflammatory rheumatism, and laid in bed for nearly five weeks. During that time, Susan offered to care for and nurse her. Following her recovery, Fletcher, who once espoused that "education is the key to the Indian's future," helped Susan go away to school in Hampton, Virginia, and then to the Woman's Medical College in Philadelphia.[79] Like the relations she established in Elizabeth, Susan's relationship with Fletcher served as an important part of her widening circle of friends and acquaintances in the East that provided the entrée for her cultural brokerage later on.

So Susan left her family and tribe once again, and this time she was away for nearly five years. Her knowledge of the world broadened to encompass advanced western learning. She mingled with students from other tribes and learned of their common fate as objects of "de-Indianization."

Several years before Susan left for Hampton, the federal government had embraced a shift in its Indian policy. Rather than simply tinkering with its long-standing concentration policy, through half-hearted efforts in education and allotment of land, the government began to aggressively assimilate Native Americans into mainstream life and culture after 1879. Eventually the government sought to end its responsibility for maintaining reservations and protecting the interests of Indians.

This "Americanization program"—to be accomplished through education, allotment in severalty, and citizenship—grew from a series of deeply held assumptions, about the nature of the American experience and image of Americans, held by members of Euro-American society in the late nineteenth century. One of these assumptions was the desirability of a homogeneous populace. In the period after the Civil War, dramatic economic expansion wrought massive political, social, and demographic change. As spatial and socioeconomic boundaries between communities blurred, general consciousness of racial and ethnic differences became intensified. The ability of the American national identity—one rooted in abstract democratic ideals of equality and freedom—to hold the republic together, was called into question. A movement to forge a homogeneous, national identity based on Anglo-Saxon culture soon took flight, and the successful integration of "aliens" (whether Indians, or European and Asian immigrants) would validate that homogeneous image of the United States.[80]

New theories of social evolution also undergirded the Americanization policy. In the later third of the nineteenth century, social evolutionary ideas, rooted in Charles Darwin's "survival of the fittest thesis," infused the intellectual commentary on the course of human history of anthropologists like Lewis Henry Morgan. According to those social scientists, all peoples passed through three critical stages of evolutionary progress: from savagism, to barbarism, to civilization. The process of attaining civilization was linear, irreversible, and predetermined, but it took hundreds of thousands of years to complete. Euro-American humanitarian reformers—ministers, politicians, upper-middle-class women social activists, even anthropologists—found evolutionary progress, or gradualism, far too slow and difficult to reconcile with the power of Christian philanthropy to effect social change. Thus, reformers in the 1880s preached that private ownership of land and education would rapidly stimulate Indian industry and civilization.[81]

They believed that Anglo-Americans, who had already attained civilization, had a moral obligation to shape the development of those beneath them, such as American Indians. This unquestioned form of paternalism, propelled by unshakable faith in the interconnected power of Christianity and Anglo culture, shaped reformers' and the government's efforts to "Americanize" Native Americans. Susan's life and bicultural identity reflected these currents of social thought.

Equally important in the process of Susan's education was her exposure to and interaction with Euro-Americans. Her experiences at Hampton and the Woman's Medical College shaped the course of her life for years to come. In her own words, she would "come from the tepee to civilization."[82]

CHAPTER THREE

"Home is the Foundation"

In an undated letter Susan La Flesche wrote to her sisters from Hampton Institute, Susan assured them that she was "doing pretty well." She played tenpins with Walter, one of her classmates, and he had taught her how to skate. In a separate letter to her sister Rosalie, Susan revealed that she also took lessons in piano and drawing. She enjoyed drawing so much that she took additional lessons from non-Hampton instructors. Preoccupied with academic work and extra-curricular activities, Susan seldom wrote to her relatives, but she had not forgotten her family back on the reservation. "The days are flying fast," she wrote, "but I want to see you all so much."[1]

Separated from her family for nearly two years (1884–1886), Susan must have been hit by occasional pangs of homesickness. She was now surrounded by lush foliage, a wind-swept seacoast, and the Chesapeake Bay instead of grassy, hilly prairies. At the youthful, impressionable age of nineteen, Susan left familiar faces behind to meet people of all colors and moved from a modest frame house to live in monumental brick and stone buildings. At Hampton, Virginia, a new cultural mélange awaited the young Omaha woman, and encounters there would further hone her ability to move with sensitivity among different peoples.

Founded in 1868 during Reconstruction as a normal school for the industrial education of black freedmen, Hampton expanded into Indian education in 1878. The parallel that reformers drew between the needs of black ex-slaves and those of Indians, in terms of preparing them for full participation in American society, made it logical to provide room for Indians as well as blacks at Hampton. In admitting Indians, Hampton provided the impetus for the development of off-reservation government boarding schools. The well-known Carlisle Indian Industrial School and other similar institutes grew out of the belief that education was the panacea for solving the "Indian Question." It was believed that the complete separation of Indian youth from their aboriginal home environment would break bonds of family and ethnic identity and, in so doing, would facilitate the young peoples' rapid and complete absorption of white ways. With their "Indianness" destroyed and their successful transformation into self-sufficient individuals accomplished, these youths included, would in theory be ready to integrate fully into mainstream society. Life on the reservation would come to an end, and the conflicts of the past would be relegated to the pages of history.[2] Or at least that was how the reformers envisioned the process.

At Hampton, the "war" for the Indian's "mind, heart, and soul" began in 1878 with a group of seventeen ex-prisoners from St. Augustine, Florida. In the next decade the enrollment climbed steadily to 120, and it remained constant to the turn of the century. As a contract school, Hampton received financial aid from the federal government, but most of its funding came from philanthropic support and from the state of Virginia. For example, Susan's education was sponsored, in addition to federal monies, by a Smith College missionary society and a benevolent humanitarian.[3]

Susan arrived at Hampton sometime in early August 1884. Her elder brother, Francis, then already a federal employee in Washington, D.C. (and soon to become an accomplished ethnologist), brought Susan, her sister Marguerite, her stepbrother Cary (1872–1952), and ten other Omaha children to the school. All were reported by the school physician to be in "fair physical condition." Following the examination, Susan moved into Winona Lodge, the new $30,000 girls' dormitory—

built with funds that, taking advantage of her national prominence, her sister Susette had helped to raise. Winona Lodge was homey; instead of huge halls, students lived in groups of twos and threes in small, private rooms.[4]

Being an older, educated student and coming from a stable, acculturated family, Susan adapted well to Hampton. She continued her ties with Christianity and became acquainted with Euro-American popular culture. At Winona, Susan enjoyed the company of other female Indians, as indicated in one of her few surviving letters from Hampton. "We are having very good times," she reported. Games were played in the evenings—checkers, dominoes, and tenpins. Susan and the other young women also organized and participated in Saturday socials, which were open to fellow male students and featured literary and musical diversions. On Sunday mornings the young women gathered for prayer service and, later, drew around the piano to sing hymns. In the afternoon, they joined the rest for Sunday school and regular church services. In Susan's words, Winona Lodge was her "second home"—the place where she re-created close supportive ties of family and community, the site where a fluid sense of "Indianness" prevailed.[5]

Susan wrote home that she had joined Hampton to find "happy seekers after knowledge." Fortunately for her, there was plenty of such company, including young women. In the year Susan arrived, females made up two-fifths of the Indian student body. The founder and principal of her new school, General Samuel Chapman Armstrong, believed in equal education for both sexes. General Armstrong expounded that both men and women should be trained to experience "improvement in mind and heart." Educated Native Americans would then return to the reservations to play mediatory roles as teachers of "civilization" and Christianity to their own peoples. As bearers of new knowledge, they would teach others to acquire temperance, responsibility, education, and "Bible truths." In short, ex-Hampton students had the awesome burden of transforming their communal-based peoples into "self-independent" citizens.[6]

Echoing the prescriptive ideology of true womanhood, Armstrong promoted the training of Indian women students for family life and

Christian benevolence. Armstrong contended that educated Indian women would prevent their spouses and families from "returning to the blanket." They would help their husbands move from hunters or pastoralists to farmers in the convoluted climb up the cultural-evolutionary staircase. As mothers, Indian women could influence tribal society and shape the future by nurturing their children. In short, young Indian girls were being imprinted with certain class and gender constructions. Armstrong once wrote: "On the Indian girl, as upon women everywhere, depends the virtue, the true value of the red or of any race."[7]

Implicit in Armstrong's viewpoint was the belief that Indians could be elevated, that they "were low, but not degraded." Though clearly a proponent of environmental determinism, Armstrong also subscribed to social-evolutionary progress. However, unlike most reformers, he believed it would take considerable time before Indians could attain the level of "civilization" of white Americans. Armstrong once wrote that "a well balanced mind is attained only after generations of improvements."[8]

Like government Indian schools, Hampton Institute served as the laboratory for the Indians' planned social evolution. Thus, would-be graduates received instruction in industrial education, with emphasis on manual labor and vocational skills, so that they could impart to their peoples a "whole circle of living." Male students learned farm labor, while females honed their household skills. According to one scholar, this emphasis on physical training reflected racialistic conceptions of the intrinsic connection between uncivilized minds and undeveloped bodies. It was believed that by shaping the body, changes in mental habits and discourses would follow suit and that only after Indians had mastered such basics could they move on to acquire the finer elements of mainstream culture. This step-by-step approach permeated the curricula.[9]

Yet students were not forced to give up completely their Indian languages or to abandon traditional arts. Out of fear that Indians would backslide, the OIA proscribed the use of native tongues both in and out of the classroom. But in a departure from the common practice at such schools, Hampton officials placed no restrictions on vernacular languages, so long as they were not used during instructional periods. Susan attained a high level of English proficiency but never lost her command of the Omaha language, which later became an essential tool for mediatory work on the reservation. At Hampton, officials insisted that they never resorted to any sort of punishment to induce the use of English. School officials also drew attention to Indian arts and crafts; classes were offered and fairs organized to show off student-made goods. This paradox of the "civilization" process was explainable: with their tribal skills intact, students could make a living back on the reservations. But implicit in this attitude of acceptance of Native American cultures was also sanction for segregation and accommodation, not assimilation. This stance was also reflected in the curtailment of social intercourse between Indian and black students. They were separately quartered, ate at their own tables, and, for the most part, they were taught in separate classrooms. Rationalized as necessary because Indians, unlike blacks, had yet to learn the value of labor, such segregation was out of step with the government's attempt to integrate Indians into mainstream society.[10]

Hampton Institute's ambivalence toward absorption of Indians into the dominant society meshed well with Susan's heritage of partial acculturation, and continuity marked the years at Hampton as Susan maintained ties with her people and tribal culture. Susan's stepsister, Lucy (1865–1923), and her husband, Noah, were close by. The couple lived in one of the institute's Indian cottages, which allowed Native American couples and families to emulate white, middle-class household arrangements. Susan and her sister Marguerite often joined them for festive occasions. When a devastating tornado swept through their reservation, Hampton's Omaha students offered money and sent clothing to their suffering tribespeople. Like other Indian students, Susan probably participated in traditional arts and crafts sessions. Hampton students were encouraged to display their articles during holidays and open days. Susan's senior class once put on a living tableau of Native American life, complete with a realistic tipi and appropriate costumes.[11]

However many other school activities reminded Susan of her cultural middle ground—of her developing ambiguous, bicultural identity. She attended meetings of the Lend-a-Hand Club, which promoted the sense of benevolence. Students in the club collected gifts for the poor and taught Sunday school. After graduation, in a letter Susan wrote to Hampton's principal, she admitted that she missed the "prayer meetings, the church, all the different forms of good work . . . Lend-a-Hand, temperance, social, and missionary work." Apparently, Susan also attended meetings of the Temperance Committee, and she probably spent time visiting the sick and helping with the spiritual and physical needs of the poor. She also joined the Christian Endeavor Society, and later in life she established a chapter on the Omaha reservation to promote catechismal precepts. The Hampton years offered ideas for the roles Susan would play later among the Upstream People.[12]

Young Susan now clearly began to identify with the new order. Looking back on her years at the institute, she appreciated the labors of her white teachers, who had done so much to "cheer, comfort, and help" her and others. Grateful for the guidance of her Hampton teachers, Susan forged relationships with them based on respect and obligation. In a letter written immediately after her graduation from Hampton, Susan said she considered herself to be one of the many "daughters" who had entered the missionary field to exert her "individual influence." And in a letter written to a teacher during the summer of 1885, while she was still attending Hampton, Susan reverentially called her women teachers "Mothers" and openly declared that she missed them during the summer vacations. She ended the letter with a prayer for her teacher's well-being and safe journey back to Hampton.[13]

Like her teachers, Susan had faith in the reformability of Indians. In a letter to Rosalie, she recounted the story of how Sam, a male Omaha schoolmate, became involved in some mischief and was subsequently disciplined. Though disheartened, Sam still "wants to learn so badly," argued Susan. She requested that Rosalie ask their father to write Sam and give him some words of encouragement. Susan believed that, like any other Indian, Sam could be as good as whites.[14]

In another letter written just after she left the institute, Susan praised the cottage program. She felt it had "awakened" many Indians to the merits of "civilization." Even the "non-progressives" were coming around, she wrote. Susan clearly distanced herself from the traditionalists; she may have felt a slight hint of embarrassment since some members of the Omaha tribe still adhered to the ways of the past. "The little wave," she added, "that started will be productive of much good to my people." Susan thought that the Indians' potential might be dormant, but it existed. And yet, by using the personal adjective "my" in her letter, Susan clearly identified with her people.[15] Partly elicited by her teachers, this range of conflicting emotions—youthful enthusiasm, gracious gratitude, guilt, and racial ambition—would spur her to edge toward the role of cultural broker.

Proud of her people, Susan did not show contempt for traditional ways. In fact, probably tired of whites' condemnation of their so-called "brutish" ways, Susan once wrote that "it is a characteristic trait, too, of the Indians to love their homes." Influenced by her father's heritage, Susan tried to find a cultural middle ground—one where both Omaha and white cultures could meet at some level of mutual understanding. At the very least, identification with the teachers' message did not lead Susan to totally abandon the past. After all, Hampton was only her "second home"; the real one was her "own dear Western home."[16]

Susan obviously internalized the civilization-savagism paradigm, but seemingly conquered the self-hatred and cultural self-loathing that paradigm suggests. This should not be surprising, since her tribe's concept of nationhood had always been in flux and could accommodate innovations. For Susan, it is probable that the incorporation of selective white ways was simply part of the long-term process of forging a personal and tribal identity. By maintaining some distance from total acceptance of either white or Omaha ways without experiencing cognitive dissonance or cultural conflict, Susan was able to develop the ability to make certain life choices that were necessary for maintaining the balance between cultures.[17] Perhaps, in turn, such mediatory work confirmed Susan's self-worth, even as she wrestled with her tentative Indian identity.

At Hampton, Susan absorbed western knowledge that prepared her for the role of a cultural broker, one who would selectively introduce more white ways to her people. She learned to set aside the Indians' cyclical concept of time, which was process oriented, and instead took on the western view that time was result oriented and linear, with an end and a beginning. This understanding of time undergirded the OIA acculturation policy and came into conflict with traditional Indian beliefs. Furthermore, instead of existing in a mythologically defined world, Susan's world was now one governed by the rationality and predictability of science.[18]

Susan's regimented daily schedule, goal oriented and task specific, usually began at five-thirty in the morning. After chores and calisthenics Susan and the other girls, dressed in uniforms of dark calico and muslin dresses, would join the boys (and black students) for classes at nine. At Hampton, Indians with little exposure to white education began in one of the Indian Department divisions (almost thoroughly vocational in nature), then moved into a full-day advanced class (also called the Indian School), and finally into the biracial Normal course. Since Susan had already spent some years in the classroom, she could bypass all the preparatory classes and enter the apex of Hampton's academic work. Because Susan was at Hampton for only two years, she must have undergone an abbreviated version of the three-year Normal course. She probably skipped the junior, or first, year and proceeded straight to the second, or middle, year. In her middle year, she studied literature, physical geography, arithmetic, physiology, and the Bible. She also had to master reading, English composition and grammar, and elocution.[19]

In her senior year Susan took civil government, history, political economy, physics, natural history (biology), and again, literature, reading, English composition, and arithmetic. Judging from a letter she wrote in the summer of 1865, she also went through a stint of summer teaching—a required component for all seniors.[20] This aspect of her education suggested the path the federal government envisioned for Indian graduates. Like almost all Indian students of the time, Susan received little, if any, formal exposure to Native American culture or history.

The long weekday usually ended at four in the afternoon. Most of the time the young women had the late afternoon to themselves, but once a week they learned to prepare and serve Anglo-American meals. Susan also took sewing lessons, as evidenced in a letter she wrote home. When the clock chimed six o'clock, all students filed into the dining hall. It was suppertime. Prayers in the chapel followed. Students then put in a couple of study hours before retiring at 9:30 P.M. The next morning, they began the whole routine again.[21]

However, that regimented schedule applied to only four days of the week. Sunday was a rest day. The other two days of the week Susan and the other students worked in the laundry rooms, kitchen, and other Hampton facilities, for which they received token wages. School officials believed that such work would make Indian women and men self-reliant and independent. Susan apparently used her wages to pay for piano lessons.[22]

Sometime just a few months before commencement, probably in February 1886, Susan must have made up her mind to apply to the Woman's Medical College in Pennsylvania. A letter from her teacher dated March 3, 1886, and addressed to Alice Fletcher revealed that Susan had received her information packet from the medical college and was in the process of writing her letter of application.[23]

Of course, Susan's decision to enter medical school was long in the making. A few years before she passed away, Susan recalled a time when, at the age of six, her father took her and her sisters aside and asked: "My dear young daughters, do you always want to be simply called those Indians or do you want to go to school and be somebody in the world?" "From that moment," Susan continued, "I determined to make something useful of my life."[24] Then, at the age of twelve, Susan witnessed the tragic removal of the Poncas to Indian Territory. The oppression marked her conscience; she wanted and needed to learn the white's ways and their source of power. Susan realized that higher education would open doors. Her relatively easy adjustment to life at Hampton stemmed from this keen personal ambition and kin influence—forces which clearly were driving her search for self-validation and power.[25]

But Susan's need to gain personal power also had origins in other equally transformative childhood experiences. As a young girl, Susan went through a dramatic incident that profoundly changed her life.

One day she had gone to succor a sick Indian woman. During the night the woman grew increasingly weak, and four times a messenger was sent for the doctor at the agency. Apparently he promised to come each time; but the night was dark, "and it was only an Indian, and it [did] not matter," recalled Susan bitterly. The woman died in agony the next morning. The reservation doctor railed Susan, preferred "hunting for prairie chickens" rather than "visiting poor, suffering humanity," railed Susan. In an interview she gave to a reporter, Susan credited this tragedy with shaping her resolve and giving her the willpower to study medicine and serve others.[26]

Susan could have joined the teaching profession; after all, this was one of the few professions Hampton graduates were trained to enter. But as she revealed in a letter to a benefactor, Susan felt that as a physician she could, "do a great deal more than as a mere teacher [since her] work . . . will be chiefly in the homes" of her people.[27] Unlike a teacher, whose already limited influence on the youth was often countered by kinship ties, Susan felt that as a physician she would have a direct impact on the lives of all Omahas and thus would derive more personal satisfaction from this type of mediatory work.

Most women graduates of Hampton did return to their Indian homes, but by and large they were still neither prepared to bring their families into the fold of mainstream society nor adequately trained to find paid work. A tabulation of data extracted from an 1891 school report indicates that over 80 percent of Hampton's female graduates never assumed a wage-earning job. Those who did, could only find positions with the Indian department, and even then they were placed at the most menial level—as cooks, seamstresses, nurses' helpers, and assistant matrons. Economic self-sufficiency remained fairly elusive. Those who married and established households discovered that the lessons of domesticity they had learned in boarding school rarely could be applied to a technologically impoverished environment. In short, schools did not train Indian women for the conditions they encountered upon returning home.[28]

Without further education and equipped with only vocational training, Susan probably would have returned to the Omaha reservation. At best she would have worked for a little while, married, raised a family, and then disappeared into oblivion. In this sense, the Hampton experience could be deemed a failure. Even schoolteaching would not have allowed her to make her mark on the reservation. For most OIA Indian employees, low salaries and paternalistic white supervisors often resulted in their having only marginal influence.[29]

Susan's decision to attend a western medical college was unique since, discouraged by societal attitudes, nineteenth-century women rarely conceived of medical training as an academic goal. But the fact that she became a healer was not unusual. In some western tribes, women sometimes assumed the roles played by shamans and medicine men. These native medical practitioners mastered their skills through visions and trances brought on by fasting. Medicine women and female shamans relied on herbs, medicinal plants, magical tobacco pipes, rock crystals, and special chants to help them cure illnesses. Though Indians could acquire medical skills at any time in their lives, Indian women could not practice healing until after menopause. This prohibition stemmed from the Native American conviction that during their menstrual periods women posed a potential spiritual danger to the tribe, especially to warriors preparing for battle or a hunt.[30] In setting out to earn a medical degree before that stage in her life, Susan broke with Omaha traditions.

A visit, probably in early 1886, to Washington, D.C., to see her family friend Alice C. Fletcher most likely helped Susan make the final decision about medical school. A few years earlier she had confided in Fletcher that she would like to "instruct [Indians] in the laws of health" and "minister to them in sickness." At that time Fletcher became determined that Susan should have her desire fulfilled. Fletcher had long thought about the need to train young Indians to assume positions in the OIA medical services, and in 1882 she wrote some members of congress to seek moral support for the idea. Fletcher now agreed to use her prominence as an Indian reformer to write a letter of support for Susan's college application.[31]

But Susan faced obstacles to her application for medical school. Funding was one; another was societal attitudes. The federal government had never provided Indians with financial aid for professional education. Well-known Native American doctors, including Charles

Eastman (Santee Sioux) and Carlos Montezuma (Yavapai), both contemporaries of Susan La Flesche, had relied on private aid to complete their medical studies. Certainly money was an issue. During the nineteenth century, many medical-college applicants turned down their admission because of the prohibitive cost.[32] More problematic were gender and racial prejudices. In the 1880s, women in the medical profession still faced the problem of sex discrimination. Women enjoyed a place in medicine before the American Revolution, but by the antebellum years they could not even retain their place in midwifery, a previously female-dominated field. Elizabeth Blackwell, the first college-trained woman doctor, received her degree in 1849. Some medical colleges in the West, desperate to fill their coffers, granted degrees to women as early as the 1850s. However, reputable colleges, mostly in the East, kept their doors closed. Not until the founding of women's medical colleges such as the New England Female Medical College (1848) and the Woman's Medical College of Pennsylvania (1850) did women begin to reestablish their access to the medical profession.[33]

But the fact that women like Susan had to flock to all-female medical colleges shows that few in society viewed women physicians as the equals of their male colleagues. Women physicians, or "doctoring ladies" as they were derogatorily called, were routinely denied hospital internships and residencies, and many state and county medical societies shunned them and blocked their admission.[34]

In the minds of their opponents, women physicians were simply an anathema, because they threatened the prescriptive gender roles for middle-class Americans—men at work, women at home. It was believed that with God-given nurturing qualities, women were more suited for the demands of domesticity and that women who refused to abide by those expectations threatened the survival of family life and risked engendering the masculization of the female sex. Femininity, the hallmark of idealized womanhood, was allegedly tied to the notion that biologically women were far weaker in mind and physical strength than men. In fact, many male physicians concluded that the female mind was simply emotional and irrational and not adapted to scientific thinking.[35]

Some opponents went so far as proposing that the intellectual inferiority of women stemmed from the smaller size of their brains and that biological ailments related to their reproductive organs—menstrual problems in particular—took away their physical vigor. Thus, they thought that women would fail to rise to the intellectual and physical challenges of medical training, and they implied that women who insisted on pursuing higher education risked tampering with their reproductive ability. Many eminent physicians and scientists believed, in accordance with the theory of the closed-body system, that the mental strain of college life would weaken the development of the female's reproductive organs. Consequently, white racial suicide would follow suit. Though opponents of female education never applied their theories about the dangers of higher education specifically to Indian women, their collective voice on the matter was strong enough to proscribe higher education for all women, Indian or otherwise. Then there was the economic question. Already in stiff competition for limited patients, male doctors feared that the entry of women into their profession would further pull down the wage scale.[36]

Fortunately for Susan there were just as many supporters of medical training for women as there were opponents. In essence, the supporters turned the arguments used against them around. While opponents argued that certain traits made women unfit, defenders of female medical training contended that the same idealized feminine traits—purity, nurturance, and domesticity—made women "natural" healers. The supporters contended that with medical knowledge and skills, women could protect their homes and families.[37] Dr. Clara Marshall, the Dean of the Woman's Medical College of Pennsylvania from 1888 to 1917, argued that women's "delicate organization . . . of the nervous system" and their keen sense of self-control made them highly qualified for medical training and practice. Graduates, she wrote, could use their knowledge of preventive medicine to help protect their own homes and families.[38]

This line of argument gained ground following the undermining of the heroic image of the physician. The discovery of anaesthesia in the late 1840s challenged the need for "manly detachment" (the courage needed to perform painful procedures), which, opponents to female medical training argued, women could not achieve. However, the use of ether and chloroform severed the idea of inflicting pain on patients from the image of physicians, and that, in turn, "feminized" medicine. Finally, defenders also argued that female modesty, which was often cited as a factor for barring women from the profession, instead demanded that women be cared for by only female physicians.[39]

In sum, allowing female entry into the study and practice of medicine was seen as part of the larger effort to adapt prescriptive concepts of womanhood to the demands of the unstable, rapidly industrializing American society. It was believed that female influence, exerted via medical work, would temper masculine individualism, rationalism, and competition.[40]

One of the graduates of the Woman's Medical College of Pennsylvania was Dr. Martha M. Waldron. After the completion of her training in 1881, she returned to Hampton Institute, where she had previously taught for a number of years. For the next thirty years, Waldron held the position of the school's first resident physician. Keenly aware of the range of maladies Indians suffered from, Waldron expounded the need for well-educated Hampton graduates to take home proper hygiene techniques and appropriate health standards.[41]

Waldron had encouraged Susan to master academic subjects, and she also considered her capable of earning a medical degree. Waldron probably was responsible for the selection of the Woman's Medical College of Pennsylvania as Susan's alma mater. On March 20, 1886, Waldron wrote to Alfred Jones, then the secretary of the executive committee of the college. In her letter, she asked on Susan's behalf for a scholarship. Jones's reply disappointed Waldron and Susan. According to Jones, all available funds had already been allocated for the year, and a "free scholarship" was simply "out of the question." He indicated that if Susan still wished to apply, she needed to turn in a handwritten application, outlining her health, character, and educational qualifications.[42]

Susan must have conveyed this disheartening news to Fletcher, because Fletcher then took it upon herself to find other sources of funding. She talked with OIA officials who were acquainted with her work with the Omaha Indians. In a letter dated April 24, 1886, Fletcher shared the good news with Susan: the "government has promised to help you." But, always distrustful of bureaucrats, Fletcher warned that "government contracts are queer." Probably as a backup, in case the Indian Office failed to completely honor its pledge, Fletcher claimed to have secured the support of "some ladies in Connecticut."[43]

The ladies were the members of the Connecticut Indian Association (CIA), an auxiliary of the Women's National Indian Association (WNIA). The WNIA drew together upper-middle-class Anglo women who were interested in Indian reform. The organization expanded from drives for political petitions into work for practical improvement—mission work, home building, and education for Indian youth. Founded in 1879, the organization quickly established branches throughout the country, including the one in Connecticut. Organized in 1881, the CIA, like its parent organization, sought to provide American Indians, particularly native women, with access to industrial training, education, citizenship, and Christianization.[44]

The labors of the CIA women suggest the exercise of "maternalism." Many Euro-American women reformers harbored the conviction that they should play a motherly role in their dealings with the underprivileged, including Indians, because they needed spiritual and economic assistance. These reformers also believed that womens' work, experience, and their role as mothers enabled them to lead the crusade for social change, while it also made underprivileged mothers (or potential mothers) uniquely deserving of help. The CIA women's relationship with Susan soon took on this unequal yet female-centered dynamic.[45]

Fletcher was familiar with the goals of the CIA, and she knew that Susan's ambition dovetailed with CIA programs. As early as February 1885, the association agreed to support one deserving Indian woman enrolled in a medical college, and in the next five years they also extended financial aid to three other women undergoing professional nursing training. Apparently the initial impetus for funding higher education for Indian women, though driven in part by Christian maternalism, was also engendered by a romanticized perception of Indians' natural inclinations toward healing. The WNIA's mouthpiece, the *Indian Bulletin*, admired the Indian woman's "quiet dignity," her "eye trained to observe," her "strict obedience, [the] outgrowth of centuries of submission," and her "deft and skillful" hands and "patient, willing feet that know no laggings"—all characteristics that conjured images of the noble "Good Indian," or "Indian Princess" image. However, Fletcher, who may or may not have known about this stereotyping of Indian women on the part of the WNIA and its auxiliaries, was also acquainted with the president of the CIA, Sara Thomas Kinney. She had met this wealthy, influential woman at the annual gathering for reform groups at Lake Mohonk, New York. Fletcher either wrote or spoke to Kinney about Susan's career goals and her financial needs. For her part, Kinney agreed to bring up the issue at the next CIA meeting.[46]

There is no doubt that Fletcher cared about Susan's future. Her maternalistic attitude was obvious. When Susan's teachers, including Waldron, failed to respond to Fletcher's letter on matters related to Susan's application, she got Susan to relay her concerns to them posthaste. In the same letter, Fletcher also indirectly advised Susan to use the coming summer to brush up her knowledge of anatomy and other relevant sciences in preparation for her first term at medical school in the fall. Susan probably was flattered by all the attention.[47] Fletcher's guidance, and her ties to a white female social network, nudged Susan closer to Euro-American middle-class society.

April came and went, and Susan's stay at Hampton was drawing to an end. Commencement was just around the corner. Soon she would leave to return to Nebraska, and yet she had heard nothing from the CIA, the federal government, or the medical college. Her future seemed uncertain.

The day of commencement, May 20, 1886, began on a gloomy note; "the day dawned dull and lowering," reported the school newspaper, and soon the "threatening clouds" turned into "showers which deepened the green of leaves." But the weather did little to dampen the festivities. Fletcher, who was present, reported to Rosalie that, including dignitaries from the capital, more than a thousand guests attended the exercises. After the opening prayer and a couple of spirituals, it was time for Susan to take center stage.[48]

The faculty had chosen Susan to be the salutatorian. Her teachers once described her as "a young woman of more than ordinary mental ability and earnestness of character." The principal, General Armstrong, had "no hesitation in speaking of her as a young woman of unusual ability." On that auspicious day, Susan was dressed in a simple but "pretty, striped dress." Looking "neat" and "lovely," according to Fletcher, Susan walked up to the podium and delivered her address, entitled "My Childhood and Womanhood."[49] In her speech, she expressed anxious gratitude to all patrons and humanitarians for their "noble work" on behalf of Indians. She felt confident that she and fellow seniors could return their kindness through their future endeavors. No doubt Susan had faith in the potential of Indians.[50]

Because of a recent congressional investigation into the effectiveness of Indian schools, Susan also felt compelled to address that issue in her talk. The investigation had resulted in several bills, all of which proposed the withdrawal of appropriations from eastern boarding schools, Hampton included. This attack on eastern off-reservation schooling stemmed from the policy-makers' and politicians' perception that educating Indians in the East was not cost effective; most alumni returned to a reservation and their education background was ill-suited to reservation life. Critics of Hampton, Carlisle, and other off-reservation schools proposed on-reservation schools that would raise the general level of education, a proposal that was eventually accepted. However, just before Susan's commencement, the bills were, at least temporarily, defeated. In making reference to that issue, Susan took a moment to express appreciation to the dignitaries attending the ceremony for their continuing support of the "civilization" of her people. In so doing, Susan showed her identification with Hampton's (and the government's) mission, and she also acted as a broker on behalf of the recently criticized institute. In extending her appreciation to the politicians and OIA officials, Susan was speaking on behalf of the school administration as well.[51]

Susan focused most of the address on memories of her early upbringing in Nebraska. In a story told with much humor and literary flourish, she took her audience back to "the wilds of Nebraska . . . on the banks of a large creek" where her childhood began. She romantically evoked those early years; she remembered the "handsome, stalwart young braves looking very fine and picturesque," as they "vied with each other" during a traditional game. Susan's memories missed none of the delights of childhood but skipped over all of the sad moments. In her remembrance, the Omahas came across as happy people, contented with farming and life on the reservation. The audience heard nothing about the poverty, the loss of land, or the threat of removal. Susan had no intention of offending people who might help her in the future.[52]

Susan certainly wanted her address to sound optimistic. She pointed out that her people had made some progress, and, in language reminiscent of social-evolutionary theory, she reminded her audience that it had taken a long time for Euro-Americans to reach a high standard of civilization. She said: "Indians are only beginning; so do not try to put us down, but help us to climb higher." Susan implied that Indians were worthy of the Euro-Americans' benevolence; Indians could succeed, but only if whites extended a helping hand. Most of all, according to Susan, Indians must learn to use Euro-American laws, provided whites were willing to share the protection of those laws with the Indians. This was probably a subtle barb at opponents of the Dawes Act—then working through the hallways of Congress—which would offer citizenship and rights to Native Americans with land allotments.[53]

Susan's long-winded speech ended with an exposition on her career goals. She said that as a physician, she would "help [the Omahas] physically, teach them the importance of cleanliness, order and ventilation, how to take care of their bodies as well as care for their souls." Susan planned to parlay the influence of her womanhood for the good of her people and, in so doing, to exemplify the mediatory role to which Hampton officials hoped their students would aspire.[54] Susan admitted that she had "a long, hard struggle before" her but added that "the shores of success can only be reached by crossing the bridge of faith." Her spiritual humbleness and her belief in God's providence were clear: "I can only rejoice that the

Lord has given to me such a great privilege . . . to help in bringing them [Indians] into the light of the gospel of Jesus Christ." By covering the themes of Christian faith, Victorian morality, and selfless dedication to her own people, Susan was trying to appeal to the sensibilities of nineteenth-century Protestant Americans.[55] She did what all cultural mediators often found themselves doing—speaking the language of the "Other" in order to build bridges between cultures.

According to Fletcher, Susan spoke articulately and everyone found her impressive. After the "thundering applause," Susan stepped forward to receive from Representative General Byron M. Cutcheon (R. Michigan) the Demorest Prize, a gold medal awarded to the graduate who attained the highest examination score in the junior year. Later Susan described that moment as a "dream." Cutcheon also extolled Susan's academic success and reminded her to "live for [her] people."[56]

The next day, a few hundred miles away in Hartford, Connecticut, members of the Connecticut Indian Association met to deliberate on Susan's request for assistance. They heard a report from Seth Talcott, who had visited Susan at Hampton and was pleased with her demeanor. The president, Sara T. Kinney, reiterated what she had learned from a Hampton teacher. She reported that Susan was of sound character and had impressive academic credentials. After a short deliberation, the association voted to support her. Without this formal agreement, Susan might not have even entered the medical college, because the school required all applicants to show that they had adequate financial means to complete the program.[57]

To raise funds, the CIA placed an appeal in the *Hartford Courant*, whose editor was the husband of President Kinney. In that appeal, Fletcher wrote that Susan was "gentle, refined, conscientious and unselfish, and seems a rare character for any walk in life." Though less effusive, her Hampton principal, General Armstrong, was no less complimentary: "She is a level-headed, earnest, capable Christian woman, quite equal . . . to medical studies. She deserves every chance."[58]

The CIA also secured a letter from Susan herself. In her letter, she thanked her "many mothers" for their generosity. She also acknowledged her mediatory role: "[I am] glad to think that through me you will be helping so many people." The rest of her letter must have pleased the CIA and the readership of the *Courant*, because Susan detailed her missionary aspirations in maternal rhetoric: "I hope to go into their [Omahas'] homes and help the women in their housekeeping, teach them a few practical points about cooking and nursing, and especially about cleanliness." Trying to be humble, Susan was quick to point out she could "show them only a little," placing her trust on future generations of educated Indian women to carry on the work.[59]

But Susan also used her letter as an opportunity to defend the value of Indian culture. She asserted that "the home is the foundation of all things for the Indians." Susan made an attempt to show that, like white Americans, Indians had the utmost respect for the sanctity of homelife. For Victorian Americans, the home served as the site for a type of nurture that resulted in self-knowledge, self-realization, and even self-redemption, but it also codified asymmetry in gender roles. Susan's focus on this ambivalent construct reflected her sensitivity to the instrumentality of Euro-American culture and also to how that culture could be selectively mobilized at appropriate moments for cross-cultural understanding. Like most mediators, Susan tried to find common ground across the supposed cultural divide.[60]

Susan's seemingly Victorian aspirations neatly echoed the philosophy of the CIA. Like other women's organizations of the day, the CIA phrased its mission in terms of caring for the home and children, thus enabling women to take on wider responsibilities without overstepping existing social boundaries. In practice, through their social work, members of the CIA violated the division between public and private spheres in a age when the valorization of domesticity was becoming increasingly meaningless because of incorporation and market forces. And by giving aid directly to women, not through their husbands or fathers, CIA reformers challenged women's economic and political dependency on men. Still, these women chose to rationalize their agency or female subjectivity in the public world on the basis of the supposedly unique qualities they had mustered through their location in the private realm of home, family, and motherhood. As a result, the CIA's appeal for financial support emphasized Susan's maternalistic desire to be a "physician for women and children." At least in public rhetoric, Susan responded likewise.[61]

Sometime in July or August, Susan heard from the medical college. She had been accepted, but there was still the nagging issue of money. By then Susan was back on the reservation, helping her father tend the annual crops.[62]

It is quite possible that the CIA appeal for contributions came up short. In early September, less than three weeks before Susan was scheduled to leave for Philadelphia, Kinney wrote an urgent letter to Commissioner of Indian Affairs John D. C. Atkins requesting financial aid for Susan. Since there was no precedent for federal support of professional education, Kinney argued that money set aside for Indian youth in contract schools be used to help Susan. Kinney also appealed to the Commissioner's Victorian preconceptions; Susan, she wrote, "would minister to the physical needs of the women and children."[63]

The Commissioner replied promptly on September 8: the request was granted. But additional complications developed. The organization filled out the necessary forms and sent them back, but for weeks they heard nothing from the Indian Office. On September 16, Kinney dashed off a short note to the Commissioner, but she never received a reply.[64]

In desperation, Kinney sent her own money to Francis La Flesche for Susan's train fare. Francis, in turn, wired Bancroft, Nebraska, for the ticket. At long last, Susan would leave on the first of the month.[65]

With the issue of financial aid unresolved, Susan must have felt some anxiety as she boarded the train for the long journey across the plains and over the Appalachians. Yet she was also excited. She felt her work "as an Indian girl" was "plain before her." Susan was one step closer to fulfilling her professional ambition.[66]

CHAPTER FOUR

"Kind of Getting There"

A tired and weary Susan arrived in Philadelphia in early October. Trainsick and homesick, Susan was glad to alight and meet Seth Talcott, the chair of the business committee of the Connecticut Indian Association (CIA). Also present to welcome her was Dr. Elizabeth Bundy, an instructor of anatomy at the college. Talcott found Susan suitable lodgings at a boarding house and took her around Philadelphia to shop for clothing, books, and supplies. Talcott also served as liaison between the CIA and the medical college and helped to smooth Susan's entrance into the institution.[1]

Susan wrote to her sister Rosalie that she found her boarding place "very pleasant" and enjoyed it "so much." She reported that the proprietor, identified as Mrs. Smith, was very kind to her and that she had "nice things to eat." In her first two years away from home, Susan occasionally assured her family that she "never got hungry here." Her early, somewhat sad memories of life on the reservation had yet to fade. Neither did the medical student forget the absence of modern utilities on the reservation; unlike her, Susan's family had no easy access to clean, tapped water. With a twinge of guilt, Susan described her room as "pretty, warm, cosy." Surrounded by mementos of her parents, friends, and teachers, she felt almost at home.[2]

The day after her arrival she was off to the Woman's Medical College of Pennsylvania. Built a little more than ten years earlier, the main building—an imposing, four-story, romanesque structure—featured lecture halls, a recitation room, a museum, two libraries, eight laboratories, offices for faculty, and common rooms for students, and all the rooms were connected via airy hallways. Adjacent to the main building was Clinic Hall, erected in 1883 to provide space for clinics and dispensary service. The "splendidly appointed" college, as one visitor described it, had come a long way since its pioneer days in a cramped, rented house. Susan was probably impressed. This would be her home for the next three years.[3]

In a letter to Rosalie, she related the warm welcome she received from Dean Rachel Bodley. Much to Susan's embarrassment, Dean Bodley rose from her chair, approached Susan, kissed her, and then gave her a public introduction before the incoming class. The dean assured Susan they were "proud" of her "lineage." The enthusiasm of the dean was understandable; for a long time she had encouraged graduates to serve as medical missionaries at home and abroad. Susan's plans to return to the reservation and aid her people fell in step with the dean's personal philosophy. In return, the Omaha student complimented Bodley's warmth: "She is very nice and kind to me and always asks if I am happy here. I like her very much."[4] That same afternoon, Susan was again singled out for attention. At an assembly, Professor Bodley welcomed her before the gathered student body, which in the 1880s averaged around 160 students. For their part, Susan's colleagues crowded around her and overwhelmed her with questions and invitations to social events. Her new friends, who hailed from all parts of the United States and from Australia, Japan, and India, were "so nice and sociable," gushed Susan.[5]

A few weeks later, Dean Bodley threw a reception for Susan's class. Throughout the evening, Susan felt a little uneasy. The stark contrast between her plain calico dress and the gorgeous silk bustles and bows worn by other women was obvious to her. She wrote home that many of the "girls wore kid gloves," but she had "none." In the late-nineteenth century most women medical students hailed from upper-middle-class families. The prohibitive cost of tuition kept those of modest means away. The poverty of Indians versus the affluence of white Americans seared Susan's mind and touched her heart. She obviously saw the Indians' larger dilemma mirrored in her own physical appearance, but she quickly assured Rosalie that she "had everything" she needed.[6]

Luckily for Susan, her financial standing soon improved. After much delay, the Connecticut Indian Association, through President Kinney's persistence, secured the necessary Office of Indian Affairs (OIA) support. A misunderstanding on the exact number of copies required for endorsement of the contract between the government and the CIA had delayed the process. This was Susan's initiation into red-tape delays, which came to mark both her public and private life. At long last, on October 14, the Interior Department forwarded its approval of the contract. With that, the federal government agreed to extend $167 per annum—the exact amount offered to each Indian student in a contract school—to support Susan's higher education. In his annual report for 1886, Commissioner of Indian Affairs John D. C. Atkins hoped that, in giving "instruction in hygienic laws," Susan and others would destroy "the influence of the 'medicine men'." As instruments of change, agency physicians could assist the government in the process of overcoming the influence of native healers, who apparently were at the forefront of those who sought to preserve the old ways. For its part, the CIA promised to "clothe, feed, lodge, and care for, and educate" Susan.[7]

However, a year later the CIA had to take on additional responsibilities when the Indian Office reduced its contribution to $125.00 in the wake of budgetary constraints under the tight-fisted Grover Cleveland administration. And at the start of her third year, Susan nearly lost all her government funding when the Assistant Commissioner of Indian Affairs, an unscrupulous character by the name of Alexander B. Upshaw, declined to renew the contract. Only Kinney's appeal to Commissioner John H. Oberly saved the appropriations.[8] Without the support of the CIA and the federal government, Susan would have found it difficult to complete the program. Tuition fees were high because medical colleges of that day received little, if any, aid from state governments and federal aid was nonexistent. Most colleges relied heavily on private gifts and matriculation fees.[9]

Despite budgetary limitations, Susan's college offered a fairly rigorous curriculum. A graded curriculum had been in place since 1869, and in 1881 all students had to complete two terms of courses each year for a total of three years. The institution not only kept abreast of the latest developments in the field but, in fact, often led the way. As late as the mid-1870s it was the only school, besides Johns Hopkins, to require mandatory work in the physiology laboratory. It was also one of the earliest colleges to offer internships as an alternative to private preceptorships, an unsatisfactory system in which the quality of the training hinged on the proficiency of the assigned mentor. But since 1861, the students at Susan's school had taken their clinical training at the college-sponsored Woman's Hospital of Philadelphia.[10]

The college also had obvious weaknesses— some over which it had little control. Entrance requirements were not rigorously applied since, like most medical schools, the Woman's College had only a small pool of applicants. Even in the late-nineteenth century, medicine remained a less than prestigious profession and thus did not attract bright, motivated students. The packed three-year program at the Woman's College offered little room for additional clinical work. Students also felt the burden of mastering a large quantity of materials and skills within so few years. Not until the early 1890s was the program lengthened to four years. Following graduation, the new doctors had few internships to choose from, because many area hospitals still kept their doors closed to women physicians. Much of the local problem stemmed from the Philadelphia County Medical Society, which excluded women until 1888.[11]

During her first term, Susan took mainly foundation courses. Her classes included chemistry, anatomy, physiology, histology, materia medica (pharmaceutical sciences), general therapeutics (general medicine), and obstetrics. In addition she learned how to dissect cadavers, observed clinical practice at the Woman's Hospital, and took weekly examinations in chemistry, anatomy, and physiology.

Following a set of comprehensive examinations at the end of that term, Susan returned the spring term for intensive work in the chemistry, physiology, and biology laboratories. Her observations of clinical practice continued and so did her classes in anatomy and obstetrics. Again the Omaha student completed examinations at the end of the term.[12]

In her second year Susan attended lectures on chemistry, anatomy, physiology, general pathology, the practice of medicine, surgery, and gynecology. Special emphasis was placed on female ailments since the school authorities predicted that graduates would serve mostly women patients. Susan took weekly tests in chemistry, anatomy, and physiology. She also did clinical work at the school's hospital and at surrounding health facilities, which included the Philadelphia and Pennsylvania hospitals where male students also trained. Her heavy schedule intensified in the spring. Practical work in all fields was required—pharmacy, surgery, obstetrics and gynecology, and general medicine. Susan also picked up courses on the diseases of the eye, ear, throat, and skin.[13]

In her final year, which was made up of only one term, Susan enrolled for classes in materia medica and general therapeutics, general pathology, the practice of medicine, surgery, and gynecology and obstetrics. She spent most of the final term in clinical training in hospitals and studying for the comprehensive final examinations.[14]

Susan's schedule during the first year involved only four days a week, with no classes on Wednesdays, Saturdays, and Sundays. In the second year she faced a more hectic timetable. Monday through Saturday, her day began at nine in the morning and ended no earlier than seven in the evening. Even the lunch hour was blocked out for clinical rounds. In a letter to Rosalie, Susan explained that though she and her fellow students were not required to attend class, all of them did so. Because of the weekly tests and because the passing mark was ninety, few could afford to miss any of the lectures.[15]

Susan seems to have adjusted well to her new surroundings, despite some initial qualms. She found the first year difficult since so much of it was new to her. Exacerbating her predicament was home-sickness. Her first few letters home dwelt on the exact number of days and months before she would see the familiar landscape again. At one point, fed up with the rigorous work, she bemoaned that she "didn't want to grow old and quiet before [her] time." In fact, Susan fared relatively well. Some of her fellow students could barely cope, since a number of them entered medical college without having met the prescribed requirement of three years of preparatory education.[16]

By the second year she wrote that she was "very much interested" in her studies. In fact she relished some subjects, particularly anatomy. In one letter to the family, she admitted that she liked her "studies very much and [I] don't mind the dissecting room at all. We laugh and talk up there just as we do anywhere." Then she described the process in detail: "Six students take one body . . . and [it] is divided into 6 parts. Two take the head . . . 2 the chest. . . 2 the abdomen and legs. Then we take off little by little." Then the students examined the skin, tissues, muscles, arteries, and veins. With almost childlike excitement, Susan related that it was "interesting to get all the arteries and the branches . . . everything has a name from the little tiny holes to the bones. It is splendid."[17]

Susan had a good sense of humor. In one letter, she told Rosalie that she was "going to wield the knife tonight—not the scalping knife, though." During the course of a coed clinical demonstration on another occasion, she watched in glee as one male student, who had earlier teased the supposedly fainthearted "doctoring ladies," swooned during an amputation. Susan later boasted to Rosalie that she "wasn't even thinking of fainting."[18]

Susan also enjoyed her studies at the Woman's Medical College because she was in the company of some of the best physicians of the time. They included Clara Marshall, professor of materia medica and general therapeutics; William H. Paris, professor of anatomy; and William H. Keen, professor of the principles and practice of surgery. Susan drew special attention from Keen. He extended a warm welcome to the Indian student and made it clear that he was very supportive of Susan's plans to return to the Omahas to practice medicine.[19]

Early in her studies, Susan received surgery-room tickets to watch Keen perform two operations. Fascinated by what she saw, she described her experience in a letter to her sister Rosalie. During the first operation, which took no more than ten minutes, Keen removed "a tumour as big as a small apple from the neck or below the ear of a colored girl." In the second procedure, which lasted only two and a half minutes, he extracted a needle from the thigh of a young woman after etherizing the skin and making a half-inch incision. "It was wonderful," Susan gushed, and "they [the students] clapped, but he stopped them."[20]

But Susan also wrote home that she experienced moments when the reality of pain and death, of suffering and loss, gave her pause for reflection. The clinical lectures she attended brought her in contact with female patients who were afflicted by such serious ailments that she "could never [have] imagined what suffering . . . there could be." Sitting in the large, crowded amphitheater, which accommodated up to three hundred, Susan could sympathize with the patients' plight and was thankful that her family remained healthy. Her description of the sessions ended abruptly when she realized that her sister might find it unpleasant, even somewhat morbid, reading.[21]

Motivated by a sense of "mission" and endowed with a good mind, the diligent Omaha made steady progress in her studies. When examinations for the first year drew near, Susan cheerfully wrote that she did not "dread them very much though." On the exams, she found chemistry "much easier" than she thought it would be, while she "got on swimmingly" in anatomy.[22]

Second-year examinations were more challenging. Susan confided to Kinney that she had dreamt about being quizzed by her professors and that by the morning of the first test, she felt as if she remembered her name, but little else. The initial panic passed once she entered the hall and discovered the "examinations were delightful." Then came the agonizing wait for the results. Days later, close to midnight, she received the news. Stunned by what she read, she could "scarcely realize it." "Multum in parvo—passed in all," she telegraphed to the CIA. Her very brief letter to Hampton Institute conveyed her excitement: "Passed!!!!!."[23]

Alone and saddled with the burden of her training, Susan found comfort and company in her fellow students. She bonded well with Jane Reid and Martha Emily Garner. A missionary who had labored among the Cherokees of North Carolina, Garner took walks with Susan and also shared her cookies, candies, and favorite songs with Susan. Equally interested in Indians, Reid puzzled over physiology with Susan. Another friend, Sarah Lockrey, lent Susan her notes after every chemistry lecture. Just before each major exam, Susan and her equally harried friends sat down and tried to anticipate the questions. In an obvious departure from the Victorian image of the invalid female, Susan and the rest took calisthenics and lifted light weights for pure physical relief. Such sports—designed to strengthen, beautify, and correct various parts of the body—constituted physical culture, which was the most widely approved form of female physical activity. Susan boasted that when she finally went home she would be able to swing an ax or harness the horses, and she dubbed as "splendid" her times dressed in blouse waists and short trousers in the gymnasium.[24]

Susan's interactions with a mostly white student body brought her further along on the journey toward acculturation. The ways of Euro-Americans rubbed off on the impressionable young Omaha woman. Susan filled the position of secretary of the Young Woman's Christian Association. She also went to the meetings of the college's Christian Endeavor Society, and every Sunday she attended student religious services in the hospital. She took part in all the school's social gatherings, shared a room with a white colleague, and even dressed like the white students. When asked by fellow students to wear her hair in a bun on top of her head, Susan happily complied.[25]

Acquaintances in Philadelphia who fast became friends also kept the Indian woman within the orbit of the white world. Interested in Indian reform, the W. W. Heritage family took Susan under their wing. With Mrs. Heritage and her daughter Marian, Susan attended church services and sat through temperance lectures. Susan often dropped by their home for tea or dinner and sometimes stayed the night. The Heritages took such a liking to Susan that they not only gave her Christmas gifts, but also sent some to her family. On another occasion, Susan spent a weekend at the home of one wealthy benefactor. There she marveled at the handmade comb and brush, the sumptuous breakfast, and the fancy silver coffee set.[26]

Yet Susan never forgot her origins and racial background. Invited to speak before missionary societies, she focused her talks on the plight of the Indians and their wants and needs. She expressed support for the General Allotment bill (passed in 1887), which would provide Indians with titles to their land. She also urged her white audiences to donate reading material to reservation Indians so that they could become acquainted with "civilization." Finally, she promoted the idea of building a hospital on the Omaha reservation. Some of these reflections were probably drawn from a letter which was meant for publication that she wrote to Susette in order to raise public awareness about Indian reform. Shy and a little withdrawn, Susan had been a reluctant public speaker, but with practice she gained confidence. She also shed her meekness. At one particular gathering, she insisted that the young girl who modeled traditional Omaha garb take off the irrelevant feather headdress. Her sense of humor always intact, Susan was much amused when the girl kept it on.[27]

Susan spent considerable time with the Indian boys at the Educational Home in West Philadelphia and with the Indian orphans at Philadelphia's Lincoln Institute. Hardly chores, these were pleasurable visits during which she often attended religious services and enjoyed student concerts. The attractive Susan captured the eye of more than one young man at the Educational Home. "One young gentleman from Dakota" who sat right next to Susan during Sunday services was so "attentive" toward her that she became a little concerned. At the Lincoln Institute, she became reacquainted with an old Indian friend, Mary Tyndall, who apparently served as an assistant teacher. Aware that Tyndall had excelled in school, Susan encouraged her to pursue a medical degree at the college. Later Tyndall chose to enter nursing school.[28]

When the Hampton and Carlisle school bands stopped at Philadelphia on their respective swings through eastern cities, Susan attended their concerts and proudly told Rosalie, in a demonstration of tribal patriotism, that "the Omahas have high standing at both schools." During holiday seasons Susan visited other Indians at their schools. She had forged particularly close ties with those she left behind in Hampton. Once she told Rosalie that though she had secured a summer position waiting on tables at a seaside resort, she would much prefer, "next to going home," to "go down to Hampton . . . to teach."[29]

While proud of the achievements of the Omahas at Hampton and Carlisle, Susan also took pleasure in the attention she had garnered. "Poor things they think so much of M [Marguerite] & I," Susan wrote to Rosalie as she struggled to maintain her modesty. A few lines later in the letter, she abandoned all pretense: "You know my name has been in the Carlisle paper as the smartest at Hampton, etc."[30]

Susan apparently served as a source of inspiration for many Indian students. Both Hampton and Carlisle school publications kept abreast of her academic progress and extolled her character. In one Hampton student publication of August 1889, Susan's accomplishments were singled out for praise. The article cited her success in medical school and her accomplishments, and the author reminded all that, though few could emulate Susan completely, it "wouldn't hurt us to try and be as good."[31]

Although Susan never ignored the needs or wants of her family back in Nebraska, the letters she wrote lay bare her sense of guilt. While Rosalie had stayed home to take care of their parents and manage family matters, Susan had moved away to study medicine and visit exciting new places. Though unavailable to share familial responsibilities and racked by guilty feelings, Susan tried to make herself useful.[32] She tried to help by doing what she knew best: Susan dispensed medical advice and prescribed medicine through the mail. Enthusiastically she asked Rosalie to "always hand me as many cases as you can." When Rosalie became pregnant, Susan reminded her not to lift heavy items or work too hard and advised her that plenty of exercise, fresh air, and sufficient sleep would ease her pregnancy. Susan also told Rosalie to relax more often and just enjoy the company of her other children. After the birth of one of her children, Rosalie suffered from continuous bouts of coughs and colds, and Susan insisted that Rosalie see a physician.[33]

Susan advised Rosalie to tell her husband, who was then recovering from some unknown illness, that he should take less quinine and set aside "more time for his meals." "I am going to write him a letter some day . . . a sisterly doctorly letter," Susan promised Rosalie. When her mother complained of a sore on her hand and an aching foot, "Dr. Sue," as she sometimes called herself, quickly sent a packet of castile soap and carbolated vaseline. She told her mother to use the latter on her aching foot and not to walk about shoeless. When her father came to the East to be fitted for a new prosthetic leg, Susan kept tabs on its production and sent it to Nebraska. Aware that good nourishment would lead to better health, she sometimes parted with her extra cash so that the family could buy meat and chicken. In her own small ways, Susan demonstrated an early interest in preventive health care, which later became part of her Indian reform agenda.[34]

While Susan's correspondence belied selfless loyalty to her family and tribe, it also revealed love found and love lost. While still at Hampton, Susan caught the eye of a fellow student named Thomas Ikinicapi. A full-blood Sioux, Ikinicapi was a fragile and sickly boy who eventually died of tuberculosis at an early age. But he had a congenial personality that exuded warmth and kindness. Apparently Susan was attracted to those qualities, as she was to his physical features. Unabashedly she described him as "without exception, the handsomest Indian I ever saw."[35]

Their feelings for each other reached a climax during one Christmas visit to Hampton. Susan went there partly because T. I., as she called him, pleaded with her to come. For her part, Susan found T. I.'s loyalty and faithfulness endearing. But just after she arrived on campus, a tiff broke out between the two of them. Mutual jealousy of the time each spent with other friends was the source of the silent war. They made up, but both sensed that this was "the last time."[36]

Susan found it difficult to reconcile duty with love. She knew that medical studies demanded all of her time. Her training and her professional ambition took precedence over almost everything else, perhaps even T. I. Furthermore, the CIA had made her promise to remain single for a year or two after the completion of her studies, so that she could devote all of her time to medical work. The women of the CIA subscribed to the late-nineteenth-century middle-class aversion to married women in the work force. Moreover, the demands of practicing medicine were seen as not compatible with the rigors of establishing a household.[37]

There was also a question of class compatibility between Susan and T. I. Though brushed aside initially by Susan, the disparity in their educational achievements became obvious. One of her Hampton teachers pointed out to Susan that she was "too good" for T. I. In a time when middle-class Euro-American women were told to avoid working-class men or those with a less than stellar background, Susan's teachers must have imparted this ideal to Susan. Though Susan had left the protective security of Hampton, the dynamics of the fictive daughter-mother relationships she had established there continued to play out.[38]

Under pressure, Susan reluctantly broke off the relationship. An emotional T. I. could not even bring himself to see her off when she left Hampton, and Susan later wrote to Rosalie that she found it "so hard to leave." However, her friendship with T. I. did not end. They continued to write to each other. Susan recovered partially from the breakup, but apparently T. I. never did. Emotionally scarred by the experience, Susan became resigned to the notion of being a "dear little old maid."[39]

However, many of Susan's letters home were filled with news of daily diversions from the rigors of medical school. Susan regaled her family with stories of her adventures, almost all of which few nineteenth-century Indian women could ever hope to experience, in the "City of Brotherly Love." It is no wonder that the new sights and sounds fascinated and impressed Susan. She attended recitals and operas at the well-known Philadelphia Academy of Music. The spectacle of Gilbert and Sullivan's *The Mikado* enthralled Susan, who was musically inclined. Another time, she saw Lily Langtry perform in *Wife's Peril*. One Christmas season she took in *The Messiah*; always appreciative of the sacred, Susan described the music as "grand." At the Philadelphia Academy of Arts, she enjoyed the diversity of visual arts displayed.[40]

After she had learned the routes of the streetcars, Susan toured Old Swede's Church, Independence Hall, and Philadelphia City Hall, thus taking in the historic ambience of the city. With friends, Susan tromped through Fairmont Park, collecting wild flowers and pinecones along the way. Curious and intrigued, they walked across the park on one cloudy, rainy day to the all-male Girard College and saw close up the daily military drill parade, which they had glimpsed from the windows of the medical school.[41]

Once Susan attended the Mummers' Parade, a New Year's Day event in Philadelphia, with her brother Francis. She noticed that some of the masqueraders wore makeup and feathers. Sarcastically, she commented that they "saw some of the parade—they dressed up as Indians too and they looked pretty well for Indians." Later it was Susan's turn to be gawked at; she and Francis drew so much attention at Independence Hall that, though laughing on the way out, they fled from the site. These two related incidents reveal Susan's awareness of visible "Indian" characteristics, which often set them apart from Euro-Americans and frequently impinged on their lives in potent ways.[42]

Amazed by the size of one department store she visited, Susan counted the number of rooms and facilities—eighteen altogether. And she noted that for effect the store displayed "real" orange trees and a gushing fountain. During this outing, Susan went in for a dress fitting. After her first humbling experience at Dean Bodley's reception and with the help of CIA members and some new dresses, Susan had become, in her own words, "a lady of fashion." Proudly she told Rosalie that she was "kind of getting there." Yet in the same letter that described her visit to the department store, Susan admitted that she missed wearing moccasins and requested that Rosalie ask their mother if she would mind making her a new pair. Susan was just as comfortable in traditional garb as she was in trendy outfits.[43]

During her years away at college, Susan must have found it difficult to get through the holidays. She spent the first Christmas with Marguerite at Hampton. Her sister graduated in June 1887, so Susan remained in Philadelphia for one Christmas. Short of money, she spent her first summer break working at Hampton as an assistant housekeeper.[44]

The next summer break, after a short stop at Hampton to attend the annual commencement ceremonies, Susan returned home. Familial responsibilities weighed heavily on her mind; her ailing parents and an untended farm had drawn her back. Engrossed in her work, the warm season flew by quickly. Upon her return to the reservation, Susan had written a detailed letter to "Mother" Kinney. Proud of her western roots, Susan wrote: "I can tell you one thing and that is a Western woman has to know how do [sic] everything that man does besides her own work, for she had to be ready for any emergency that may occur when men are not around." That shimmering summer Susan balanced household, field, and medical work. She cooked, sewed, measured land for a fence, ricked hay, harnessed horses, and, of course, nursed the sickly.[45] The range of her activities contradicts any notion that Susan subscribed to the Victorian ideal of the languid countenance of the "true" woman.

By the time Susan arrived home, many Omahas had fallen ill—victims of a severe measles epidemic that swept through the reservation. Families were ravaged, and lives were lost. Susan argued that the tragedy of the epidemic could have been ameliorated if more Indians had accepted western medicine. She experienced great difficulty in convincing her people of the efficacious nature of the medicine she brought with her. Susan was clearly frustrated with the Omahas' resistance to "progress." To remove any lingering doubts, she quite often had to ingest the medication herself. Susan did succeed to some extent—a fact she proudly attributed to her racial ties with the patients. She also handed out delicacies that friends back in Pennsylvania had sent for the ill; she would increasingly draw upon the resources of the female network of benevolent reformers she had come to know. But Susan lamented that her labors did not come easy, because the Indians lived "so far apart, that sometimes [she] could visit only ten families in one afternoon, going 25 miles for the purpose."[46]

Late in the summer of 1888, Susan's father, Iron Eye, passed away. There is little surviving evidence regarding the circumstances of his death. Apparently he caught a serious cold and was ill for about two weeks before he died, surrounded by his children. His funeral was attended by Indians and non-Indians—a testament to his ability to cross the cultural dividing line. The funeral procession was the largest ever held in that part of the state.[47] Susan did not leave behind any written reflections on her father's death. However, it is possible that his demise reminded her of his commitment to serve the Omahas, a calling that she surely embraced and actively practiced in the coming years.

Susan realized that her people had a long way to go before health conditions improved. In a somber tone, she wrote: "If one wants to accomplish much work they must go out every day. So much can be done, by going to see them and while you are there tell them how to tidy up or show them how, which is still better." In fact, Susan reported that "these Omahas" needed help in many aspects of life— "business, land, money, and horses, what kind to buy and all."[48] By using phrases such as "these Omahas" and "them," Susan chose to distance herself from her tribespeople and to draw a blatant distinction between herself—one who had successfully moved from "tipi to civilization"—and tribal members who still seemed impervious to the concept of linear time. She probably also hoped to close the gap between herself and white reformers, who still saw her as subordinate to them.

That summer Susan played the mediatory role she had promised to fulfill in her Hampton commencement speech. The summer-long experience strengthened her resolve to work even harder in the future for the betterment of the Omahas' physical health. Susan felt that Euro-American ways would save the Omahas. But embedded within her letter to Kinney was also a tinge of contempt for, or at least disapproval of, traditional ways that hindered the Omahas' climb up the ladder of social evolution.

Convinced of the value of the Euro-American culture, Susan gave her endorsement eagerly when the CIA offered to put Marguerite through nursing school. Still, Susan realized that perhaps Marguerite was "not strong enough for such work." Torn between concern for Marguerite's well-being and a need to be truthful to her "missionary role," Susan finally justified her support as an attempt to give her sister "a lift." What was good for the CIA would be good for Marguerite as well. But in the end, following her stint at Hampton, Marguerite turned the offer of nursing school down for marriage and a quick return to the reservation.[48]

In her dealings with the CIA, Susan played the role of cultural broker to the hilt. Grateful for the care and the many presents she received from her "foster mothers," she was more than happy to return the favor when she was asked to visit Connecticut towns and speak in support of CIA's efforts on behalf of the Indians.[49]

In early October 1887 Susan's highly anticipated week-long visit began. She visited an asylum for hearing-impaired girls, then she spoke at a church in the town of Meriden. The *Hartford Courant* reported that "all who met her are charmed with her modest ways and her evident earnestness in the work she had chosen."[51]

The highlight of the visit was an afternoon lawn party, complete with tents, Chinese lanterns, flowers, a full orchestra, refreshments, and, of course, Susan herself. CIA members took the opportunity to draw attention to the group's work and to raise some money. For her part, Susan took a moment to thank her "foster mothers." In her remarks before an estimated audience of three hundred, she praised the work of the association, particularly the home-building project on the Omaha reservation. Through this project, Omaha families secured low-interest loans from the association and used the loans to build frame houses. Susan could not ignore the benevolence of the CIA toward her people.[52] However, most of her address was a rehash of her Hampton commencement speech—her goals, her aspirations. Susan did add that she had an advantage over a white physician because she knew the Omahas' "language, customs, habits, and manner of living." Susan understood well that the process of "Americanization" would founder without the active participation of the Indians themselves. Though used or manipulated by the CIA for their ends, Susan also knew how to turn the tables on her benefactors. Her mediation may have seemed at times to have been commandeered by Euro-American reformers, but she was always cognizant of the direction of her brokerage. Over the next several decades Susan would center her energies on her own people and recast her knowledge of the "Other" in the form of a tool to help her tribe maintain a degree of autonomy. Susan's education and subsequent labor was for the good of her own people—not just to satisfy the conscience of white reformers.[53]

By early March 1889 Susan had arrived at the last hurdle in her education. Her final examinations were just around the corner. Kinney confided to a friend that Susan was "shaky," since she had to study and still be on call at all hours. However, Susan seemed to hold up well under the pressure. In the midst of her examinations, she assured a benefactor that she was "alright," though not without a hint of anxiety.[54]

On March 14, 1889, in the presence of members of the CIA and the faculty of the college, Susan graduated. She had made it through the long years of medical training. Along with thirty-five other students all dressed in caps and gowns, Susan received her doctorate of medicine from T. Morris Perot, the president of the board of corporators (trustees). James Walker, M.D., professor of the principles and practice of medicine, delivered the address to the graduating class. In his remarks, Walker lavished praise on the first Native American woman physician. He said that La Flesche had conscientiously pursued her ambition. Her "courage, constancy, and ability," he waxed, had brought her this far in the fulfillment of "a desire to see her people independent" of the inefficient OIA medical services. In future years, Susan often found herself at the receiving end of the OIA's slow-moving bureaucracy.[55]

Following commencement, Susan took a competitive examination. She had decided to compete against eleven other candidates for one of six internships available at the Woman's Hospital. Despite the keen competition, she won a spot. Susan would spend the next year serving as an assistant to the resident physician.[56]

Exhausted from the tensions of the last few months, Susan heeded the advice of friends and left for Hartford, Connecticut, for a short vacation. Once there, she found herself the object of adulation, as Indian reformers toasted her success at a grand tea reception with several hundred people.[57]

At the behest of CIA members elsewhere in Connecticut, Susan agreed to a whirlwind speaking tour. She visited association branches at Hartford, Waterbury, Winsted, Farmington, Guilford, Norwich, and

New Britain. She shared with each audience—in eloquent, emotive language—her childhood memories, her academic success, and her plans to help her tribe on the reservation and assured them that Indians were not impervious to the ways of "civilization." Since these gatherings were also designed as membership drives, Susan dwelt on the positive impact of the association's work among her people and urged potential members to join the Indian cause. Much to the delight of the CIA, Susan's efforts paid off. The membership of the branches rose quickly, and according to the CIA annual report of 1889, Susan's occasional visits over the years "stimulat[ed] interest in Indian work and strengthen[ed] the bonds of mutual sympathy." Like her sister Susette, Susan seemed to project the "Indian Princess" image, which drew Euro-Americans to become interested in the CIA's agenda, and Susan capitalized on that appeal in order to serve the needs of her people.[58]

After her triumphant speaking tour, Susan returned to Philadelphia. Right away, she was caught up in the drama of hospital life. Daily, from eight in the morning until past the noon hour, Susan tackled the heavy load of outpatient cases at the Woman's Hospital of Philadelphia. She spent her afternoons assisting with and observing operations or preparing medications ordered for patients by senior physicians. Before supper she dropped by the outpatient clinic and did follow-up work on former inpatients.[59]

Sometimes in the evenings, Susan accompanied the resident physician on her house calls in some of the most run-down neighborhoods of the city. These home visits, in addition to the work she did at the hospital, must have impressed upon her the wants of the poor, which in turn reminded Susan of those she had left behind in Nebraska. Still, in a letter to her "Connecticut friends," Susan described her "life here [as] intensely interesting."[60] The house calls were probably Susan's best learning experiences, since most pre-internship training in the nineteenth century offered somewhat limited clinical practice. This period was also a turning point in her life in another sense; the phrase "Connecticut friends" would be substituted henceforth in Susan's letters for "foster mothers" or other similarly maternal phrases. It seems that, having fulfilled her obligations, Susan saw no need to maintain the rhetoric of the mother-daughter relationship; she was gradually asserting her selfhood and moving out of the shadows of white benevolence.

Perhaps restless and eager to return to the reservation, Susan decided to apply in June 1889 for the position of government physician at the Omaha Agency Indian School. Aware that theoretically Native Americans had priority in the Indian service, Susan identified herself as "an Indian girl" and "a member of the Omaha tribe" in her letter to the new Commissioner of Indian Affairs, Thomas Jefferson Morgan. She gave her educational background, and then she ended her application on a confident, almost boastful, note: "I feel that I have an advantage in knowing the language and customs of my people, and as a physician can do a great deal to help them."[61] Fortunately for Susan, Commissioner Morgan believed that talented Indians should have access to higher education and professional careers. "Young Indian men and women should be encouraged to prepare themselves . . . for work among their own people as physicians and nurses," Morgan wrote in his annual report.[62] Less than two months after Susan had filed her application for the job, she received an offer. On August 5, 1889, she accepted the position.[63]

As a Hampton student, Susan had once written a brief article on the works of Helen Hunt Jackson, the writer and Indian reformer. Susan praised the novel *Ramona* (1884), in particular, for both its literary qualities and its tragic plot. Her piece ended with a call to all Indians to keep on "living and working for our people" so the tragedy portrayed in that novel would never be repeated in reality. Now, in her own way, Susan was prepared to answer that call.[64]

CHAPTER FIVE

"My Work as Physician Among My People"

"When I saw her I did not think she could live through the day," Susan told the captivated audience at Hampton Institute. Already enfeebled by "consumption," or tuberculosis, a patient now suffered from "la grippe," or influenza. In heavy snow and sub-zero temperatures, the Omaha physician had driven six miles across rough country to the sick woman's ramshackle home. There she found the entire family crowded into a one-room house. Lying in one corner was her patient, a former Hampton student. When recounting the episode for her Hampton listeners, Susan pointed out that the woman's "clean and neat" room—adorned with sheets, pillowcases, photographs, and a clock—bore testament to the impact of a Hampton education. But her patient "had had no food for four days." Susan prescribed stimulants that revived the sickly woman, and later she returned with milk, eggs, and beef. She went daily to check on her patient for the next two weeks. Once when she was preoccupied with illness within her own family, Susan missed her usual routine visit. That day the Indian woman passed away.[1]

Susan recounted this dramatic but tragic story during an address at Hampton Institute's May 1892 commencement ceremonies. In her talk, "My Work as Physician Among My People," Susan shared tales

SUSAN LA FLESCHE PICOTTE, M.D.

of medical ailments, sufferings, and losses. The Indians' progress toward "civilization" also received coverage. Always an advocate of her people's potential, Susan rarely missed an opportunity to showcase their advances. She made it clear that she was glad to be back with "the people of [her] own tribe." Susan took much delight in seeing the high hills and rolling prairie once again; "it is beautiful out here," she exclaimed in a letter to the Connecticut Indian Association (CIA).[2]

Amid this familiar landscape, she practiced medicine among her people. In carrying out her medical duties, Susan found the context in which to escape the maternalism of white reformers and develop her independence. In so doing, she was to gain even more of the necessary confidence to speak and act on behalf of the Omahas. Her brokerage moved increasingly in the direction of helping her own people, and less in that of simply promoting the dominant society's agenda. Unlike her contemporaries Charles Eastman and Carlos Montezuma, who supported the Society of American Indians' pan-Indianism movement, Susan's activism revolved around local affairs. Like many educated Indians, Susan probably conceived that this was a good time to use her white skills and knowledge to help her race while claiming a place for herself in the tribal society.[3]

Susan's efforts to gain some stature in the tribe began at a modest level. The Office of Indian Affairs (OIA) had appointed her to a newly created position—physician to the government boarding school situated near the agency complex. According to OIA directives, like all school physicians, Susan had "oversight of all sanitary matters." She was expected to "give the students simple, appropriate talks on elementary principles of physiology and hygiene," and more advanced students were to receive instruction in "nursing and care of the sick." However, Susan was not obligated to serve the larger Omaha population.[4]

When Susan joined the school, she found conditions there intolerable. OIA inspector Frank C. Armstrong visited the school in November 1889, just two months after Susan's return. He found the "school grounds, condition of rooms, beds, dormitories, etc." in "bad order and not properly attended to." Armstrong placed the blame squarely on the superintendent and matron, both of whom apparently had been remiss in their duties. But the inspector praised La Flesche and called her a "good influence with the pupils" and "a good e.g. [example] to employees and pupils."[5]

Because of the state of disarray, Susan found plenty of work at the school with which to occupy herself. At her new workplace, she kept office hours in the morning, afternoon, and evening. The instruments and medical books the CIA sent her came in handy.[6] During this period the Indian Department neglected much of the medical services, and often doctors were left to their own devices to secure needed supplies. Luckily for Susan, she had the support of eastern benefactors; the relationships she had fostered with supporters in the East now could be called upon to service the needs of the Omahas.[7]

The young Omaha physician found her work "very pleasant" and she "enjoyed it exceedingly." True to her sense of humor, Susan wrote much about the antics of her young charges. The children "are exceedingly willing to be dosed," she chuckled; so much so that she had to "almost hire some of the invalids to keep [them] away from me." Once a week, Susan paid a visit to the local Presbyterian mission school, by then an all-girls school. There she kept track of the health of some thirty pupils and periodically left instructions for the school nurse.[8]

In the evenings, Susan played more the role of a teacher than that of a physician. At the boarding school, she delivered informal talks in physiology and hygiene and sometimes gave students English and arithmetic lessons. Singing hymns, making scrapbooks, telling Euro-American folktales, and practicing marching skills were some of Susan's other school activities—all legacies of her Hampton days. Adhering closely to her bicultural identity, Susan played her part in the Americanization of the Omahas.[9]

Though Susan admitted that her wards were "backward"—she still distanced herself from the "uncivilized" past—she also sought to convince her white supporters of the value of Indian culture and mores. In one letter to the CIA, she educated them on Indians' traditional respect for their elders. She cited the example of her students rising from their seats whenever she walked in. True to her mediatory role, she wedded Indian mores with Victorian mannerisms.[10]

Over time Susan's efforts at the boarding school paid off. In his 1890 annual report, Indian agent Robert H. Ashley wrote of the vast improvements in that school: the old building was gutted and a new one erected; the student dormitories and staff living quarters went through extensive renovations; and a system of waterworks, previously nonexistent, was put in place. Since government officials had been less-than-complimentary about the superintendent and matron, Susan probably deserved much of the credit for initiating these changes.[11]

By 1893, Susan reported that, besides nutritious food, "good drainage and ventilation, [and] cleanliness" had contributed to maintaining the "good physical condition of our school children." The school superintendent echoed that conclusion in even more succinct terms, reporting: "Not a child in bed on account of sickness" for the entire year of 1892. The inspector who visited that year commended Susan for being "faithful in her work." "She appears," he continued, "to understand the duties of her position."[12]

But Susan wished to serve Omahas who were not privy to the services she rendered at the school. Inaccessibility of medical services was a common characteristic of turn-of-the-century reservation life, and before she had returned from the East the nearest physician had been located almost eighteen miles from the reservation.[13] In the winter of 1888, the year before Susan came home, a devastating measles epidemic swept through the reservation and claimed many lives. Almost ninety Omahas died—a significant toll for a population of less than twelve hundred people.[14] Help did come from surrounding doctors, but, as one missionary put it, "the Indians [are] not very receptive to western medical intervention." Since the Omahas figured the disease came from whites, many were suspicious of western remedies.[15]

Still, both field officials and local missionaries lobbied the Indian Department for a reservation physician. There was no response, and no one came, at least not until 1888 when the Women's National Indian Association (WNIA) established a mission on the reservation headed by a trained physician, Dr. Lawrence M. Hensel, and his wife (identified as E. B.). Together the husband-and-wife team struggled against language and cultural barriers and ministered to the physical needs of the Omahas. They also received instructions from the association to proselytize the Word among the Omahas. However, the mission failed—the victim of insufficient resources and inadequate funding. A government physician did arrive shortly before Susan came home, although he served two reservations—the Omahas' and Winnebagos'—and in fact operated from the Winnebago reservation.[16]

Because the government physician's office was located ten miles from the Omaha reservation, Susan found herself inundated quickly by calls for medical aid.[17] But she first had to prove her capability to skeptical, "non-progressive" Omahas, and that opportunity came with her initial case. An eight-year-old Omaha boy came in with a childhood ailment, and Susan duly prescribed the treatment. The next day, feeling a little apprehensive about her diagnosis, Susan rode on horseback eight miles into the country to the home of her young patient. Relief came over her when she spotted him "splashing in a nearby creek . . . and having an immense amount of fun." This rapid recovery apparently won her "no end of fame," to borrow Susan's immodest declaration. Omahas soon began to flock to her clinic for succor and comfort.[18]

Susan told Amelia S. Quinton, president of the WNIA, that she had "almost more work to do among the adults, for they come to [me] almost every day." Much to her delight, even the "non-progressives" or traditionalists sought her out for professional aid. Cognizant of sex discrimination against women physicians back in the East, she assured Quinton that the Indians had "not shown the least prejudice so far towards women physicians."[19]

In Indian societies, gender figured less in determining an individual's status than age, kinship networks, and personal contribution.[20] Ironically, Susan received the benefit of this traditional attitude from her people while trying to foster the ways of Euro-Americans in the same group.

Susan was so popular that within three months of her arrival, she had taken over most of the OIA physician's caseload. She attributed this success with the Indians to the fact that she "understood their language, and they felt [she] was one of them." Her personality, kinship ties to the Omahas, and demonstrated knowledge and skills contributed to her influence with the Indians. Particularly, Susan was able to reach out to Indian women, supposedly the major focus of her CIA-defined mission. Susan reported that she had more work "among the women than [she] ever thought [she] would have." She explained that Indian women came to her because they were reluctant to approach a white male doctor. By 1891 some physicians in the area were even losing some of their white patients, men and women, to Susan.[21]

Though Susan served slightly more women than men, she largely failed to fulfill the mission the CIA had outlined for her—in sum, to be "physician to women and children." Through "daughters" like Susan, the CIA had hoped to transform "heathen" women into paragons of Victorian womanhood. In theory, following their adoption of domesticity, Indian women would parlay their influence for the good of their families and tribes. From homes more like those of white Americans, Indian women would be able to serve as spiritual and moral bulwarks against "primitiveness."[22]

But Susan was too busy with her medical duties to carry out such high-sounding goals, as well-meaning as they may have been. She was barely able to make time for weekly services and interpreting work at the local church. Now and then she showed a few women how to sew, but aside from that, she did little else to share domestic skills.[23] Saving lives was her primary concern, and at this stage in her life, she remained steadfastly on course. Susan was hardly the formal educator the CIA had hoped she would become. In fact, Susan even defied the nineteenth-century convention—and the prediction of the medical school authorities—for women physicians, most of whom set up practices at home that catered almost exclusively to women and children. Clearly, Susan did not follow that norm.[24]

When the physician for the combined Omaha and Winnebago agency left at the end of 1889, Susan applied to the Indian Department for permission to serve the Omaha population. Besides, she shrewdly argued, the supplies that the OIA had already sent for use with the adult population of the reservation would go to waste if unused. Less than two months later, the official reply reached her and permission was granted. In her follow-up letter, Susan assured Thomas J. Morgan, commissioner of Indian affairs from 1889 to 1893, in a confident tone that, despite taking on additional responsibilities, she would still "give just so much time as" the Indian students in the boarding school needed. Susan was hardly in an anomalous situation; most OIA physicians worked both in the schools and the reservation. Soon Susan found this challenge to be an uphill battle. She became so engrossed in her medical work that within the year she gave up her evening teaching role.[25]

"My office hours are any and all hours of day and night," a weary but smiling Susan told Sara Thomson Kinney when Kinney visited the reservation in 1891. In a letter to his superiors dated March 3, 1891, Agent Ashley lauded Susan for having "done a great amount of work for the Omaha Indians." Susan had given "every moment" to her people, he continued. The OIA field inspector Arthur M. Tinker was more succinct, stating that she was "very popular." Both Tinker and Ashley agreed that Susan had much influence on the tribe and was taking the place of the medicine men.[26]

Susan prescribed medicine and dispensed advice from an office in one corner of the school yard. As Kinney described it, the twelve by sixteen foot plastered-and-painted frame building looked like a miniature drugstore, with a small counter, weighing machines, and shelves lined with drugs of all kinds. Through donations contributed by WNIA branches, Susan filled cabinets with magazines, pictorial books, scrapbooks, and games. The office functioned almost like a community meeting place. Omahas often dropped by to visit with Susan, to chat with other friends, or simply to make use of the games and reading material.[27]

Susan was fortunate. Most OIA physicians worked in decrepit surroundings. When assigned to his first clinic at the Yankton agency Charles Eastman, a contemporary of hers, discovered that it "had all the charm of a large corn crib, and was about as effective in blocking the chilly winds."[28]

Susan told her Hampton teachers that many Indians came to her office not only for medical care, but also for help in daily business affairs of various types. Quite often, she translated and wrote letters and documents for them. Faced with the pressures of serving a larger population, Susan found it a little difficult to balance medical work and the mediatory role of translator and letter writer. In the latter capacity, following the passage of the General Allotment or Dawes Act, Susan had to inform and instruct Omahas on their responsibilities and rights as citizens of the republic. In this role, Susan translated not only a language but also a culturally prescribed world view and its expectations. Land allotment and its attending legal complications began to consume much of her time.[29]

Susan was quick to point out to the Connecticut Indian Association that the Omahas were worthy of "civilization." She boasted that Omahas were "improving very fast in many ways." Very few lived in tepees, most owned machinery and farming implements, and, except for a few, Omaha men had adopted "the civilized style of dressing." Educated Indians filled positions ranging from store clerks to farmhands in outlying towns.[30] Susan glossed over the fact that most of these dead-end jobs paid poorly and the vast majority of Omahas still lived in poverty. Her intercultural role sometimes led her to shade the truth in an attempt to create an imaginary bridge between disparate worlds. She implied that Indians deserved whites' benevolence and respect.

The obligation that weighed heaviest on Susan's mind was to provide medical succor for the tribal population. As an agency physician, she not only attended to those who called at the office, but also visited "the Indians at their homes" and did her "utmost to educate and instruct them in proper methods of living and of caring for health," as detailed in OIA directives.[31]

Making home visits was no easy task. Omahas were scattered over an undeveloped, undulating terrain that was thirty miles long by fifteen miles wide. Most of the so-called roads were little more than poor dirt tracks, which were so bad that a single horse could not pull a wagon on them. "After trying for some time to go about on horseback," Susan bemoaned, "I broke so many bottles and thermometers that I had to give that up."[32]

A team and buggy would have helped, but the Indian Office provided none. Even as late as the first decade of the twentieth century, physicians had to struggle to secure funding for transportation. Susan first tried hiring a team but that proved to be expensive, and so she used the services only when necessary. If the distance Susan had to travel was only a mile or so, she walked. After several years she purchased a team and buggy.[33]

To make matters worse Susan, like most physicians of that time period, could not rely on OIA supplies. Often the supplies that arrived were either old or broken, and delays were not uncommon. Once WNIA donations ran out, Susan frequently had to fall back on her own financial resources in order to purchase additional medicines and related necessities.[34]

For all her trouble, Susan received meager compensation. Initially she received a salary of $500.00 per year. In 1891, at the recommendation of an impressed field inspector, she earned a two-hundred-dollar raise. However, the additional money was drawn from the tribal funds. Her paycheck paled in comparison with that of army and navy physicians who earned twice as much. The estimated average yearly earnings for a doctor in the late nineteenth century was $1,200. Fortunately for Susan, the WNIA also paid her $250.00 per year for her role as their medical missionary.[35]

In the late-nineteenth century, OIA physicians laboring in the field received little attention from the Indian Department in Washington. Occasionally the Indian Department recognized the inadequacies of the system of delivering medical services. In his 1890 report, Commissioner Morgan admitted that there had been "a large degree of needless suffering and hundreds of deaths that might . . . have been prevented." To his credit, Morgan did raise the issue again and again, but to no avail; Congress came up empty-handed on appropriations to expand the existing services. Morgan's successor, Daniel M. Browning, made little reference to the subject during his tenure (1893–97). Commissioner William A. Jones, who served for nearly a decade (1897–1905), maintained a complacent attitude. However, the shocking findings of the early 1900s regarding conditions in Indian schools eventually forced him to confront reality. Until then the OIA, engrossed in allotment in severalty, would not turn its full attention to the problems in the boarding schools.[36]

Meanwhile, agency physicians suffered the indignity of living in decrepit, cramped quarters. They made do with blunt and old instruments and put up with constant delays in the shipment of supplies and equipment. They had to turn in countless periodical reports on diseases treated and the improvement of sanitary conditions. And they traveled many miles each day in order to see a few patients.[37]

Unlike Susan, her colleague Charles Eastman was never able to afford a team. Suffering the discomfort of riding on horseback, he traveled between fifty and seventy-five miles on a normal day. Eastman complained bitterly of the poor quality of the drugs supplied to the agencies by unscrupulous contractors. Like Susan, Eastman had to dig into his personal savings to buy supplementary medicines.[38]

Because life-threatening epidemics frequently swept through the reservation, Susan often ran low on supplies. The Omaha doctor treated a range of acute and chronic ailments, including influenza, dysentery, cholera, and eye-related disorders. The most serious sight disease Susan treated was trachoma.[39]

By the early 1910s, when accurate statistics became available, an estimated 33 percent of the Omaha population suffered from some form of eye contagion. Compared to the affliction rate for the general Indian population—which stood at roughly 27 percent in 1910—it seems that the Omahas were hit slightly harder than other tribes.[40] After one serious epidemic in the early 1890s, Susan instructed her patients to use separate towels and basins.[41] Without the benefit of chemotherapeutic agents, such as sulfanamides and tetracycline, and a clean water supply, recovery from this type of eye contagion was slow, and if untreated, the disease could lead to partial or total loss of sight. Further handicapped by incomplete knowledge of the etiology of such diseases, nineteenth-century doctors had to emphasize prevention.[42] Susan taught her patients to understand that "isolation is prevention" and instructed them not even to "touch articles touched by the afflicted one."[43]

Sadly, though some physicians like Susan were well aware of preventive methods earlier, it was not until 1895 that the Indian Office issued its first directive on preventative measures. The roller-towel system was condemned in the directive, but little else resulted from that official memorandum.[44] The OIA did not push for specific appropriations to fight against the disease until 1908, when an outbreak of trachoma cases at the Phoenix Indian School in Arizona drew national attention.[45]

On the Omaha reservation influenza was the most serious malady of the late-nineteenth century. During her tenure as OIA physician, Susan examined many such cases. The reservation was hit hard by two epidemics of "la grippe," during Susan's first winter as a doctor. However, except for the death of two young babies, no other fatalities were recorded.[46]

The low death rate that year could be attributed to Susan's labors. She cited the winter months as the busiest time of the year. In the winter of 1891 she saw an average of more than one hundred people each month. Each day of that season she left home early in the morning and returned late at night. Susan reported that the influenza epidemic raged "with more violence than during the preceding years; some families were rendered helpless by it, sometimes all the family but one or two being down with it." In December, with the mercury hovering between fifteen and twenty degrees below zero, she was still out making house calls.[47]

In that month, only one patient died. Already very ill with tuberculosis, the woman succumbed to the influenza epidemic. Susan wrote that the patient turned so weak that "every breath she drew was in agony." She "was too weak to even whisper," Susan continued. The Omaha physician made her patient comfortable, but there was little else she could do. The sickly woman died two weeks later.[48] Nevertheless Susan treated many Indians successfully. One "man was so ill that the family did not expect him to live, and Indian medicine had been of no avail," Susan wrote. She gave him some medication, and he rallied around. In a few days he had recovered.[49]

Many of Susan's patients became easy prey for the influenza epidemics once tuberculosis had worn them down. At the turn of the century, tuberculosis took a heavy toll on Indians. But the Indian Office, ignorant of the origins of the disease, did little until the late 1900s to control and eradicate the contagion. Commissioner Jones believed that tuberculosis was hereditary and that Indians were predisposed to succumb to the malady. Although that viewpoint reflected the general public's view, physicians knew better. William Osler, whose medical textbook educated two generations of American physicians, offered an in-depth analysis that refuted the hereditary and the unfavorable climate and sedentary living arguments. Osler argued in favor of the discovery in 1882 that the disease was spread by a pathogen, the tubercle bacillus. But it was more than twenty years before the reductionist assumption that a specific organism could be responsible for the manifestation of a particular disease became a part of public discourse.[50]

A 1904 OIA survey conducted on field physicians finally brought the attention of the authorities to the pathology of tuberculosis and its prevention. The conclusion drawn from that survey read: "Tuberculosis is more widespread among Indians than among an equal number of whites." The rate of affliction among the Omahas was about 50 percent higher than that of whites. But between 1904 and 1909, lassitude still characterized the official response to the pestilence. OIA officials in the capital, especially Commissioner (1905–1909) Francis E. Leupp, played down its prevalence. Only when Commissioner Robert G. Valentine, who served from 1909 to 1913, appointed Joseph A. Murphy as the first medical supervisor of the entire Indian service was there concrete action.[51]

In the field, physicians like Susan did the best they could. In her 1893 report, she wrote that tuberculosis was on the increase in the tribe and most of the tribal deaths in that year had resulted from the contagion. The advice Susan dispensed was "plenty of fresh air and sunshine."[52]

While commonsensical and ameliorative, that advice did not eradicate the pathogen. An individual could be infected by inhaling the tubercle bacillus in fresh droplet nuclei or via dust particles in the air. Without the benefit of antibiotics, discovered in the 1940s, recovery from tuberculosis was slow and sometimes impossible. Doctors in the late-nineteenth century relied on cod-liver oil and arsenic, but these did little to kill the pathogen, which can quickly spread throughout the body.[53]

Susan herself attributed the transmission of the disease to three factors: diseased meat, instead of fresh game; poorly ventilated homes, instead of airy tepees; and consanguineous, instead of exogamous marriages. In this matter, she hinted that she had some misgivings about the costs of "civilization." Her sister Marguerite once wrote: "Sometimes I am sorry that the white people ever came to America." Susan may have shared those sentiments. She had once written about the beauty and practicality of the tepee and mud lodge, and she could appreciate the value of her native heritage.[54]

With the exception of May 1892, when she left to attend the Hampton commencement and visit friends in Philadelphia, Susan had worked continuously since returning to the reservation. By late 1892 the hectic schedule and the weary miles of traveling began to take their toll on her. The frail young physician had never enjoyed robust health. In her second college year she had complained of breathing difficulties and a "kind of numbness." But she brushed the symptoms aside, attributing them to mental and emotional stress.[55]

In early December 1892, she was bedridden for several weeks. In a letter to Francis, Rosalie related that Susan had pain in the head and the back of her neck "constantly" and that her ears also troubled her "very much." By the first week of the new year, Susan had recovered and could return to work.[56]

Despite her emaciated condition, Susan declined few calls. But the "hard rides were exhausting," she lamented. They were also dangerous. One spring day, while riding in a storm, she was thrown from her carriage. Internal injuries kept her house-bound for a prolonged period. Enfeebled, Susan had to turn down an invitation from Alice C. Fletcher to speak at the World's Fair of 1893–1894 in Chicago.[57]

When fall came, Susan fell ill again and left the school to return to her mother's home for nearly fifty days. During that interval, her mother, Mary Gale, suffered a serious decline in her health. Another unnamed member of the family also needed medical attention. Still somewhat weak, Susan returned to her workplace when her mother recovered. But soon a student whom the Omaha doctor had been treating died and, in her own words, Susan "broke down." In a letter to Indian agent William H. Beck, Susan explained that she left for home again "in order to be able to get enough strength to resume school duties."[58]

Beck was unconvinced. Apparently the OIA physician should have applied to him for a leave of absence, and he threatened to recommend a reduction in her salary as a form of disciplinary action. However, Beck recanted once he accepted the circumstances surrounding her departure.[59]

So Susan returned to her duties, but not for long. One day in mid-November 1893, she came home very late in the evening. According to Rosalie, Susan was shocked to find Mary Gale sprawled on the floor "almost dead." Earlier Susan had pleaded with Marguerite to take care of their ailing mother. For unknown reasons, Marguerite refused. Now a crisis, both personal and familial, had developed.[60]

Susan's career goals competed with familial obligations. According to Rosalie, Susan "hated to give it [her work] up." Presumably, the Omaha doctor not only hesitated to abandon her medical work, but also the public honor that came with it. However, she probably reminded herself that she had forsaken familial responsibilities while away in medical school. This was the opportunity to assuage her guilt. In the end, Susan chose to give up her job and conserve her limited strength in order to use her medical skills for her mother's sake.[61] Of course, her own health probably played a part in Susan's final decision. Apparently, despite the earlier disagreement, Agent Beck valued her services, and he gave her two months to reconsider. The Omahas also pleaded with her to withdraw the decision.[62] But Susan's mind was made up; personal ambition had to take a backseat to kinship ties.

With public life behind her, Susan now took stock of her private life. In the spring of 1894, with hardly any warning, Susan surprised her family and friends with an unexpected announcement: she had met someone and had accepted his marriage proposal. With the memories of her experience with Thomas Ikinicapi still lingering, Susan's family was caught offguard. Her friends in the East greeted the news with dismay. Through its official organ, *The Indian Bulletin*, the Connecticut Indian Association told members that they "must bury regret at [their] loss." It hinted that Susan's "bright, intelligent spirit" might go to waste following matrimony. The Heritages, friends from her Philadelphia days, wrote in a disappointed tone that they "can't send congratulation." Their daughter with whom Susan had spent many happy moments, Marian Heritage, raised objections about Susan's "poor health" and "the quality of the man she's marrying."[63]

Marian Heritage was probably referring to the "colorful" background of Susan's fiancé and the class difference between them. Not too much is known about him. A Sioux Indian from the Yankton agency, Henry Picotte was born in 1860 and was the son of an OIA interpreter. As a young man Henry had apparently worked at a circus sideshow. Sometime before the mid-1880s, he married Victoria Hedges, and together they had three children. Then in 1892 he hurriedly left South Dakota for the plains. His brother Charles, who was already married to Marguerite La Flesche, needed him. Stricken with tuberculosis, Charles now relied on Henry to tend to his farm and financial matters. By all accounts, Henry faithfully fulfilled that role. Before long Henry had set his roots in Nebraska, and he soon divorced his wife.[64]

Probably impressed by Henry's dedication, Susan found herself falling in love with him. After all, as described by a close friend, Henry was a "handsome man with polite, ingratiating manners, and a happy sense of humor." Many years later, after Henry's demise, Susan confided in a friend that she had loved him "very much," even though they seemed "utterly unlike" each other.[65] Since marriage and marital status were not important markers of gender identity in Indian most societies, Susan probably married for love. Then again, sickly and jobless, she may have felt insecure. Matrimony may have appeared to be the avenue to personal fulfillment in a Victorian style. As an individual with a fluid, bicultural identity, Susan conceivably could have accepted this argument.[66]

She certainly never gave up her desire to be a mother. During her college days, she wrote that motherhood was a "privilege." She told Rosalie it was a shame that, for medical reasons, some women could not bear children. In another letter, Susan hinted that she would like to have a husband and family even after she embarked on her career.[67]

For whatever reasons—societal conventions or personal, intimate ones—Susan probably deemed it the right moment to marry. Almost thirty years old and having fulfilled her promise to the CIA, Susan now chose to revoke her pledge to remain a "dear little old maid." On the last day of June 1894, with Marguerite as the witness, she married Henry Picotte at the local Presbyterian church.[68]

After their betrothal Susan and Henry moved into a house across from that church, located almost twenty-two miles from the agency in the town of Bancroft. Soon Susan began seeing patients from her new home, which was not uncommon for women physicians of that period; it gave them the flexibility to maintain a professional career and a household. But for Susan, this new path was still strewn with unexpected thorns. Within a year after her wedding, she suffered the symptoms of that unknown ailment again. "Susie has been very sick," Rosalie told Francis. Rosalie also reported that she "had given up all hopes of her when she commenced to improve."[69]

That illness must have complicated Susan's first pregnancy. Still she carried the infant to full term, and Caryl Picotte came into the world a healthy, eight-pound baby boy. Judging from a letter to the CIA, Susan seemed to relish motherhood. Proudly she described Caryl: "He has thick black hair, and his brilliant black eyes follow us all over the room." But childbirth weakened Susan considerably. A tender and loving man, Henry came to her rescue. Apparently he had good fatherly instincts. For the first few weeks after the delivery, he "staid up every night and took the entire care of him [Caryl]." Even after months had passed, he occasionally rose at night to check on their infant son.[70]

Despite motherhood, Susan continued practicing medicine. Being self-employed, she enjoyed enough flexibility to balance work and home life, although it did involve some effort. Sometimes Susan took Caryl with her when she had to make house calls. Once Caryl went along on an eighteen-mile ride through rough country. However, Susan felt guilty about taking her baby along and soon chose to leave him behind with family members and friends.[71]

Apparently Henry was a very supportive spouse. When a call came one night for Susan to aid an Omaha woman and she hesitated, Henry insisted that she respond. He said: "It won't take long, only three hours to go, and you can relieve her." Henry drove the buggy, but halfway there it gave way. Somehow he fixed it, and they arrived in time to save the sickly Indian woman. In the daytime, Susan often left their baby in Henry's care. Sometimes she would be away all night, and in the morning, with his son in his arms, Henry would go looking for their loved one.[72]

When their second son, Pierre, was born in early 1898, Henry was equally supportive. However, Susan had to take Pierre with her more often on house calls, since Henry was busier with his stock and crops. Pierre and Caryl were the only children Susan ever had. Like most women doctors of that time, Susan had to keep the family small in order to integrate her domestic obligations and career demands.[73]

Though Susan enjoyed a flourishing practice and followed a hectic schedule, she never gave up the hope that someday she would return to her old job as school physician. Financial needs might been another motive; she had taken out a loan from the CIA and had yet to settle any of that amount. As a general practitioner laboring in an isolated, somewhat impoverished part of the country, Susan probably earned only a meager income.[74]

When the physician at the Omaha boarding school left in the spring of 1896, Susan submitted an application for the position via the Indian agent William Beck. For nearly three months she heard nothing. In mid-June, Alice Fletcher wrote to Rosalie and told her that there was little news on the application. Fletcher also matter-of-factly conveyed the information that Susan would have to sit for the civil service examination before she could be considered for the appointment. Following the restructuring of the Indian medical services in 1890, physicians had been placed in the classified civil service and all potential employees had to pass a competitive examination designed to end the spoils system. This unpleasant news spurred Susan to action.[75]

The Omaha physician resubmitted her application, and this time she wrote directly to Commissioner Browning. Making full use of her identity, Susan reminded the Commissioner that the civil service regulation did not apply to Indians like herself. Fearing that her health might have caused her original application to be ignored, she assured Commissioner Browning that she had recovered fully from her fall in

1893. As proof of her professional competence, the shrewd doctor mentioned her practice among the white people of Bancroft. Susan also knew that in the late-nineteenth century the OIA still barred married women from high-ranking positions in its services, but she asked to be given an exemption since she had successfully balanced a career and a family. Finally, she told the Commissioner that she could "help in many ways" if allowed to work among the Indians.[76]

To back up her claim, she appended a petition from the Omaha tribal council. The petition noted that since Susan had a proven record and knew the Omaha language and customs, the council had "great confidence in her," and they asked that she be appointed to the vacant position. Agent Beck echoed the council's stand and recommended that Susan be appointed. Beck wrote that Susan's racial origins and the fact that she "is quite successful as physician and gives satisfaction to Indians" were strong enough reasons to give her the job.[77]

Much to her dismay, Susan was denied the appointment. In a letter reprinted in *The Indian Bulletin* she explained that money was the problem. However, since there is no evidence that Susan ever took the civil service examination, her application probably was rejected almost immediately. No physician was ever appointed to the school, a fact which suggested that budgetary constraints remained a stumbling block in the OIA's effort to improve the delivery of medical services on the reservation.[78]

Despite the disappointment, Susan continued to practice medicine among both Indians and non-Indians. Gradually, she even won the respect of white doctors in the surrounding towns. Once an emergency call came from Lyons, a town nine miles away. In a gathering storm, she rode out and met the two local doctors. Their patient faced complications in childbirth, but with Susan's help they saved both the mother and child. After the ordeal, one of the attending physicians quipped that their success was "thanks to the skill of Dr. Susan."[79]

In the summer of 1897 an already emaciated Susan succumbed once more to the unknown ailment that had troubled her earlier. She was so ill that her family was prepared for the worst. This experience left a profound impression on the barely thirty-two-year-old woman. In a letter to a Hampton teacher, she recounted how deeply moved she was by the show of emotional support from both Indian and white neighbors. They brought her flowers, fruits, food, and words of comfort. The many expressions of congratulations she received following recovery gave Susan a great deal of moral encouragement. "When I felt a little depressed," she confided in her ex-teacher, "I would think there was not much use in trying to help people, that they did not seem to appreciate it but this summer taught me a lesson I hope I'll never forget." She ended that letter by vowing "to do right and live a better life." Susan's focus on emotional satisfaction was rather telling of her motivation for mediation; the gratification she felt from such labor propelled many of her life choices.[80]

By the turn of the century the Omahas' struggle to preserve autonomy and territorial integrity had forced many educated tribal members to enter the political realm, and Susan was no exception. Her entrée into politics seemed inevitable, but she was also impelled by personal reasons. Highly cognizant of her mortality and family problems, and later troubled by bureaucratic inertia, she threw herself into temperance work and the politics of allotment in severalty. The former gave Susan the image of a Victorian reformer, while the latter earned her the role of a tribal leader. In carrying out those roles, Susan found herself roving back and forth between cultures, and this must have caused her some stress. Maintaining an in-between ethnic role was probably not an easy challenge, but perhaps the difficulty was cushioned by Susan's growing realization that her mediation was gradually beginning to promote the wants of her people over the aggressive demands of Euro-Americans.

CHAPTER SIX

"This Curse of Drink"

"For four years, from 1889 to 1893 I worked among the Omahs [sic] . . . At first I went every where alone . . . and felt perfectly safe among my people," Susan wrote to Commissioner of Indian Affairs William A. Jones. "But intemperance increased," Susan sadly recalled, "until men, women, and children drank; men and women died from alcoholism, and little children were seen reeling on the streets of the towns."[1] Written in 1900, this letter offers a glimpse into one of the pressing social maladies that afflicted the Omaha reservation. Well aware of the impact of alcohol, Susan tried to eradicate this social disease through political lobbying, secular improvement, education, and moral persuasion. Her actions revealed both the spirit of evangelical Protestantism and that of the turn-of-the-century social gospel movement. The latter emphasized the attainment of a perfect moral order through social reform, while the former prescribed salvation through the "sanctification" of individuals via conversion. However, both movements drew their origins from Christianity. Late-nineteenth century reformers believed that alcoholism inhibited religious witnessing, and it was even seen as a symbol of moral pollution. The proposed remedy thus zeroed in on pietism as much as it did on social benevolence, although the latter would receive more emphasis than the former as the century drew to an end. In the fight against drinking, the conversion and salvation of Indians was believed to be just as important as their worldly uplift.[2]

Susan's anti-drinking stance must have been honed by her father's position on this issue. Joseph La Flesche's proscription that "drink is bad for the red man" had been passed along to his children. While still a medical student in Philadelphia, Susan had attended temperance lectures delivered by leading crusaders such as Harriet Whitehall Smith and Francis Willard. Such women reformers often saw alcohol abuse and related crime and injustices done to women, as a symptom, not a cause, of poverty. Environmental determinism, and by its extension a secularized understanding of causation, was increasingly taking center stage over the belief that alcoholism was caused by a biological predisposition.[3]

For women temperance advocates, heavy drinking symbolized a distinctively male culture outside the orbit of female influence and antithetical to the sanctity of the Victorian home. Alcohol abuse also reminded women of their vulnerable, dependent position within the family. Susan never articulated this protofeminist "home protection" theme, although she did express concern about the disintegration of Omaha families and of the tribe and how that decline was engendered by shifting conditions on the reservation. However, like many of her religiously inspired and educated peers, Susan later became a temperance speaker, lecturing on the spread of alcoholism among her people.[4]

Of course, heavy drinking was nothing new; the problem could be traced back to the apogee of the fur trade during the early nineteenth century. The drinking problem on the Omaha reservation seemed to be under control during Iron Eye's lifetime, but the Dawes Act set in motion a series of events that revived this social disease.

Many social problems arose among the Indians again following the introduction of liberal land-sale and leasing policies. Although the Dawes Act prohibited leasing of Indian allotments during the trust period of twenty-five years, eventually in 1891 policy makers allowed those Native Americans who, by reason of infirmity or other disability, could not work their land to lease it for three years for farming and grazing purposes or ten years for mining. Before the end of the century, this lease option was also extended to able-bodied Indians who could not or would not use their land.[5]

On the Omaha reservation, leasing policies wrought disastrous results. Rather than promoting self-support and industry, leasing policies encouraged Indians to live off land rentals, which were often the first step toward the sale of Indian land. The first signs of trouble surfaced in 1891. Robert H. Ashley, the OIA agent, reported that preoccupation with leasing had caused some Omahas to "have badly neglected their crops," while "whiskey make[s] sad havoc."[6] The next year Ashley alerted his superiors to the "alarming extent" of the use of intoxicants.[7] By early September of that year the OIA inspector William W. Junkin reported that the majority of Omaha Indians had leased their land and were "in the condition of idleness and poverty."[8] One unidentified Omaha made the following comments: "Nearly all of the land is leased, and most of the Indians have scarcely a thing to show for the rent they receive. . . . Leasing is ruining the Omahas in every way."[9] Dr. Susan La Flesche wrote that the destitution on the reservation stemmed from the fact that the Omaha men used their lease earnings for liquor, while "no machinery was bought, no household improvements were made, and complete demoralization . . . prevailed." She recalled that Indians who leased their lands "lived only from day to day" and "made no provision for the future."[10]

Quite often, Indians leased land to whites in payment of debts or in order to secure loans and credit. For most Omahas, leasing their land was unavoidable; with little cash to buy seeds and equipment for farming and no collateral to secure loans, many Omahas had to choose this route to survive. Some Indians were so desperate that they even leased land to whites without obtaining Indian Office approval. Others, egged on by their prospective lessees, occupied unallotted land and rented it out in clear violation of OIA regulations. Unattuned to the intricacies of a money economy, many Indians quickly raked up more debts and eventually had to sell their land.[11]

The level of Indian dispossession rose dramatically once the safeguard of inalienability surrounding trust allotments had been removed. In 1902 Congress allowed heirs to sell trust estates. Not long after, owners of allotments whose trust period had to yet to expire were allowed to dispose of their land through the provisions of the Burke Act of 1906. After 1907, sick, disabled, and incompetent Indians were also offered the option of selling their land interests. Euro-American speculators or their lawyers often gained power of attorney over the lands of these so-called incompetents and eventually persuaded them to give up their landholdings.[12]

Often, frequently through the use of alcohol, land grafters also maneuvered Indians into fraudulent land transactions. Susan recounted one story of an Omaha Indian, Louis Levering, who had lost his land after he signed away the title while still in a state of inebriation. She charged another Omaha, Thomas Sloan, a mixed blood of dubious tribal affiliation, with perpetrating the crime. Apparently Sloan, an attorney, had been working in collusion with an Anglo-American real estate company interested in taking control of reservation land. Susan also claimed that a partner of Sloan, W. E. Estill, bore responsibility for plying Victoria Wood Phillips with whiskey in order to induce her to sell her land. Estill apparently also had deceived Phillips on the exact amount she was to receive for the transaction. Additionally there was the case of Henry Parker. Estill had offered Parker whiskey, and while Parker was inebriated, Estill had persuaded him to sell forty acres of his land. To make matters worse, Estill defrauded Parker of a portion of the purchase price and gave him a worthless promissory note.[13]

Francis La Flesche attributed the general tragedy of Omaha dispossession to his people's "lack of business training and experience," while his sister Susan acknowledged that their people did not know how to effectively use the land accruements.[14] She admitted that Indians had to pay "dearly" for the teachings of "civilization." Yet she argued defensively that the cost arose because Indians did "not understand all the ways and methods of the white man." According to a story Susan related, one Omaha sold his entire heirship holdings for a mere six thousand dollars. Then he held a celebration where whiskey flowed freely, and he distributed money to his guests. He also bought himself a few buggies. Within the year, he had spent all the proceeds of the land sale.[15]

Indians who lost their land were deprived of more than just natural resources. Since land represented existence, identity, and a place of belonging and not merely real estate to be bought and developed, Omahas found that their whole way of life was now under full assault. Their culture and religion had already been discredited by the Americanization policy. Now, finding their land and economic resources gone and citizenship and political autonomy meaningless, some Omahas resorted to alcohol abuse.[16]

Contemporary scholars argue that heavy drinking is used as a means of coping with unpleasant emotions or situations and that it serves escapist functions. Alcohol may have given some Native Americans a sense of superiority and confidence, albeit ephemeral in nature. One scholar even argues that by participating in drinking as a shared recreational activity, Native Americans were engaged, in the absence of other means, in an attempt at "asserting and validating" their Indian identities.[17] However, heavy drinking also exacerbated health problems and sped the unraveling of societal structures, giving the Indians even more reasons to seek escape. On the whole, the Indians' deep feeling of inadequacy and inferiority, growing from their relations with Euro-Americans, is considered to be the most important factor in the rise of alcoholism among some American Indian tribes.

In the long run, the availability of intoxicating beverages became a key element in the Indians' cycle of land sale, low self-esteem and morale, heavy drinking, and continued poverty. After more than a decade of such dissipation, Francis observed, in a 1901 letter written to a nephew, that leasing, land sale, and the illicit peddling of liquor "have done them [the Omahas] more harm than anything that happened to them in their history." Though rampant drunkenness might have offered some a brief escape from dispossession and cultural disruption, it also expressed the despair and dependence of a conquered people.[18]

During her years as a government physician, Susan had witnessed the depth of the effects of alcoholism as a social disease. When Sara Thomson Kinney visited her in 1891, Susan told her that at the start of her tenure she had received repeated calls for camphor. Soon she discovered that the acidic substance served as a substitute for whiskey, and she quickly removed camphor from her stock.[19] In her letter to Commissioner William A. Jones, Susan recalled that in the course of making house calls she often witnessed "drunken brawls in which men were killed . . . and [that] no person's life was considered safe."[20] Years later, during her testimony before an inquest, Susan recalled that in the 1890s some inebriated Indians met their death through accidents. One Indian had been run over by a train while he was drunk. And she remembered that Furnas Robinson had drowned in the Missouri River after a drinking bout. Another Omaha had fallen from his buggy one night and had been found frozen to death the next morning. In dramatizing the cause of temperance by retelling numerous anecdotal accounts about the baneful effects of heavy drinking, Susan replicated the approach Euro-American women temperance advocates took in that period.[21]

Susan and some other educated Omahas believed the self-inflicted violence and dissipation that alcohol caused were unacceptable. They sought to end the tragedy through prohibition and religiosity. When signs of trouble first appeared in 1891, she and a few other tribal members organized a law and order committee that provided names of whiskey traffickers and bootleggers to the reservation agent for subsequent legal action. In her 1891 visit to the reservation, Sara Thomson Kinney observed: "Their efforts are meeting with some success . . . several offenders have already been brought before the courts through the efforts of this committee."[22]

Though Susan supported coercive methods, she also embraced persuasive ones, and in so doing she took a slightly different course from most turn-of-the-century temperance women, who now tended to emphasize secular social reform over pietism. Susan hoped the appeal to piety and higher morals that she employed would effect a change for the better. From her office at the agency, she ran a reading room, which offered games and reading material that she hoped would provide a diversion from "harmful amusements," including heavy drinking. Beyond that, in her capacity as unofficial tribal advisor and leader for the Omahas' Christian Endeavor Society, Susan must also have addressed this issue with tribal leaders.[23]

In that same year, Susan and other educated Indians lobbied for a vote on prohibition for Thurston County, the area with the heaviest concentration of Omahas. By that time what was taking place in Thurston County was being repeated all across the country, especially in the West and the South, as the push for county local-option laws became the rallying cry of national temperance organizations, particularly the Anti-Saloon League. A single-issue pressure group inspired by the social gospel movement, the Anti-Saloon League lobbied for laws that would strike a practical blow against liquor traffic. By attempting to decrease the supply of liquor, the league hoped that labor productivity and general social good would triumph. In this sense, the goals of Susan's crusade were no different from those of the larger movement. Back in Thurston County, she led the preelection campaign to educate tribal members on the voting process and its larger social and moral significance for the tribe.[24]

In a letter to the Women's National Indian Association (WNIA), Susan claimed that all Omahas wanted the saloons in the surrounding towns to close down, but few could read the ballot ticket. Liquor dealers took advantage of this, and with the help of their representatives, tickets with "Against Prohibition" stamped on them were issued to the Omahas. In response, Susan and her assistants went around the reservation and enlightened Omahas about the possible misuse of the tickets.[25]

The temperance advocates' educational work continued right up to voting day, but the liquor interest groups had the edge. The liquor promoters told the Indians that since they had become citizens of the republic, they had the same rights as Euro-Americans and thus could drink as much as they desired. The laws against the sale and distribution of liquor to Indians—the Trade and Intercourse Acts—no longer applied to newly enfranchised Indians. A sufficient number of Indians ended up voting against the local prohibition option to keep the county wet. Thus, Susan and fellow temperance supporters met defeat in spite of strong Omaha support. Though highly supportive of the Dawes Act and its granting of citizenship rights to Indians, she reluctantly admitted that American citizenship had also given the Indians the right to buy whiskey.[26]

For her part, Susan exonerated those Omahas who chose to vote against prohibition. Defensive of her people, she also indirectly hinted that whites should forgive Indians, since they did "not understand all the ways and methods of the white man." In a typical mediatory attempt to soften potential misunderstanding, Susan assured Euro-American reformers that without the manipulation of bootleggers and liquor dealers, the Omahas would stand behind the prohibition platform if they were given another opportunity to vote.[27] However, she seemed ignorant of, or perhaps chose to ignore, the fact that some Omahas had literally sold their votes to the whiskey peddlers in return for cash.[28] As always, Susan sought to find common ground across the cultural divide. This stance also revealed her growing sense of tribal patriotism, which encouraged Susan to attempt to distance her people from the rapacious behavior of Euro-Americans.

In 1892 Wajapa, a successful Omaha farmer and a friend of the La Flesche family, held a large gathering at his home that was attended by leading "progressive" Omahas, including Susan. During the meeting, rousing speeches were delivered. After the meeting, Wajapa passed a petition around within the tribe that asked the Indian Office to set up a fund to enforce existing anti-drinking laws. The financial resources for this fund were to be derived from some of the proceeds of the leasing of unallotted tribal land. This proposal received the endorsement of the Indian agent, but the OIA did not offer a response. Thirteen years passed before the OIA secured the first appropriation from Congress to support efforts to stamp out the sale of alcoholic beverages.[29]

"Drinking is still going on among our people," lamented Susan in an 1893 letter to the WNIA. With hardly any restrictions, saloons in Bancroft openly sold whiskey to Indians. Liquor was also available on the reservations. Susan blamed white people who leased Indian land for the flow of liquor into the reservations. She described one unlicensed saloon as akin to "a fountain, and the liquor wells from it as if from a spring."[30]

In the same letter to the WNIA, Susan demanded more vigorous prosecution of the law. She must have been referring in part to the enforcement of the 1892 revised federal statute prohibiting the sale of liquor by both non-Indians and Indians on all reservations. The law also proscribed the sale of such beverages to Indian allottees who had land still held in trust by the federal government or to any Indian who was a ward, or under the guardianship, of the United States. Susan may also have been alluding to the law, passed in 1891 by the Nebraska legislature, which prohibited the sale of alcohol to‘ non-citizen Indians.[31]

But enforcement of these laws was no easy task. Some Omahas, citing their right to drink whiskey, declined to testify against liquor dealers. Fearing undue publicity or bodily harm, local officials and residents of the surrounding towns also refused to testify. Even when convicted, liquor peddlers received little punishment; the penalty of a fine of twenty-five dollars plus court costs deterred few and emboldened some. Further, drunken Indians were rarely incarcerated for long; after the Standing Bear decision of 1879, Indians technically could obtain a writ of habeas corpus against anyone, including the government, endeavoring to confine them.[32]

Susan recounted woeful tales of Omahas who had died after drinking bouts, and how one inebriated Indian had smashed a buggy and beaten a woman and her child. Aware that her people could not make "any true progress in any direction with this curse of drink among" them, she implored the WNIA to use its moral and political leverage to help lift the bane of alcohol. To drum up more support, Susan apparently also sent a copy of this letter to the Hampton student newspaper, *Talks and Thoughts*.[33]

But the onslaught of the social contagion associated with liquor continued unabated. In a passionate letter to *The Indian Bulletin*, published in May 1894, the Omaha physician railed that intemperance was worse than it had ever been. Just a few weeks before, a young man had frozen to death while under the influence of alcohol. But this was not the first death; intemperance had led to the loss of lives in all of the three preceding years.[34]

Highly disturbed by this pattern of destruction, Susan lashed out at white Americans who defended the Indians' right to drink as citizens of the republic. Perhaps more uncharacteristic was her rejection of the argument that the "cure must be placed in his [Indian] soul." To accept that argument, she said, was to "have no cure at all."[35]

Susan hinted—now echoing the stance of mainstream reformers— that she believed remonstrance and moral appeals had made little headway against the drinking problem. After all entire families, including mothers and young children, had fallen under the sway of alcohol. The moment for more coercive methods had arrived. "Every time an arrest and imprisonment has been made," Susan argued, "it has had a salutary effect on buyer and seller." To back her argument, she quoted from Indians who told her that "if you could only take it away from us; we would not drink . . . if the white people would only shut it off from us we would be forced to get along without it." Susan downplayed the Omahas' involvement and instead placed the blame at the doorstep of white America. She implied that the Omahas were only victims of manipulation by non-Indians.[36]

But thus far inadequate funding and a shortage of enforcement officials had derailed the prosecution of the guilty parties. The Omaha doctor now pleaded for both, and she promised to write to the state-level WNIA auxiliary for support in political lobbying. "The help of the law would be a substantial plank to stand on," she ended the letter confidently.[37]

Susan's efforts and her sense of urgency ran almost parallel to those of the Omaha tribal council. In 1894, the council submitted a request to the OIA to help revive the Omaha tribal police force, which had been disbanded following Joseph La Flesche's death in 1888.[38] The next year a grave tone pervaded the council's early summer meeting with the visiting OIA inspector. The council pleaded with the inspector to find a solution to the Omahas' "demoralizing state." Members also asked for a law or rule by which the "alarming state of drunkenness . . . may be corrected." Finally, they repeated their request for the establishment of a police force to check this social disease. The tribe offered to contribute five hundred dollars toward this effort. Although the inspector concurred in his report with the council's proposals, the Indian Office ignored the recommendations.[39]

However, anti-liquor sentiments persisted among Susan and other Omahas. The Meiklejohn Bill, sponsored by Nebraska Third District Representative George D. Meiklejohn, sought to curb the alarming increase in alcohol use by Native Americans and the intensified liquor traffic. On January 31, 1896, leading Omahas—51 women and 183 men, most likely including Susan—signed a letter to Commissioner Browning urging him and all "friends of the Indians" to secure the passage of the bill. In their letter the Omahas acknowledged "the impossibility of restraining . . . Indians from its [alcohol] use." Apparently they believed that only coercive methods would work.[40] The bill, which became law on January 30, 1897, made it unlawful for anyone to sell or supply alcohol to allottees whose land was still held in trust, or to any Indian supervised by the government. The penalties for trafficking ranged from imprisonment for not less than sixty days to fines of up to two hundred dollars.[41]

The law clearly negated the citizenship provisions in the Dawes Act that had technically ended federal powers of guardianship over the Indians.[42] Supporters of the Meiklejohn law argued that this inconsistency was unavoidable, in light of the fact that a number of federal district courts had ruled that the 1892 revised statute prohibiting the sale of alcohol on reservations was inapplicable in cases involving Indian allottees.[43] Two years after the passage of the Meiklejohn law, Commissioner of Indian Affairs William W. Jones reported that "the [liquor] traffic . . . has been decidedly interfered with."[44]

But on the Omaha reservation trouble surfaced again in 1899 when the U.S. deputy marshals, who had been sent to the reservation in 1897 to eliminate bootleggers, were removed by a budget-conscious Indian Office. Bootleggers from Sioux City quickly swarmed the reservation holdings in search of potential customers.[45]

Within a year the situation on the reservation had become so serious that Susan wrote to Commissioner Jones imploring him to reappoint the marshals. "Of what use will be the money saved . . . if our people are to be demoralized, mentally, morally and physically?" she asked. "The Indians are drinking all the time again," she cried, "and the towns are filled with drunken Indians." When she admonished some of the intoxicated Omahas, they retorted: "The Government says we can drink again." Apparently many Indians interpreted the pullout of the deputy marshals as the end of anti-drinking laws.[46]

This incident also served as evidence of the intratribal conflict engendered by Susan's crusade. On another occasion, the Indian

Office had fired a field official who Susan believed had performed well in the struggle against liquor. The inspector who removed the official called his defenders factionalists. In her letter of protest, Susan offered a sharp retort: "The so-called 'factional fight' was between Right and Wrong." She also made her position clear: "I knew I shall be unpopular for a while with my people, because they will misconstrue my efforts but this is nothing, just so I can help them for their own good."[47]

Her superior attitude and her actions very likely infuriated tribal members who favored freedom of choice. She probably irked imbibing husbands when she gave shelter to their abused wives and children. At other times council members had consulted Susan before they submitted names of drunken individuals to the tribal attorney for federal prosecution, which must have placed her at odds with the pro-drinking faction. By speaking in support of politicians who wanted to prohibit the sale of liquor and extolling the efforts of OIA officials who arrested the whiskey peddlers, she invited the wrath of "non-progressive" Omahas.[48] Although Susan was fairly silent on the animosity she encountered, published OIA reports recounted many cases of Omahas' evasion of the anti-drinking laws. Their repudiation of the laws served to spur Susan to action, which placed her even more at odds with the tribal faction that favored freedom of choice when it came to alcohol.

But Susan was no stranger to factionalism. Her father, Joseph, had championed unpopular causes, ranging from frame houses to temperance, on the reservation for a long time. Convinced of the moral approbation of her crusade, she minced few words and probably riled many people on and off the reservation.

Some of the resentment directed against Susan most likely reflected resentment against her family. As an OIA field matron in the 1890s, her sister Marguerite La Flesche Diddock had challenged traditional Omaha marriage patterns and pressured the Indian agent to suspend entitlements to those who resisted Euro-American conventions. Another sister, Rosalie, and her husband, Edward Farley, had faced charges of mismanagement of tribal land and had been embroiled in a bitter, protracted lawsuit with other leading Omahas and white businesspeople, who sought profit from the leasing of tribal land. All three women were daughters of the man who had earlier convinced the tribe to surrender their lands—an event that most traditionalists saw as a betrayal of Omaha autonomy. The family's half-blood origins and their ties to the white world only served to deepen the rift between the progressives and traditionalists.[49]

Susan's promotion of Christian civilization or, in this case, temperance among her people sometimes placed her on the razor edge of the cultural border. She could choose to respect the rights and freedoms of American Indian citizens, or she could labor to impose Euro-American behavior on them. Either way, she would end up promoting dissension on the reservation.

In a letter written in 1900, when alcoholism had reared its ugly head on the reservation again, Susan recalled how the Meiklejohn law had brought peace because "immorality among a notably moral tribe is checked." Children had no longer suffered abuse at the hands of their parents, and homes in "danger of being wrecked were built up again." In her opinion, the law had previously effected an obvious transformation for the better. Susan also implied that Indians could be as good as whites if they were given the opportunity. She argued that the logical solution to the drinking problem would be to enforce the law to its fullest extent.[50]

Harry L. Keefe, the attorney for the Omaha tribe, largely agreed with the Omaha physician but parted ways on the issue of recent enforcement. In a letter to the commissioner, Keefe suggested that the doctor had exaggerated the efficaciousness of the Meiklejohn law. In sum, he noted that very few cases resulted in convictions, while the penalties imposed on those found guilty were not "commensurate with the offense under the law"—arguments Field Inspector William J. M. Connell echoed in a 1900 report to the Indian Office.[51]

Keefe repeated these arguments in his letter to Representative George D. Meiklejohn. Susan had also written to Meiklejohn, and so Keefe felt compelled to issue a correction. Keefe wrote that "in her [Susan's] zeal for the welfare of her race . . . she has forgotten or overlooked some of the abuses that existed under the mode of prosecution." The fault lay "not in the law but in the execution of it," he said. It is entirely possible that in her almost evangelical desire to rid her people of the social malady of alcoholism, Susan shaded out parts of the reality associated with the enforcement of anti-drinking laws.[52]

To generate support for her cause, Susan sent a copy of her letter to the WNIA's official organ *The Indian's Friend* and also to Herbert Welsh, the executive secretary of the Indian Rights Association, an Indian reform organization. In the cover letter, she asked Welsh if he could render "assistance in this matter." Obviously she had hoped that Welsh would use his clout and political ties to influence the Indian Office. No reply from Welsh has been found; perhaps, he never sent one. Her plea for help from the Indian Office also drew silence, possibly because of the lack of funds.[53]

The failure of the Meiklejohn law was obvious. In 1902, the Omaha Indian agent bemoaned that "simple fines and jail sentences have little terror to those engaged in this business." Other critics of the law complained that it did hardly anything to deter habitual drunkards. The final blow for the Meiklejohn law came in 1905, when the Supreme Court ruled in the decision *In The Matter of Heff* that the 1897 law was unconstitutional as applied to Indian allottees. After this decision, the superintendent of the Omaha agency reported an increase in alcohol consumption.[54]

With the failure of federal punitive measures, Omaha Indians now returned to the idea of prohibition at the local level. Through the good offices of the Presbyterian Board of Home Missions, Susan lobbied the Indian Office once again. In her 1905 letter she called for an outright ban on intoxicating beverages in new towns created from ex-reservation lands. She expressed confidence that such a ban would be legal since the Supreme Court had recently deemed such prohibition constitutional.[55]

In true Progressive-Era fashion, Susan then singled out the railroad company developing the ex-reservation land—one owned by the magnate James J. Hill—as the champion of the liquor interest group, which she believed would "erect saloons and sell liquor in these new towns [and] render the situation among my people doubly horrible." She offered a specific solution: deeds conveying Indian land to the railroad for the establishment of new towns should carry a clause that prohibited the sale of liquor and the erection of saloons.[56] Indeed liquor was already flowing freely from fledgling new towns into the reservation. In his 1903 annual report, the superintendent of the Omaha and Winnebago agency claimed that 90 percent of the alcohol imbibed on the reservation during the last year had originated from Homer, which was only a few miles north of the Winnebago reservation.[57]

Susan's call for action was followed up in the next year by the lobbying efforts of an Omaha delegation to Washington, D.C. Meanwhile, back in Nebraska, the Omaha doctor took to the lectern, imploring her mixed audiences to support prohibition. According to poet John G. Neihardt, an acquaintance of Susan's and a local resident, Susan was an eloquent speaker. At a high point, she would suddenly stop speaking and stand still for several moments. "She vibrated as she stood," remembered Neihardt, "and a change came over her face. Then she would speak the final words and the effect was great indeed."[58] Susan had finally shed her innate shyness as she found the inner courage to wage the battle against insobriety.

Liquor had "degraded the Omaha Indians," she declared. She placed the blame squarely on saloon keepers and claimed that the Indians were simply innocent victims who truly desired to abandon their drinking habits. Inviting her audiences to join the fight to terminate the licenses of the saloons, she pleaded with them to quit "straddling the fence," but instead, "vote for the right." The additional trade created by the saloons was not worth putting up with the "evils," the Omaha doctor argued. Susan reportedly said that the man who voted to license the saloon was "just as guilty of the blood of his brother man, who is ruined by the saloon, and is just as much responsible for the evils . . . as is the saloonkeeper." She seemingly had lost patience with both Indians and non-Indians who refused to testify against bootleggers and liquor suppliers. Shortly after this passionate speech, citizens in Bancroft outlawed the saloon—both Susan's implorings and the national trend had finally made an impact.[59]

When Superintendent John M. Commons arrived to assume control of the Omaha agency in 1906, the situation on the reservation took a turn for the better. By then "a wholesome social reaction from within the Indian himself" had developed, Susan said in a public hearing. The Omahas' sense of self-reprobation, coupled with the efforts of Superintendent Commons, had turned the tide, at least for a while. In part, some Indians found it imperative to abandon their habit; otherwise, Commons would hold up their annuity monies and rents from leasing the lands—a course of action supported by the tribal council. In dealing with habitual drunkards, Commons insisted that they turn in their monthly allowances from land sales at the local stores for necessities. Commons would then conduct a follow-up check on the items purchased. Commons not only monitored the behavior of those with drinking problems, but also took a personal interest in them. He visited their homes and gave them lessons in kitchen gardening.[60]

Susan praised Commons as tireless and relentless in his fight against bootlegging on the reservation. She also claimed that previous agents had never come close to matching his labors. Once the Indians became interested in "anything that might assist him [them] to climb upward again," Susan said, "they began to go to church." She declared that religion and Commons had saved the Omahas. Her implicit endorsement of the agent's coercive methods no doubt exacerbated the strife between her and imbibing Indians.[61] By 1908 Commons reported that there was "growing sobriety, industry, and proper living in every respect" and that only a minority of the Omahas remained alcoholic.[62]

Shortly after 1905, Susan's struggle against heavy drinking among her people had become perhaps more personal than political. Out of fear of being attacked or molested by imbibing Indians, she had been forced to limit her movement around the reservation. Her brother-in-law Noah La Flesche, who had taken their family name when he married her step-sister, Lucy La Flesche, drank more than Susan thought he should. Her sister Rosalie had been threatened once in her own home by a drunken man, and eventually her husband, Edward, also took to the bottle.[63]

But the most painful agony for Susan had been watching her own husband decline in health, in part because of tuberculosis but also due to heavy drinking. In a letter written to a friend immediately after his demise in 1905, Susan lamented that she missed him so much she wished that she could "turn time back a little." She confessed to having such "a longing" for him "that sometimes" she could "almost go wild." Despite his flaws, she had loved him very much. Perhaps Susan felt that her loss could have been averted if Henry had drunk less. Like some other temperance reformers who were motivated by the loss of loved ones, her public mission now turned into a personal one.[64]

Through moral exhortations and political lobbying, Susan and other leading Omahas drew the attention of their fellow tribal members to this social tragedy. As early as 1907, a special liquor agent reported: "There is less real drunkenness among the Indian than formerly."[65] In a letter dated November 15, 1907, addressed to the commissioner of Indian Affairs, Susan echoed that comment. She described her people as "drinking much less," "working better," and "beginning to get interested in the church." The Omahas should be given another field matron, "since they are beginning to climb up," she argued.[66]

Created in 1890, the field matron program strove to promote the assimilation and Christianization of American Indian women through the introduction of Victorian domesticity and mores. Like the OIA and its field matrons, Susan obviously hoped that once Omaha women had adopted certain white-American gender roles, they would influence their husbands to give up drinking. In her role as cultural broker, she echoed somewhat the theme of turn-of-the-century Americanization.[67]

"Real missionary work," which the new OIA official would carry out, she hinted, took time and used indirect methods. "You can't rush at the Indians with an open Bible any more than you can the white people," Susan wrote matter-of-factly. She implied that the Bible-thumping approach could not produce success on its own. In taking this pragmatic position, she demonstrated a keen sense of under-standing what was necessary to reduce the chasm dividing the two cultures. The OIA's reply must have disappointed her; citing the lack of funds, the Indian Office turned down her request.[68]

To a large extent, Susan had made that request because of her own failure to carry on the work. In her own words, she "had broken down from overwork." Hospitalized for several weeks in Sioux City, Susan was told that she would have to forgo her routine for at least six months.[69]

Despite her feeble state, Susan did her part to try to eradicate the social "evil" of drinking. The well-known special anti-liquor agent William A. Johnson gave her due credit for her invaluable assistance. Johnson secured information on liquor dealers and recalcitrant Indians from Susan, who received such information from other cooperative Omahas. "Mrs. Picotte, the missionary here, does a lot of good," he declared.[70] Presumably, Susan's efforts further widened the rift between her and Omaha traditionalists.

Sometime in 1906 Susan had agreed to take up "work" with her people. The Presbyterian Church had offered her the role of Indian missionary among the Omahas, and she had accepted. This offer developed in part through necessity. For almost two years, since 1905, the local Indian congregation—the Blackbird Hills Church—had been forced to make do without a pastor, and the number of attendees had dwindled to a handful.[71]

The Presbyterian Church's offer dovetailed with Susan's strong personal interest in evangelization. In traditional Indian cultures, women had always played an active role in religion. Following the arrival of Europeans, more Indian women than men had been active in Christianity. Church-related activities served as a natural extension of their traditional role as transmitters of knowledge and faith. As a woman with an Indian identity, Susan inherited that legacy.[72]

But it is also conceivable that since Susan had white cultural ties, her missionary work served as an avenue for personal fulfillment, a choice made by countless Euro-American women of that period. At forty-one years of age, bereft of her husband and unable to regain her government physician position, Susan might have seen missionary work as a good opportunity to make something of her approaching middle-age years. Additionally, by the time she received the offer, the still unknown degenerative disease from which she had suffered for years was gradually making her deaf and the pain now extended down into her back. Cognizant of her mortality, Susan probably realized that time was running out. Though she had largely fulfilled her father's dictum that along with power and privilege came a responsibility to care for the poor and the weak, she thought she could do more. After she accepted the appointment, Susan moved to the agency at Macy so she could be closer to the Omahas.[73]

In a 1907 letter to Commissioner Francis E. Leupp, Susan shared some of the fruits of her new labor. She explained that her medical education had come in handy for her missionary work. Whenever Omahas came to her for medical advice, she would speak to them about the Word of God. As a result, "they are drinking less and making more," she proudly told the commissioner. Susan seemed to make good use of her stature as a respected physician to try, through moral persuasion, to influence tribal men and women to discard their drinking habits. Though earlier she had moved away from this approach somewhat, she now came back to it. Perhaps she felt that a two-pronged strategy was required; after all, some temperance advocates embraced coercion and persuasion and saw no contradiction in adopting both simultaneously.[74]

As a Presbyterian missionary, Susan was expected to submit occasional reports to the church authorities. One such report, published in a 1908 church periodical, indicated just how well Susan fit the role of cultural broker. Her report began with an overview of the Omahas' progress toward "civilization" that stated: "We had two railroads, the telephone, the telegraph and other conveniences." Her people "always had a very high standard of morality; they live a moral life," she declared emphatically. With some exaggeration, Susan claimed that the Omahas had never known what thievery was, nor had they ever committed any murders. Not only had the Omahas proved their potential for receiving "civilization," she suggested, but they had also traditionally shown the highest respect for morality. She believed all that had changed when "the white man came to us and brought us . . . whiskey."[75]

In this way Susan seemed to have a slightly simplistic view of the causal link between alcohol abuse and the socioeconomic plight of her people. Like some other contemporary Euro-American advocates of Indian reform, she seemingly traced tribal degradation and dissipation uniformly to the influence of liquor. But her earlier comments that suggested Indian alcoholism grew out of the practice of leasing and land sales imply that, unlike Euro-American reformers who were removed from the immediate surroundings of the reservation, she understood that the cause-and-effect relationship of alcoholism could be more complex.

"The history of the past twenty years among my people is a black one," Susan wrote sadly in a 1908 article. Alcohol abuse had resulted in their complete demoralization. But the situation changed once she took over the Blackbird Hills Church, Susan boasted. In the beginning she conducted lay services for only two or three Indians. But within a few weeks the attendance had risen to twenty-five, and six months later, to ninety.[76]

In the church, attendees followed services in the Omaha language. Susan read the Bible in her native tongue and interpreted the hymns, and she held Christian services for the deceased. She also encouraged couples destined for matrimony to undergo a Christian ceremony, complete with a license. Susan wrote that she kept her layperson services simple and emphasized the redemptive power of the Christian God and the belief that there is "hope for all sinners."[77]

In her article, the Omaha physician recounted stories of Indians whose lives had taken a turn for the better once they had accepted the Word. She told of one elderly man who "drank very hard," but then "came very regularly to church" and soon asked to be baptized. Susan noted that in the previous two years she had witnessed less drinking. "The women are drinking much less, and are taking care of their homes and of their children," she reassured the church authorities.[78]

For some Omahas Christianity seemed to have offered deliverance from a life of insobriety. Eventually some chose to enter into the fold of Presbyterianism. In early December 1907 twenty children and another twenty adults were baptized. In February 1908 forty-five adult Indians joined the church and twenty-two received baptism. By freely using the Omaha language to preach, Susan reached out to more Omahas than had her white predecessors. She very likely deserved all the credit for the growth of the Omaha congregation. A news item covering the baptisms of 1907 concluded: "This was not the result of a revival but is the culmination of the missionary work of Dr. Susan La F. Plicotte[sic]," who had given "the sympathy and help of one Indian to her own people." Self-described as the church's "pastor, janitor, organist, and clerk," Susan took much pride in her role as promoter of the whites' religion.[79]

In fulfilling that role, she probably saw the conversion of Omahas as the route toward tribal revitalization. Ironically, Christianity could serve as a powerful binding and healing power for the Omaha Nation even as these native people struggled against the juggernaut of white civilization. The parallels between their traditional beliefs and Protestantism allowed the Omahas to find various convictions in the catechism that were compatible with the structures of their faith. Traditional fatalism was compatible to the providence of the Christian God, while Omaha rituals of self-sacrifice and mutilation resembled the effects of Redemption in terms of creating a bond with supernatural powers. Not least important was belief in the power of the Word (ritual words) and the efficacy of prayer—both of which were fundamental to Omaha traditionalism.[80] There is little evidence that Susan actively sought to exploit these parallels, but presumably she knew of them.

Even after a pastor arrived sometime in late 1908, Susan continued to play an active role in the church. Every sabbath she ran the Sunday school class at the Blackbird Hills Church and, in the afternoons, held Christian Endeavor meetings at her new house.[81] After her husband's demise, she bought a lot in the town of Walthill, which was located on former Indian land. This move away from Macy, where many Omahas lived, to a white-dominated area probably was prompted by the leasing of her reservation land and her plan to build rental properties in Walthill (see chapter seven). She had a modern home complete with a fireplace, furnace, large windows, and an indoor bathroom built on the lot.[82] Susan, her two children, and her frail mother moved in as soon as the home was completed.

The Omaha doctor gradually became part of the leadership structure of the white-dominated Presbyterian church in Walthill. She served as the president of the church missionary society. The organization held a monthly study circle during which guest speakers delivered talks on a diverse number of topics including the social integration of Mexican and black Americans, Hampton Institute, and the immigration question. To raise funds for missionary work, the society put on concerts. Susan and other members of the group also solicited the aid of the local merchants and townspeople of Walthill. Between 1910 and 1912 she also spent much time raising funds for the renovation of the Walthill church. And in her capacity as president of the missionary society, she periodically attended gatherings of the general assembly of the Presbyterian church and also delivered talks at religious meetings on topics ranging from the new Bible-study movement to missionary work in Latin America.[83]

Even as Susan moved into the social circle of the non-Indian community of Walthill, she maintained her ties with the Omaha tribal population. In 1909 she defended their welfare when the Indian Office transferred Agent Commons to another agency. She wrote the Indian Office that Commons had "been tireless and constant in his fight against bootlegging on this Reservation and the result is that it is almost eliminated." To prevent this "evil" from returning, she implored the Indian Office to reinstate Commons. She also presented her case in writing to President Theodore Roosevelt. Susan failed to stave off the removal; a few months later, Commons left Nebraska.[84]

In the same set of letters, she made a reference to an earlier request for deed restrictions prohibiting the sale of liquor in all towns that had once been part of the reservations. Again this was as much a personal as it was a public issue for Susan. One of the targeted towns was Walthill, where she resided after 1907. Susan and other members of her family successfully persuaded the Indian Office to withhold deeds for the lands until the matter could be resolved to the Omahas' satisfaction. Sometime in late 1906 or early 1907, the secretary of the interior finally approved the temperance provision.[85] The *Heff* decision had left the government with no way to keep liquor peddlers away from Indians with land allotments. The temperance provision, however, would check the supply of liquor on the outskirts of the reservation, and thus, hopefully, it would help keep the reservation dry.

In a letter written after the provision was approved, Susan asserted that she, her nephew Caryl Farley, and an unnamed individual "were instrumental in securing, through protests in [the Indian] department," the deed restrictions.[86] No doubt Susan led the political lobbying on the issue, but this method of attempting to mandate temperance was nothing new.

On October 28, 1905, all Indian agents received instructions to include a temperance provision in deeds for inherited Indian lands. But because the provision proved to be unpopular with land buyers, the Indian Office withdrew the restriction less than four months later. The OIA also realized that the restriction would probably leave little impact on liquor traffic since it pertained only to heirship lands.[87] Though Susan and her supporters did not conceive the idea of deed restrictions, they certainly deserved credit for reviving it, expanding it to cover more types of Indian lands, and lobbying for its reintroduction.

The revival of deed restriction received strong support from towns bordering the reservation that had already refused to license saloons or had licensed them with the condition that they sell no alcohol to Indians. Many Euro-Americans in Nebraska supported the provision because by then the temperance crusade was picking up momentum. Since 1906 a state law prohibiting the sale of liquor to Indians, minors, and habitual drunkards had been in place, although enforcement was hampered by the lack of adequate funds. Thus the federal restriction became necessary. Aside from creating public sentiment against drunkenness, the immediate result of deed restriction was to make it more difficult for Indians to obtain intoxicants.[88]

The temperance proviso, however, did not cover at least five nearby towns, such as Bancroft, Pender, and Homer, which sat on largely non-reservation lands. Licensed saloons existed in all of them. Bootleggers and their Indian "runners" sold high-priced whiskey to Omahas while white merchants looked away, since drunken Indians were big spenders. Thus, alcohol still flowed from the saloons into the reservation. Later, as automobiles became more common, such temperance restrictions proved completely unworkable.[89]

Contemporary research indicates that prohibition generally does not eradicate the propensity to drink, although it does reduce overall consumption.[90] For some Indians, religious traditions provided a reason not to seek out liquor. Before World War II some Native Americans successfully combated alcoholism through revivals of traditional spiritual movements such as the Sun Dance and the Handsome Lake Cult, and through shamanic healing.[91]

A number of western tribes, including the Omahas, discovered peyotism, an aboriginal religion, notwithstanding its superficial syncretism with Christianity. In the Omaha version, though adherents invoke the name of Jesus Christ and use Christian symbols—such as the cross, copies of the Bible, and a heart-shaped fireplace representing Christ—as part of the ritual, the etiology of peyotism is based upon traditional beliefs. Adherents use native paraphernalia, such as gourd rattles, feathers, a staff, and pipes, and consume parched corn in sweetened water, fruit, and dried sweetened meat, reminding them of their ancestors' mixed economy. More important, peyotists ingest buttons of the peyote cactus in an attempt to attain visions of shamanic images with healing powers.[92]

Looking back, Susan said that the peyote religion arrived on the reservation in 1907; ethnologist Melvin R. Gilmore placed it closer to late 1906.[93] Peyote had been used in pre-Columbian Mexico, and its ritual use spread northward to the present-day American Southwest in the early eighteenth century. By the 1870s the Kiowas and Comanches had helped spread peyote use to the Great Plains. In the early 1890s the Comanche peyote-religion leader Quanah Parker visited the Otoes, who eventually amalgamated Christian elements into peyotism. An unidentified alcoholic Omaha visited the Otos in the winter of 1906–1907 and was informed that the plant and its attendant rituals would cure drinking. Upon his return to the reservation, he and a few other alcoholic Omahas formed a mescal society.[94]

Initially, Susan saw peyote as a "great evil" and supported federal efforts to suppress its importation from Mexico into the United States. Susan once said during an interview that the "mescal bean" was no less baneful than alcohol. She believed that if Indians could just deprive themselves of these habits, then they "would progress rapidly."[95] In this sense, Susan echoed the position of the OIA, which opposed peyotism because it negated Americanization. The Indian Office believed that peyote was addictive, and that its use led to the "loss of physical and mental vigor" and encouraged "idleness."[96]

Susan's misgivings about the peyote religion probably had much to do with the fact that it quickly surpassed Protestantism in terms of popularity and the number of followers. In 1914 OIA officials estimated that one-third of the tribe was using peyote buttons. This might have been a conservative estimate, because Gilmore maintained that by 1911 peyotism had been adopted by at least half of the tribe. Traditionally a people open to new ideas, the Omahas rapidly took up this promising panacea. Meanwhile, the Omaha Presbyterian congregation remained small; in 1913 only about fifty had formally joined the church.[97]

In a diary she kept between 1910 and 1911, Susan recorded a few occasions when Omahas shared with her the positive impact that peyotism had had on their lives. By 1914 Susan was willing to admit that the "mescal" or peyote button had "helped them [adherents] to keep sober." The buttons served as "a physiological antagonist to liquor," she explained. As a result adherents of the religion gave up drinking, and they "began to build up their homes, to save their money and became more thrifty," she continued. In 1912 sixty-six members of the Omaha Mescal Society, who had signed a petition to the OIA pleading for the end of the ban on importation of peyote buttons, claimed that the peyote religion had "made a wonderful difference and change for the better."[98]

Late-twentieth-century research has shown that peyote has little, if any, physiological effect in curbing the appetite for alcohol. Like other nineteenth-century Americans, Susan was unable to understand the chemical properties of the buttons. Some present-day psychologists, however, are convinced that peyote and the rituals surrounding it could possibly serve as an effective form of indigenous therapy.[99]

By moving along the "Peyote Road," or the ethical code of the peyote religion, followers learned restraint, responsibility, and the avoidance of destructive practices, including the use of alcohol. In so

doing, Omahas also restored their "Indianness." Once they redis-
covered spiritual communion and faith in Indian religious values,
they also regained part of their native identity, which they had lost in
the process of Americanization. Thus, peyotism offered more than
just an escape from alcoholism; in fact, it allowed adherents to
spiritually reconnect with some of their religious traditions.[100]

Susan never publicly acknowledged that peyotism had restored
some aspects of tribalism. To do so, she would first have had to
disavow cultural conformity and the goal of Americanization. In
effect, she would have had to accept a "return to the blanket." In a
typical mediatory attempt to close the gap between cultures, she
chose to interpret peyote use as another way to temperance.

In a letter written to Francis just before her death, Susan reported
that "members of that new religion say that they will not drink," and
"indeed have quit drinking." She credited this behavior to the fact
that "they pray intelligently, they pray to God, they pray to Jesus."
According to Susan, the Omaha followers also prayed for the
children and that God would "bring them up to live sober lives." She
chose to see peyotism as an Omaha variant of Protestantism, although
in actuality it was an indigenous religion. To interpret it as even a
partial return to tribalism and old ways probably would have been too
much of a negation of her labors and commitment to progress for her
to accept. Omaha peyotists, like other Indian peyote adherents,
continued to lobby the OIA to sanction their purchase and use of
peyote. In 1918, three years after Susan's death, an Omaha pro-
peyote delegation appeared in Washington to testify before a sub-
committee of the House of Representatives regarding a pending
antipeyote bill. At the hearing, Francis La Flesche spoke glowingly
about the peyote religion and quoted Susan's letter to augment his
position. Together with other American Indians and their supporters,
Francis and the rest of the delegation helped defeat the bill.[101]

In 1914, just a year before her demise, Susan had made another
effort in the war against insobriety. By then, the superintendent of the
Omaha Indian School reported: "The liquor traffic seems to be in a
flourishing condition." Peyotism had left a positive impact, but Susan
explained that since the issuance of more fee patents after 1910, "a

few men have fallen away" each year, because the sale of unrestricted land had given them money to squander on alcohol. She wrote to Commissioner Cato Sells and urged his office to prevent the liquor traffic. Susan told the commissioner that several weeks earlier a young Indian man in an intoxicated state had killed an elderly Omaha during the course of a brawl. Later, the accused committed suicide. In a sharp tone, she wrote that "the white man who sold [the alcohol] being well known—nothing has been done about it."[102]

In the same year Susan served as an expert witness during an inquest of an Omaha man who had died from alcohol misuse. As always, she took the opportunity to expound on the debilitating effects of liquor. "We find the Omaha Indian before the advent of the white man a fine specimen of manhood . . . [but] with liquor, we find . . . physical degeneration of the Indian," she said. Alcohol tended to reduce Indians' resistance to disease, Susan argued, and so they became highly susceptible to contagions. She bluntly stated that the Indian had been reduced to "a weak puny specimen of humanity."[103]

Susan blamed the tragedy on the federal government. The OIA, had made "no concerted persistent effort," she charged. Lessees who openly sold liquor to Indians often escaped prosecution, and special agents had accomplished little in the struggle against bootleggers and saloons, she added. Susan hinted that the fault lay in the character of the agents, and she urged that anti-liquor officials appointed to the reservation should be impartial, moral, and above corrupt behavior.[104]

Until the end of her life, Susan continued to wage the battle against intemperance. It could be argued that she adopted this crusade to halt the erosion of tribal identity. Through the call for prohibition and exhortations for temperance, she tried to check liquor traffic. She did help to reduce the level of alcohol consumption, but a resounding success eluded her. Due to limited funds, the Indian Office could not help her translate good intentions into acts of faith. Often, the intransigence of the Euro-American business world derailed her efforts. The continual opposition of some segments of the tribe to her interference also played a part in her failure. Ultimately, Susan's crusade was flawed; it did little to address the fundamental cause of the malady—the sociocultural losses that Omahas confronted by the turn of the century.

But the last fifteen years of her life were hardly a complete failure, and she never was ostracized by a significant number of Omahas. Her involvement in the land allotment issue would remain a significant contribution to Omaha history and would help Susan to claim the stature of a tribal leader.

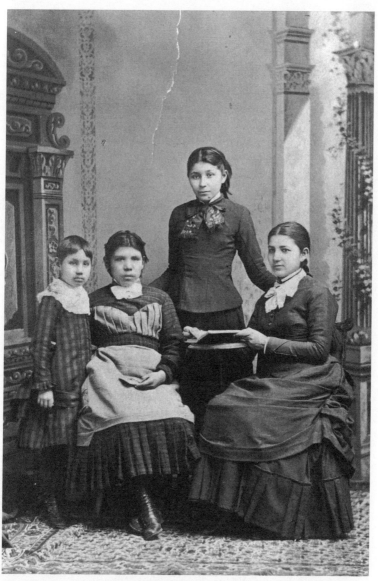

From left to right: unknown, Mary Tyndall, Susan La Flesche, and Marguerite La Flesche in their adolescent years, ca. 1880. Courtesy Nebraska State Historical Society.

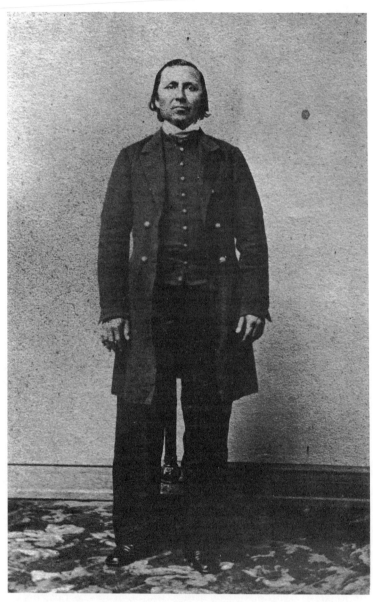

Joseph La Flesche in Euro-American garb, 1854. Courtesy Nebraska State Historical Society.

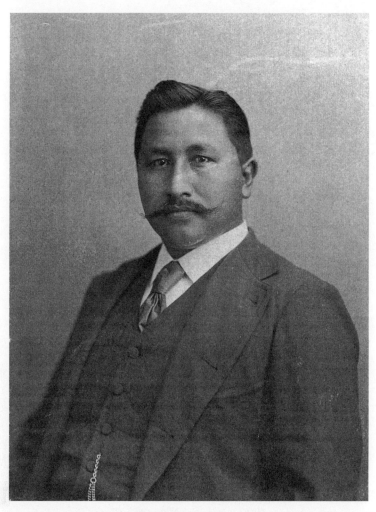

Susan La Flesche's stepbrother, Francis La Flesche, possibly ca.
1900. Courtesy Nebraska State Historical Society.

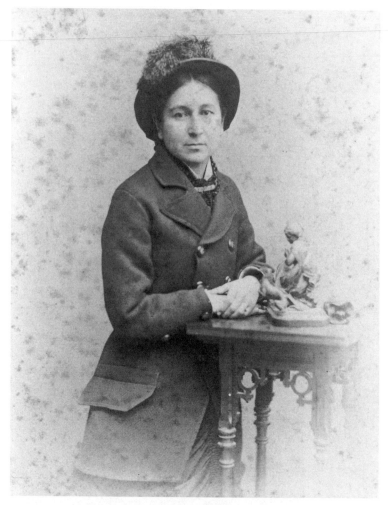

Susette Tibbles, Susan La Flesche's oldest sister and a well-known activist, ca. 1890. Courtesy Nebraska State Historical Society.

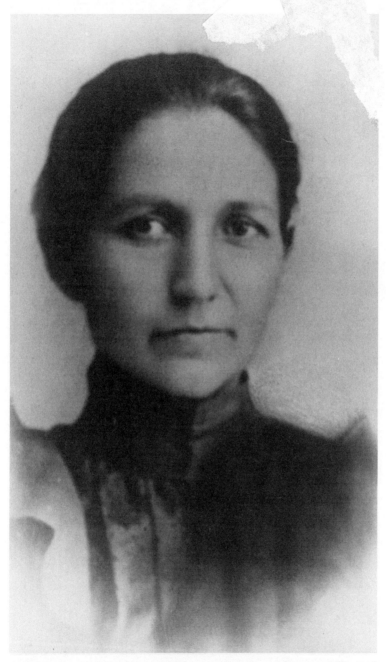

Marguerite La Flesche Diddock, who once served as an Office of Indian Affairs matron, ca. 1895. Courtesy Nebraska State Historical Society.

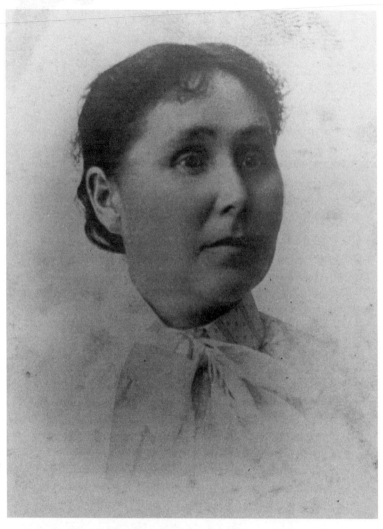

Rosalie Farley, another La Flesche daughter, ca. 1860s. Courtesy Nebraska State Historical Society.

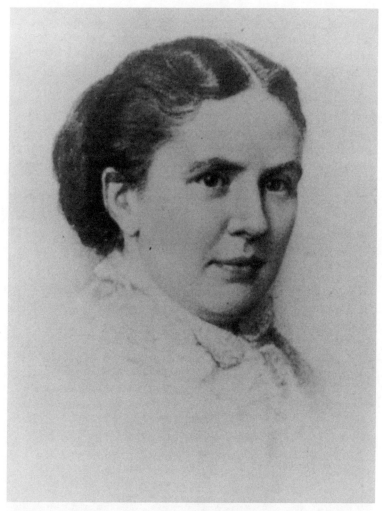

Alice C. Fletcher, Susan La Flesche's mentor and a close family friend, possibly ca. 1890. Courtesy Nebraska State Historical Society.

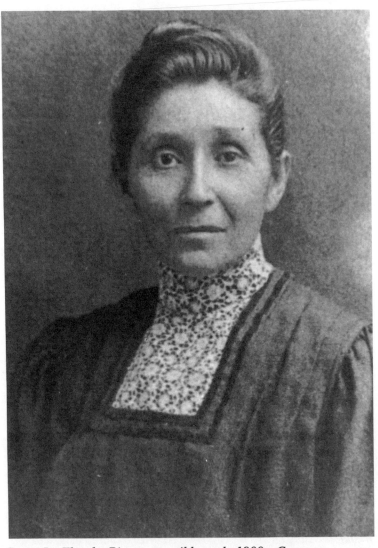

*Susan La Flesche Picotte, possibly early 1900s. Courtesy
Nebraska State Historical Society.*

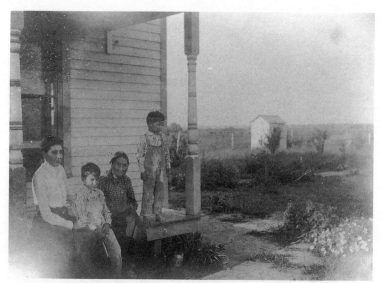

Dr. Susan La Flesche Picotte with her mother, Mary Gale, and her sons, Caryl and Pierre, at home in Bancroft, Nebraska, August 1902. Courtesy Nebraska State Historical Society.

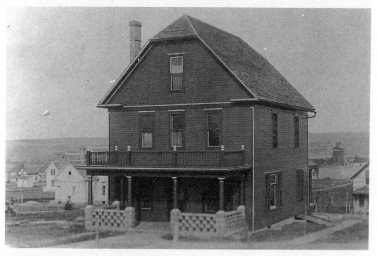

Susan's house at Walthill, Nebraska, date unknown. Courtesy Nebraska State Historical Society.

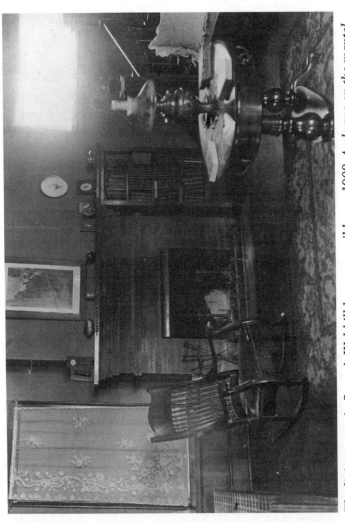

The living room in Susan's Walthill house, possibly ca. 1908. A plaque on the mantel reads "East . . . West." Courtesy Nebraska State Historical Society.

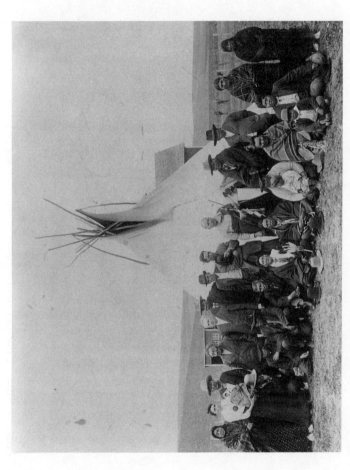

Susan La Flesche Picotte (second from left) at a peyote religious meeting, date unknown. Courtesy Nebraska State Historical Society.

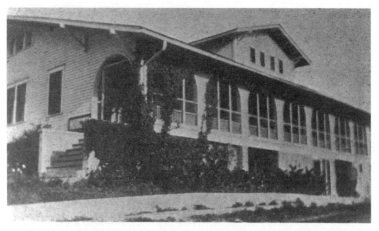

Hospital at Walthill, date unknown. Courtesy Nebraska State Historical Society.

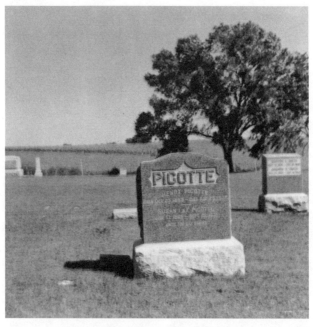

The final resting place of both Henry Picotte and Susan La Flesche Picotte, date unknown. The epitaph on the marker reads: "Until the Day Dawns." Courtesy Nebraska State Historical Society.

CHAPTER SEVEN

"A More Liberal Policy"

In July 1907 Susan wrote to Commissioner Francis E. Leupp that her deceased husband, Henry Picotte, had left her and her children some allotted land, about one hundred and eighty-five acres in South Dakota, but she complained that the disposition of the land had run into numerous complications. These problems sowed seeds of doubt in her mind about the paternalism of the federal government. Complications arose because at the time of Henry's death his allotment was still held in trust by the federal government, a common predicament faced by Indian heirs at the turn of the century. Since the land was part of a larger inheritance, which included children from his first marriage as heirs, partitioning or leasing it was unfeasible. Like most Indian heirs of small land parcels, Henry's heirs agreed to sell all of it in accordance with the provisions of the May 27, 1902, act.[1]

But the sale of the heirship land had taken years to conclude, because the process was protracted and time-consuming. The 1902 law delegated to the government the responsibility of appraising all tracts for sale and establishing a minimum price. Since, like all allottees, Henry could not include trust lands in his will, his heirs had to prove their respective competency—ability to manage their own affairs or support themselves—in order to receive the fee-simple patents. Those who were still minors—including Susan's children, Caryl and Pierre Picotte—had to find a legal guardian who resided within the jurisdiction of that inheritance to oversee their interests. In accordance with OIA procedures, the issuance to Indians of fee patents, or deeds of ownership, for their land was the last stage in "freeing" the Indians from government control. Only after the fee patents had been issued could the final sale proceed at a designated public auction. The OIA established multiple regulations in order to protect the Indians from losing their lands to whites, but the regulations also reminded the Indians of their status as wards of the government.

When the disposition of the land finally did move through the legal maze, the Omaha physician encountered obstacles in trying to secure the money due to herself and her children. Suspecting that the agent at the Yankton reservation, R. J. Taylor, had been behind the delays, she told Leupp that the field official had "shown a strange reluctance to have this money leave the state of South Dakota." "My recommendations and applications for the money lay for weeks in his office," she continued bitterly.[3] Susan subscribed to some aspects of Euro-American culture, but now she slowly discovered that allotment in severalty was, like alcoholism, another less-than-enchanting phenomenon introduced by whites into the Indian world.

Susan's letter to the Indian Office was not the first she wrote on this subject. After the land had been sold in late 1906 for over eight thousand dollars and the necessary papers drawn up, there had been a delay of almost four months in securing the Indian Office's approval for the transfer of the deed. The approval finally came in mid-February.[4] Then two months passed, but the money was nowhere in sight, even though the transaction had been made in cash—an Indian Office requirement. Puzzled by the delay, Susan wrote directly to the Indian Office in mid-April. To prove her competency, she had enclosed "many letters of recommendations from business men of integrity." Although she did not reveal the contents of those recommendations, they were probably testimonials to her industry and ability to make a living, the major criteria for competency during Commissioner Leupp's administration. An astute woman who understood the ways of Euro-Americans, Susan would have made sure that she had left nothing to chance.[5]

In the follow-up letter, Susan disclosed that her inheritance would be used for a new house and the children's education—intentions which technically departed from the Indian Office's original plan that all proceeds Indians received from heirship lands should be used to improve their allotments. But, though evidence is unavailable, it is doubtful that the Indian Office would have used this divergence against her. At the height of the allotment-in-severalty program, in order to replicate the "separate spheres" ideal, the OIA deliberately encouraged men to engage in cash crop farming and wage work and women to labor at home. In an attempt to create gender hierarchy and promote masculine individualism, the OIA rarely gave Indian women any technical assistance in farming and other related work. Further, all the annuities and other monies due to the tribe went to male heads of households. As a result, often women were either dependent on their spouses' earnings or left to fend for themselves by leasing or selling their inheritances.[6]

Following the death of her husband, Susan had leased out her own land parcels in Nebraska, which totaled 640 acres, at two dollars per acre. By leasing with the consent of the government, Susan, like so many Indians, made a mockery of the original goal of allotment in severalty. Her application and recommendations for the heirship proceeds were then passed on to Taylor, who was expected to determine her competency to receive the disbursements. But she never received a response.[7] By then, nearly two years had lapsed since Henry's death and more than eleven months since the district court in South Dakota had determined the division of the inheritance among his heirs.

On May 13, 1907, having heard nothing from Washington and hoping for some sort of clarification, she chose to contact Taylor. Susan's letter, which did not survive the passage of time, must have been short and blunt, since his reply was equally brusque. The abeyance stemmed from the fact that the local banks "are full to the utmost capacity of their bonds," Taylor explained. He told Susan that he would have to write to the Indian Office for further instructions.

Satisfied that he had little control over the situation, he offered no apologies.[8]

Since Taylor had made it clear that the matter was out of his hands, Susan now turned once again to the Indian Office in Washington, D.C. In her letter to Leupp, she asked him to "cause some encouragement" that the checks be deposited "right away." She suggested using another bank, if indeed the regular depositories could not accommodate the transactions. Throughout the letter she maintained a polite tone but minced few words. Employing the Euro-American rhetoric of the day, she wrote that she and her children would consider it a miscarriage of justice should the money remain unused. She intimated that the money would be employed for worthy endeavors; she would use it to build a "good home" and give her "boys the privileges of a good education." At this juncture she attributed Taylor's lassitude to the fact that she was "entirely unknown to" him. As a result, she feared Taylor was going to recommend that her share be withheld. To prevent that, Susan got her brother Francis to hand deliver copies of the recommendations and application to the Indian Office.[9]

The Indian Office promptly took action on her complaint and demanded an explanation from Taylor. Defending himself, Taylor claimed that the money was deposited in a bank on May 16, 1907— the same day he wrote to the Omaha physician and told her that there was little he could do in lieu of further instructions! He further claimed that on May 23—the same day the Indian Office wrote to him—he had decided on Susan's competency. He recommended that she should receive all of her inheritance in one lump sum. Clearly Taylor had been remiss in his duties; at the very least, he was guilty of procrastination.[10]

Sometime between the end of May and early July, Susan finally received her share of the proceeds from the sale of her husband's allotment. With that settled, she turned her attention to her children's share of the inheritance. She forwarded an application to Taylor but received no response. Having learned her lesson, Susan now wrote directly to the commissioner, with a copy to Taylor. In this correspondence, she claimed an Omaha identity for her children. Apparently they had never been on the Yankton Sioux tribal rolls and had only been on the Omaha rolls. This could be construed as a demonstration of her, sometimes shaky, Omaha tribal patriotism and a desire to pass an Omaha identity on to her children. But Susan also harbored a more obvious intention. She implied that her children's de jure identity was good enough to warrant transferring their money into her care, especially since she was their legal guardian.[11]

But Susan was not the only guardian. Since her children's inheritance lay in another state, she could not serve as the legal guardian for her children's inherited land. Peter Picotte, a male relative, played that role. But now he posed an obstacle. According to Taylor, Picotte had refused to sign the checks for the transfer of those funds. Without Picotte's consent, Taylor concluded, he could do little else.[12]

Taylor's reply did not sit well with Susan. Outraged by Picotte's behavior, Susan now tried to assail his character. In a stinging letter to Commissioner Leupp, she called Picotte a "hard drinker." An "utterly irresponsible" man, Picotte had a reputation for handing out money wantonly during times of revelry, she charged. It was "strange," she sarcastically commented, that she, "a mother . . . and bitterly opposed to whiskey . . . should be denied the right to care for her children's money, while it should be given into the care of a man who is a hard drinker."[13] Clearly the Omaha doctor was upset that her standing as an exemplar of Victorian morality now held little importance with the Indian Office.

In that same correspondence she took a swipe at Agent Taylor and claimed that he and Picotte were in some sort of a conspiracy against her. Susan offered examples of Taylor's obstructionism: he kept her in the dark about the approval of the deeds, he held up her share of the proceeds, and he never replied to her application for the children's money. Only when she wrote directly to the commissioner, did she hear from Taylor about Picotte's intransigence.[14]

Anticipating the possibility that the Indian Office might question her motives, she shrewdly laid bare her plans. She needed to prove beyond doubt that she could manage the anticipated funds. In sum, she intended to invest her children's inheritance in rental properties. Such properties would be cement block houses "on account of their cheapness, less need of repair and less danger from fire," she explained. It was obvious that Susan had given some forethought to this matter since she could also quote figures and possible earnings. She assured the Indian Office that the profits would be set aside for the children's college fund or to "start them in business."[15] Her overall plan certainly showed an awareness of the corporate capitalist mentality that pervaded the Progressive Era. Efficiency and rationalization of resources were the slogans of the day, and seemingly Susan was no stranger to them.

She made no mention of using the money to purchase another farm, even though she and Henry had run a fairly successful one before his demise. Probably her poor health precluded that option. The Omaha physician ended this letter with a request for a direct reply from the commissioner, for she "would never see it if sent to Mr. Taylor."[16]

That sharp, even acerbic, letter evoked a rapid response. On July 13, 1907, about five days after she wrote the letter, the Indian Office sent Susan a short note. According to the note, Taylor had been given specific instruction and the matter would "be attended to without further delay." As indicated in another piece of correspondence, Taylor was told to override Picotte's objection and was ordered to transfer the money to the care of the field official at the Omaha agency, John M. Commons. This was duly accomplished within the month.[17]

Following the transfer, Susan labored to get the children's money released completely to her care. Without this control, she would have had to apply for the money in small amounts via the Indian agent. In her letter of application, she repeated the money-making plan and pointed out that her investment would yield far more earnings than the paltry interest collected from leaving the funds in the bank. Luckily Susan was on good terms with Superintendent Commons, who wholeheartedly supported her request. Within ten days, the approval from the Indian Office arrived.[18]

However, her battles with the Indian Office bureaucracy were far from over. In mid-1908 her children inherited some money from their Sioux relatives. To avoid the previous entanglements, Susan completely bypassed Agent Taylor and wrote to Commissioner Leupp.

Proudly, she revealed to Leupp that she had succeeded in carrying out her business goals: already she had built a house and rented it out, and another one was in the planning stage. She mentioned that the new inheritance was also earmarked for a rental property. Again her business venture clearly diverged from the norm for self-employed women of the turn of the century. Most ran businesses directed at female consumers, such as millinery and dress-making ventures, and few owned male-dominated enterprises such as medical practices and rental properties. The Indian Office duly granted Susan's request for the inheritance, and shortly afterward a local newspaper reported that her properties were going up.[19]

Negotiations were more complicated for her husband's heirship lands, property inherited from his father and two brothers. In spring 1909, after a six-month delay, the transfer of deeds for the lands in question was forwarded by Taylor to the Indian Office for official approval. But Taylor had conveyed none of this information to Susan, much to her dismay. A year later she heard from her Sioux relatives that all the heirs had received their money—all except her and her children. By this time she had already written a few times to the authorities, but to no avail.[20]

The impediments Susan faced were not unique, since countless other Native Americans encountered them as well, and she was not unfamiliar with such obstructions. By the end of the first decade of the twentieth century, following the implementation of the Omaha Allotment Act of 1882 and subsequent related legislation, Susan's role as letter writer-cum-interpreter for her people had expanded into the area of defending the land interests of Omaha tribal members. The surviving diary that she kept between 1910 and 1911 bore testimony to her efforts to fight for Indian autonomy and to the manifold problems encountered by Omahas in their attempt to protect and manage their properties. In this capacity, Susan's brokerage attempts were less on behalf of Euro-American "civilization" and more in the interest of Indian rights. Ironically, her efforts would promote the dispossession of the Omahas.

One Omaha woman, Mrs. Dan Wolf, sold forty acres of her allotted land, but after two years she had never received a cent of the proceeds. Wolf finally approached Susan for help. Susan, in turn, called the Omaha agent and received a promise that the money would soon be remitted. Often her mediation was not enough; many Omahas, in the judgment of the bureaucracy, were incompetent and therefore would squander away their money. One couple, Luke White and his wife, wanted to withdraw all of their heirship money from the Indian Office but the local superintendent turned them down. He also rejected W. Reese Harlan's application to sell his land. Presumably both sets of applicants were considered unfit to handle the anticipated proceeds.[21]

Cases of Omahas who desired to sell their land or access proceeds being held by the Indian Office were numerous. Often such Omahas needed the money to consolidate their existing tracts or to make improvements on their houses and farms. Susan almost never denied them help, even when she herself doubted their competency. By that time the regulations for competency and sale of land had been tightened to prevent rapid dissipation of the assets. But enforcement was casual, arbitrary, and bogged down by procedures. Ironically, safeguards put in place that were designed to protect the interests of Indians may have jeopardized the Indians' welfare.[22]

A more common problem faced by the Omahas was failure to receive sufficient or even any earnings from their leased lands. Almost every other day, Susan received at least one such complaint. Sometimes the fault lay with the Indian Office's failure to forward the proceeds in a timely fashion (since the late 1890s the Indian Office had required all lessees to hand in their rental money to the field official, who would in turn disburse it to the Indian lessors). Quite often Susan would telephone the Omaha agency at Macy to enquire about a delay, and sometimes she succeeded in securing the back rents.[23]

At other times, the culprits were none other than the white lessees. According to Susan, Dan Wolf had leased his land out to Joel Turner, but the latter had not turned in any rent for nearly two years. Mrs. Cline, who did not receive all of her rental income, also approached Susan. She hoped to get the money to pay for a new house. Some outraged Omahas, fed up with the delays, went to Susan to ask that she intercede on their behalf to terminate contractual agreements.[24]

In some instances of Indian disagreements with Euro-Americans, Susan stepped in and actually tried to resolve the matters without the support of the Indian agent. Once Dall Grant had leased a "hotel" (possibly a boarding house) to a white but had left some things behind. When Grant tried to reclaim his belongings, the white lessee blocked his entry. Susan gained access, but had to return later for a few more items. When the lessee succeeded in blocking her entry, she retaliated with a sanitary notice (by then, she was a member of the health council of Walthill).[25] Occasionally Susan visited recalcitrant non-Indian lessees, hoping to convince them to help clear the backlog of debts owed to Omahas.[26]

By the end of the first decade of the twentieth century, a number of restrictions imposed on allotted lands by the Dawes Act of 1887 had been lifted. Amendments to the original legislation had opened the door to early alienation of allotments. This was particularly true after the passage of the Burke Act of 1906, which authorized the secretary of the interior to issue a fee patent to any competent Indian before the end of the trust period of twenty-five years. Then, in 1907, Congress authorized the sale of restricted land of sick, disabled, and incompetent Indians in accordance with rules set out by the secretary of the interior. As a result, the number of applicants for fee patents rose dramatically between 1906 and 1910. Not surprisingly, Susan found herself inundated with requests for the patents in fee. This was a time-consuming task, since she had to gather personal and family data for the applications and often, for the sake of verification, had to consult the Omaha tribal rolls. When the deeds arrived, Susan would convey them to the town of Pender to be officially recorded.[27]

The other matter that absorbed much of her time had to do with applications for individuals' shares of the tribal funds. In 1907, as part of the larger effort to end tribalism and promote the "civilization" of Indians, Congress approved a bill which allowed Indians to access the funds on a pro rata share basis, provided they personally applied for the money. Before long, Omahas partook of this latest source of

SUSAN LA FLESCHE PICOTTE, M.D.

funding. Susan's role in the process involved filling in the applications, making inquiries whenever a delay in payments occurred, and helping Indians who were unfamiliar with the white economic system cash or deposit their checks.[28]

In her mediations among the Indian Office, Omahas, and Euro-Americans, Susan became sensitized to the possibility of fraud and deception committed against the Omahas. This was a problem on many other Indian reservations as well. In early January 1909 the Omaha physician agreed to help the Indian Rights Association (IRA) defeat the confirmation of Z. Lewis Dalby as Indian inspector. Apparently, in a previous Office of Indian Affairs position, Dalby had badly treated Indians at two separate reservations. He was suspected of committing graft and corruption. Spearheading the movement against Dalby was Samuel E. Brosius, the IRA Washington agent, who instructed Susan to write to senators and other politicians, in addition to securing affidavits against Dalby. Presumably she carried out those instructions, because two months later she asked Hollis Burke Frissell, the principal of Hampton Institute, to inquire about Dalby's appointment. According to Frissell, the appointment had been withdrawn.[29]

A few months later an even larger issue impinged on her life. Superintendent John M. Commons, whom Susan had praised for his aggressive approach to the Omahas' intemperance, had embroiled himself in a fight against a male, white-dominated syndicate charged with plying the Indians with liquor and then cheating them of their lands and proceeds. In a series of convoluted and emotionally charged letters, Susan accused the syndicate of perpetrating those "evils." She claimed that, in an attempt to discredit Commons, the syndicate had incited Indians to complain about his job performance to the visiting field inspector. Seemingly the main complaint was that Commons was slow in releasing Indian money and land from the existing restrictions. The ultimate goal was to remove Commons so that the syndicate "can do as they please with the Indians," Susan wrote. She pleaded with Commissioner Robert G. Valentine not to remove Commons; she declared that if they removed him, the OIA would be guilty of harkening to the voice of "Evil." In addition, she wrote that

Commons stood for "decency, sobriety, and honest dealings" and had always protected her people.[30] Susan was so convinced Commons could head off the impending disaster that she wrote to Secretary of the Interior Robert G. Ogden and telegrammed a short message to Matthew K. Sniffen, the executive secretary of the IRA. She asked both to use their good offices to put a hold on Commons's transfer. But all of these efforts came to naught. Later the Omaha doctor probably regretted defending Commons, since the following year he was indicted, along with eight other men, for land fraud against the Omahas.[31]

Commons left the Omaha reservation, but the syndicate—made up of Omahas Thomas Sloan and William F. Springer, along with non-Indians William E. Estill, Llewelyn C. Brownrigg, and Garry P. Meyers—kept up their presence. Susan now took on the syndicate. She accused Sloan, an attorney and fellow Hamptonian, of having "defrauded, coerced, and exploited the Omaha Indians for a number of years." In her letter of complaint to the secretary of the interior (with a copy to the commissioner of Indian Affairs), Susan cited case after case of such duplicity.[32]

In her correspondence, she directed most of her vituperation at Sloan, who had once been indicted on charges of conspiracy to fraud. According to Susan, about a month before Grace Cox died of tuberculosis, Sloan had convinced Cox to adopt Jeannie Woodhull. Following Cox's demise, Sloan appointed himself as Woodhull's guardian and, in a suit against the natural heirs of Cox, won for her a handsome settlement. When Woodhull reached legal age, Sloan demanded 50 percent of her inheritance. In a bizarre twist, he then represented one of the natural heirs against Woodhull, who was represented by an attorney selected by Sloan himself![33]

The fraud committed against Cox, Woodhull, and the other heirs was nothing compared with that perpetrated against young minors. Sloan often got himself appointed as their legal guardian, and then for years swindled their annuities and leasing monies. Susan claimed that Sloan had also conspired with a number of her relatives, including her brother-in-law Noah La Flesche, to secure allotments in the name of deceased relatives. Once the allotments arrived, Sloan turned against his partners-in-crime; he occupied the lands for years on end without paying rent, and then tried to force the others into selling the lands to him at a price less than its market value.[34]

Susan alleged that Sloan's partner Estill also had a "very bad" record. He had induced James Wolf to sign away his land deed and had given Wolf an unsecured purchase note in exchange. Later, Susan discovered that Estill had also overcharged Wolf on the legal fees. In several other instances, Estill got Indians with allotments intoxicated and maneuvered them into bogus land transactions. Other partners were guilty of similar charges, Susan railed.[35]

In the summer of 1909 Susan felt compelled to bring these charges of fraud to the attention of the federal government, largely because on July 10, 1909, the trust or guardianship period for many Omaha allotments would expire. Without the restrictions, she feared that the Omahas would easily fall prey to the chicanery of the syndicate. To prevent that from happening, Susan urged a stay of Commons's impending transfer and, more importantly, an investigation into all of the charges.[36]

Because neither the Indian Office nor the Interior Department responded to the call for action, she wrote once again. In her July 13 letter, somewhat piqued, Susan made her position against this "injustice" clear: I "shall continue to protest until the various complaints . . . have received the merited consideration." The problem was that the Omahas still needed protection over their lands and monetary resources, she reiterated. Some "are incompetent for self protection," she bluntly wrote.[37] Seemingly, true to the confluence of cultures that shaped her life, Susan called for Victorian benevolent paternalism—an ideal promoted earlier by her sponsors, the women of the CIA.

She told Commissioner Valentine that the key to shielding Indian interests was conscientious enforcement of the regulations. Otherwise, stratagem of the kind that had lately taken place would occur again. Susan related to him that as the July 10 deadline approached, the reservation was being overrun by land speculators who tricked Indians into parting with their lands. The syndicate in question had spearheaded that land grab and stockpiled currency so they could purchase land immediately after midnight on July 10. In fact, even before the expiration date, the syndicate had signed forty preliminary contracts with various Omaha individuals.[38]

Luckily for the Omahas, a few days before the deadline, President William Howard Taft extended the trust period on nearly all of the original Omaha allotments for ten years. But Omahas judged to be competent could still be given patents in fee. That kept the door open for the syndicate, and soon it began urging restricted Omahas to apply for land titles.[39]

Susan's pleas for help went unanswered, and the warnings she issued fell on deaf ears. The 1909–10 findings of a competency commission led to the issuance of fee-simple patents to more than two hundred Omahas. The commission's intent was to remove the restrictions on the sale of Indian land and therefore placate local Euro-Americans who wanted to acquire Omaha land and also to place more of it on the Thurston County tax rolls.[40]

But about a third of those considered competent by the commission had objected to the process earlier. Convinced they were not ready to assume full responsibility, many of them predicted the subsequent land losses. Within less than five years, land grafters had maneuvered 95 percent of them, often through the use of alcohol, into surrendering their deeds.[41]

Paradoxically, right in the middle of the commission's work, Susan advocated a more liberal fee patent policy.[42] Her position seemed contradictory in light of her full awareness that some Omahas were incapable of managing their own properties and would be easy prey for unscrupulous land dealers. However, this contradiction is somewhat explainable.

In early 1910 at a meeting with OIA officials in Washington, Susan explained that most of the Omahas were competent and capable of handling their own affairs. The remaining tribal members, a minority, would "be just as incompetent as they are today" at the end of the ten-year extension of the trust, she declared. She explained that the fault lay with the Indian Office, because the restrictions placed on land and money and the constant supervision of the Indians had stifled the development of their business acumen and knowledge of the white world. "If we are incompetent today, it is because we have been kept from developing as we ought to have by experiences gained through. . . contact with the white man," she said.[43]

Here Susan clearly embraced the Euro-American reformers' notion that self-support could only come about in a non-segregated society; otherwise, the reservation system simply sapped any remaining spirit of self-aggrandizement. Ironically, by doing so she promoted the Americanization policy in the face of obstructions from the Indian Office, the agency entrusted with carrying out that same policy.

Susan's tirade about the Indian Office's restrictions began innocuously as an attempt to forestall the consolidation of the Omaha and Winnebago agencies as one administration. Before 1904 the agencies had indeed operated as one. A little before that year Susan had appealed, on behalf of the Omahas, to President Theodore Roosevelt to look into the possibility of separating the agencies to make them more efficient. That appeal was successful, and the superintendent of the Omaha reservation had offered OIA services at Macy since 1904.[44]

Ironically, six years later the Indian Office returned to the idea of consolidation. By then Robert G. Valentine had assumed control of the Indian Office. Like some Progressive-Era reformers, Valentine considered himself a student of efficiency, and he saw consolidation of agencies as part of an ongoing effort to centralize and streamline the bureaucracy. Consolidation was also conceived as the capstone of the work of the competency commission. After competent Omahas had received their respective fee patents, the Indian Office figured that there would be less to do, and so consolidation would be logical and most economical. Centralizing power in the hands of one superintendent for two reservations would also expedite official business, the Indian Office claimed. The government assured the Omahas that services would improve immeasurably.[45]

The Omahas were unconvinced. In fact, a "spirit of dissatisfaction" had swept through the tribal population. Susan was caught up in the tide of negative sentiments as well, and she decided to lodge a protest with the Indian Office. Her decision to line up with her people was not an easy one, since she had always defended government policy. In a letter to Alice Fletcher, she revealed why she chose to cast her lot with the Omahas: "I should most certainly lose my self respect were I to keep still when I thot[sic] anything was going to be done that would be to the detriment of the Omahas. I don't care an iota what the Depart[ment] thinks of me!" This was not only a question of moral choice, but also of her status within the tribal society, and on that subject she was not willing to compromise.[46]

This may have been a turning point in Susan's life; not only would she now tie her fortunes to those of her people, but also she would try even harder henceforth to escape the stifling grasp of white paternalism. She had become somewhat disillusioned with the non-Indian world. But, in her role as cultural broker, she remained cognizant of the need to direct Indian-white discourse toward a desired end or at least away from misunderstandings. She would continue to mediate the interchange of cultures, even as she interpreted the exchange of desires and promises.

In a polite but firm letter to Acting Commissioner Frederick H. Abbott, Susan admitted that when he took her into confidence in late summer and told her about the proposal to combine the agencies, she had thought it might work, though it was her understanding that consolidation would take place much later. Abbott probably saw her as a leading tribal member who could influence the Omahas to line up behind the proposal. He probably regretted mentioning the proposal, for now Susan had changed her mind.[47]

In her letter, she questioned the assumption that the Omahas would need little assistance once they received the fee patents. Though Susan believed in the high-minded goals of allotment in severalty— "industry, good citizenship, and temperance"—to borrow her own words, she had also had enough first-hand experience of the program's flaws to grasp reality. She argued that the Omahas must retain the full-time services of the present superintendent, Andrew G. Pollock, who could help competent Indians to manage their new titles, particularly in the efforts to consolidate their subdivided land and establish a "home" like those of Anglo-Americans. Pollock could also guide the incompetent to meet the criteria for competency.

SUSAN LA FLESCHE PICOTTE, M.D.

"Without such guidance and supervision it means a tragedy for many," Susan discerned. No doubt she had in mind all the troubles that the Omahas recently had experienced with land speculators such as Thomas Sloan. Pollock, who had become acquainted with the people and conditions, would and could protect the Indians' interest, she confidently asserted.[48]

Susan also reminded Abbott of the inconveniences Omahas had encountered before 1904, and of their needs being "always secondary to the interests of the Winnebagoes." Delays in the payment of monies and in the execution of their leases were common. Susan could only draw the obvious conclusion: "The consolidation must be postponed if the best interests of the Omahas are to be served," and to those ends, she repeated, Superintendent Pollock should be retained.[49]

The replies Susan received from Acting Commissioner Abbott were disheartening. In sum, Abbott rejected all of her arguments against consolidation. The additional staff—clerks and two OIA farmers—would devote their time to developing vocational and agricultural interests among the Omaha men. In fact, he claimed all outstanding matters such as leasing, land sales, schools, and morality "will be given more careful consideration" under the consolidated bureaucracy.[50]

Susan didn't know that Abbott had hastily ordered Pollock to file a report on the reactions of the Omahas to the envisioned plan. Pollock hinted that educated Indians like her were behind the incitement of sentiments against consolidation. Pollock claimed that Susan had simply refused to accept his reassurance. In a sexist manner he attributed that to her gender: being "woman like she could see it but one way," he caustically wrote.[51] Prescriptive Victorian sex roles—domesticity for women, politics for men—ideals to which Susan had never adhered, were working against her.

Pollock clearly was not on the side of the Omahas. He planned to stay away from the upcoming special tribal meeting, and he promised Abbott that he would do his best meanwhile to keep the merger under wraps. Finally, and probably much to Susan's dismay, Pollock had recently told her that he had decided not to stay, regardless of the

— *162* —

outcome.[52] Without his support, the Omahas turned to educated members of the tribe for leadership.

In response to Abbott's recent correspondence, Susan quickly sent him a handwritten retort. In the very first line of her letter, she assured him that she was not opposed to the provision of additional government farmers. The Omaha physician feared that the Indian Office might have misunderstood her and seen her as an opponent of progress. Mediation required the ability to identify with both sides of the cultural divide, or else the mediator would suffer. As always, this educated woman had to tread carefully lest she lose her links to the white world. Then Susan rebutted Abbott's arguments: "I can't very well see the economy part of it when . . . the clerical force is to be enlarged," she wrote bluntly. Since the Omahas had little confidence in Albert Kneale, the superintendent of the Winnebago Agency who would head the unified administration, she argued that it would be inefficient to remove Pollock at this precise moment. According to Susan, Kneale already had more work than he could handle, and so logically he could not take on the Omahas' interests.[53]

Susan explained that she was fighting for the retention of the agency as it was because she knew the Omaha interests demanded such a course of action. Should the Indian Office reject the request, the "Indians won't stand for it and will protest," she warned.[54]

As she had anticipated, the protest occurred soon and was loud. On December 21, 1909, Omahas gathered at what Susan called an "Indignation meeting." There they signed a petition against consolidation and asked Susan to report their reactions to the Indian Office. In her lengthy letter, she probably left the authorities with the impression that she had tried to play the role of the reconciler, or at least the interpreter for OIA intentions. At the outset of the meeting, she shared with the Omahas details of the consolidation, including the official rhetoric on its positive impact. She also urged the Omahas not to sign on to anything until they fully understood the proposal.[55]

Of course, she had already laid bare her own thoughts on this subject. But, for reasons of propriety and probably for fear of being portrayed as a troublemaker, she chose to adopt a moderate stance.

Toward the end of the report, Susan intimated that she sensed Abbott had resented "the interference of a woman in his administration." To deflect further criticism, she claimed that she was only speaking on behalf of the Omahas when she first wrote to him.[56] Clearly she was reacting to Euro-American gender sensibilities about women's "rightful" exclusion from the public sphere. In actuality the Omaha doctor was a woman who hailed from a race that believed in the equality of the sexes, and she had never been hesitant about speaking her mind. Thus far she had spoken as an individual; henceforth she would also speak on behalf of the majority of the tribe.

She reported that the Omahas were opposed to consolidation because "it would work great hardships on them." Like Susan, most Omahas remembered the last consolidation, and doubted that this one would work in their interests, especially since they now had more business to transact, and Pollock could barely keep up with the pace. Kneale could never handle the workload, the Omahas implied. Hiram Chase warned that if Pollock left, then the Omahas would rather manage their own affairs. Francis Freemont echoed that sentiment and emphatically stated that the Omahas had "the right to have a voice in what was for their wel-fare." Accordingly, Pollock was the right man to protect them "against the bad white men," Freemont continued. One speaker after another spoke in favor of retaining Pollock or having no official at all. The Omahas threatened to "to cut loose from Department supervision." The Omahas' defiance seemed unanimous as everyone present rose in a show of support for that viewpoint. The fight over temperance apparently had not destroyed uki'te, or tribal unity, for the Omahas now stood as one in the common protection of their interests.[57]

After the meeting, Susan approached Superintendent Kneale. She spared no words in letting him know exactly how the Omahas felt about the proposal and told him that because of the opposition, he would fail in his new job. When Kneale replied that God would erect a barrier if the plan was unworkable, Susan's quick comeback was that "God had put thirteen hundred Omahas in the way." She closed her letter with a challenge to Valentine to respond to the Omahas' plea for help. Shrewd mediator that she was, Susan craftily evoked the language of white paternalism: "Are you going to deny to all these people that which they know will be strength and example to them in their struggles?"[58]

In his responses, Commissioner Valentine told the Omaha doctor that the envisioned plan was just an administrative change to make it possible to carry out certain programs and that little else would be altered.[59] Still unpersuaded, Susan submitted a series of scathing articles to local newspapers in order to rally non-Indian support for the Omahas' position.

In her writings, Susan pointedly responded to each of the official arguments made in favor of the consolidation proposal. She argued that the centralization of power in the hands of one superintendent for two reservations would be a "detriment," not an expediency as claimed by the OIA, to Indian affairs. She explained that the existing Indian Office infrastructure placed heavy demands on field officials, who had to file a heavy load of paperwork for every transaction. Since the additional clerks based at the Macy agency had no discretionary powers, and since the new superintendent would be spending less than three days per week at the Omaha reservation, "inevitable delay will be the result," she asserted.[60]

Delays were already common, and Susan took this opportunity to attack the creaky OIA bureaucracy. In one article, she described some of the ways in which "the Indian [was] restricted and bound with red tape." She related a number of "ridiculous instances" in which paper work had delayed the arrival of badly needed funds. One autumn a patient of Susan's had to be operated on for appendicitis, and the superintendent telegraphed Washington for authority to admit him into a hospital. The approval did arrive—in May of the following year. In a few cases such inertia cost the lives of the sickly. "I have watched them die without it [official approval for funds]," the Omaha physician wrote. Some of those who died were even denied the dignity of a proper burial because the money for it arrived months later.[61]

More often, the Omahas had to put up with the inconvenience of lengthy procedures, even to access funds to purchase a blanket shawl or wheelbarrow. Though processed at the agency level, all such applications had to be forwarded to the Indian Office in Washington, and it might take weeks for the approval to return. In her capacity as a physician, Susan had trouble collecting payments for outstanding medical bills because of such bureaucratic red tape.[62]

"We have rules and regulations to the right of us, to the left of us, behind us; do you wonder we object to continuation of them in front of us?," Susan lashed out. The Omahas were inundated by a flood of circulars and regulations that constantly changed to "fit the ever shifting, ever experimenting policy of the department," she observed sarcastically. She claimed that as a result, the Omahas had to rely heavily on agency officials to keep abreast of the latest developments. The consolidation proposal would deny Omahas easy access to the superintendent, the only official with discretionary powers. Already the Omahas, who lived scattered all over the reservation, had to drive on dirt tracks, sometimes in inclement weather, for about ten miles in order to reach the Macy (Omaha) agency complex. If the consolidation went through, the Omahas would have to travel an additional ten miles to the Winnebago agency.[63]

These hardships seemed unnecessary to Susan, who insisted the "majority of the Omahas are as competent as the same number of white people." In the last three years the Omahas had recovered from their intemperance, and they were now "climbing steadily upward." The Omahas were certainly more acculturated than the Winnebagos, she asserted. Thus the official argument that the Winnebagos and Omahas could be ruled by the same administration was an insult to the Omahas' sense of self-worth. Using the language of Euro-American reformers of the day, she proudly described her people as "independent" and "self-reliant." "This condition of being treated as children we want to have nothing to do with," she asserted curtly.[64]

In a turnabout of judgment, Susan probably no longer considered the Omahas to be "like little children, without father or mother," a description she once shared in the late 1880s with a group of Euro-American reformers. She believed that the Omahas deserved the freedom to enjoy their property rights, instead of being held back along with the Winnebagos.[65] Her call for autonomy undoubtedly contradicted her earlier pleas for the Indian Office's protection.

Finally, Susan tackled the issue of the government farmers who had responsibility for starting a new model farm. Earlier in her correspondence with Abbott, she made it clear that she did not oppose the reintroduction of such assistance under the consolidation proposal. Now the voices of the larger population had swayed her toward their position. On January 4, 1910, more than two hundred Omaha families gathered at a meeting and voted to turn down the whole consolidation proposal, including the model farm plan and its attending officials. The Jeffersonian agrarian ideal that Susan's father had embraced had been, in fact, a mirage—a goal that had become all the more unrealistic since the implementation of the Omaha Allotment Act of 1882. Simply put, independent farming never became the basis of the Omahas' economy. By the end of the first decade of the twentieth century their income came primarily from rental fees, land sales, and wage labor.[66]

Susan was cognizant of economic realities, and now she offered a commonsensical explanation for the Omahas' present conditions: "You cannot make farmers of the Indians anymore than you can the same number of white people—some have no taste or calling for it." With this statement, she called into question the logic of continuing to foster agrarianism. To her the consequence of pursuing this path seemed obvious: the money set aside for this purpose—almost $50,000—would be wasted on uninterested Omahas. She also wrote mockingly that it was "going to be a great pity" that the model farm would be so inaccessible, being located at the Winnebago agency.[67]

This flow of reasoning brought the Omaha physician back to her original theme: consolidation promoted prodigality, not economy. She found the OIA's economic reasoning unfathomable, since all the salaries of the field officials would be raised and the staff would be expanded. Wryly she concluded that the Indian Department's calculations must be "in accordance with their other theories." In sum, she declared that the proposal should be scrapped; otherwise, the Omahas would resist to the utmost. "You can never push an Omaha down or pass a thing over his head," Susan warned, for "he will light on his feet facing you."[68]

By the first of the year, the Omahas had decided to send a dele-gation to Washington to present their case. They believed this was necessary, since the Indian Office had proceeded with its consolida-tion plan in early January. Hiram Chase, Daniel Webster, Simeon Hallowell, and Susan La Flesche Picotte—all educated, "progres-sive" Omahas—were selected to represent the tribe.[69]

But Susan had qualms about her participation. Throughout the previous spring she had been diagnosed as suffering from a severe case of neurasthenia—a functional nervous disorder characterized by profound physical and mental exhaustion. Headaches, noises in the ears, insomnia, nervous dyspepsia, palpitations, and spinal irritation were some of the common symptoms. Many of these palpable physi-cal ills were actually symptoms of other diseases, then unknown or unfathomable. This so-called "nervous disease," which became the fashionable diagnosis for middle-class women of leisure, offered reinforcement for the stereotypical image of the Victorian lady—one who was invalid, weak, and delicate.[70]

Susan probably was suffering from a serious, unknown ailment. She came close to death and had to be cared for by a nurse for nearly six weeks. She recovered in the summer, but by January 1910, in the middle of the consolidation controversy, the symptoms—lethargy and the inability to digest food—returned. Citing poor health, she declined the invitation to join the delegation. However, the Omaha delegation refused to accept the excuse, and they even threatened to carry her to the train and put her on it. Susan relented and, as she related in a letter to a Hampton teacher, she was soon embroiled in planning their presentation.[71]

Beginning in late January, Susan and the rest of the delegation met with various government officials, including Commissioner Valentine, Secretary of the Interior Richard A. Ballinger, and Attorney General George W. Wickersham. These intermittent meetings lasted into the middle of February, and by then the Omaha doctor confessed that the tense fight had sapped all her "nerve force."[72]

During meetings with officials from the Interior and Indian Depart-ments, Susan reported that the consolidation, which was then moving through its initial stage, had already posed difficulties for the Omahas.

They particularly resented the "store orders" system, whereupon incompetent Indians cashed in an endorsed bill at a designated store for approved items. Omahas also complained of the delays in business transactions ever since Kneale had taken over as the superintendent of the consolidated agencies.[73] It seemed that all the Omahas' predictions of the negative effects of combining the agencies had come true. The consolidation also opened up more complications by expanding the role of government farmers. By this time Susan had gathered enough information on the government farms to make an informed judgment. The farmers were given respective jurisdictions and operated from sparsely populated areas. Their duties included the processing of leasing applications. The Omahas, who owned small parcels scattered throughout the reservation, had to travel some distance in order to access the services of the farmers.[74]

Susan indirectly accused the government of breaking its promise to turn Indians into self-respecting American citizens. The incompetency of some Indians was the government's fault, she charged. She said that Indians lacked initiative and achievement "because [they] were deprived of assuming responsibility."[75]

In her meetings with government officials, Susan sidestepped the fact that releasing some unacculturated Omahas from restrictions on the sale or rental of their allotments might lead to dissipation and destitution. She was certainly conscious of that fact—her repeated calls earlier to Superintendent Pollock for protection betrayed that awareness. But apparently she chose to let that inconsistency go unrebutted. She certainly never attempted to reconcile the desire to throw off the shackles of white paternalism and the need for protection from rapacious non-Indians. It was undoubtedly difficult to chart an appropriate course—one that would preserve Omaha autonomy and still lead the tribe into the twentieth century. Susan recognized these pivotal goals, but her ability to identify with both sides of the dividing line sometimes trapped her in the middle. Like so many educated Indians laboring on the cultural frontier, she found that an appropriate solution remained elusive.

Susan agreed with the reformers' argument that the reservation system had demoralized rather than uplifted the Indians. She believed that only experience would lead to personal growth and the attainment of competency and that without it Indians would continue to depend on the Indian Office. That dependency concept was flawed from the start. When one government official tried to put the blame for the Omahas' deprivation on the "pernicious effect of the credit system," Susan lashed out that the conditions were "the fault of your [the Indian Office's] system, not the fault of the Indian." She pointed out that the inefficiency of the OIA bureaucracy had caught the Omahas in a bind time and again.[76]

When their requests for funds were rejected by the OIA, Omahas turned to merchants and moneylenders, who often demanded usurious interest rates. Mrs. La Cook, a patient of Susan's, put in a request for money from her trust fund to use to pay for a critical operation. The Indian Office turned her down, mainly because the bill lacked the signature of a surgeon. Mrs. La Cook had to turn to a moneylender who charged her an interest rate of 7 percent. Susan predicted that the woman would never be able to pay off her $1,400 debt plus interest. Mrs. La Cook was no isolated case. As a physician, Susan encountered many Omahas who went without proper medical attention when their applications for funds were held up. Such individuals sometimes could not even borrow money from white moneylenders because of poor credit histories.[77]

Susan insisted that the Omahas wished to live up to their financial obligations. They "want a more liberal policy; they want to be able to do their own business . . . and be able to pay their own bills," she declared. They also implored the OIA to lift existing restrictions so that they could quickly consolidate their fragmented lands, which were currently scattered all over the reservations. In short, the tribe asked for relief from rules and regulations that had circumscribed their development as competent citizens of the republic. The Omahas wanted to live like Euro-Americans rather than as wards of the federal government, Susan continued. She warned the officials that her people, "who have suffered enough," planned to "cut loose from the department" if their demands, which included fee patents, were not met. What began as a straightforward anti-consolidation movement had turned into a full-scale attack on paternalism and the underlying premise of the historical ward-guardian relationship between the Omaha tribe and the United States government.[78]

The efforts of the Omaha delegation bore fruit, albeit with devastating consequences. Against the wishes of traditionalists such as White Horse but following the recommendation of the competency commission, the Indian Office issued 244 fee patents, covering the rights to 20,199.23 acres, to 230 Indians all on the same day, March 17, 1910. Susan was singled out by one Nebraska newspaper for having helped the tribe draw "up a second declaration of independence." Within the year, however, 60 to 75 percent of the fee-patented land had been sold and half of the patentees had already wasted their proceeds. "Money in the pocket of an Indian, is like water in a leaky bucket," Superintendent Kneale wrote candidly, "it soon runs out and no one knows where it . . . [has] gone."[79]

The dissipation stemmed from the fact that even before allottees received their fee patents, land grabbers had infested the Omaha reservation and persuaded the allottees to sell or lease the land to them. In October 1910, land speculators expected the Indian Office to issue more fee patents to Omahas who had recently been declared competent. Apparently Susan had been keeping tabs on these unscrupulous local whites. Early that month she wired Commissioner Valentine and informed him of the ongoing duplicity on the reservation.[80]

In that telegram and a follow-up letter, she charged that land jobbers had offered the legal services of their Washington attorneys to help Indians speed up the approval of their fee patents. After their attorneys had pocketed the $100.00 fee charged for processing the patents, these speculators offered bribes to agency clerks to release the list of successful applicants to them before the applicants received their respective notices. They then approached unsuspecting patentees and offered them paltry sums for their land. The grafters promised their victims that the money could be applied to rent for the land should their applications be rejected. By the time the patents arrived the deeds had been transferred into the hands of those disreputable whites, and the Indians had sold their lands in exchange for wretched proceeds.[81]

SUSAN LA FLESCHE PICOTTE, M.D.

In her follow-up letter, Susan offered proof of such dissimulation. She provided the names of both the culprits and victims in four cases and cited the dollar amounts of the losses. She reported that upon examining the county records, she had discovered that the speculators had moved so fast that deeds were signed away on the day of the patents were issued, and often the land was mortgaged simultaneously. Susan argued that such fraudulent transactions could have been staved off if the OIA had proceeded rapidly with the patenting process, plugged the leaks from within, and informed the Indians on its decisions in a timely manner.[82]

Anticipating the OIA's counterargument that Indians who had been declared competent should be capable of protecting themselves, Susan offered a simple, yet appropriate retort: "I ask he [the Indian] be given an even show with the attorneys and speculators at the start." She contended that competent Indians could look out for themselves provided Euro-Americans did not have an unfair advantage over them.[83]

She also criticized inconsistencies in the criteria of the competency applications. This, however, was not a new subject. During the height of their work, the competency commission had recommended allottees for fee patents even though they did not meet the requirements—knowledge of English and the ability to support oneself. Susan offered the case of Louis Levering who, though a drunkard and of unsound mind, still received his fee patent. The outcome seemed almost predictable: while in a stupor, Levering sold all of his land at almost 50 percent less than the estimated market value.[84]

In this correspondence Susan revealed a fairly deep understanding of the problems that came in the wake of the patenting process. Although she recognized that the release of land titles did not signify that the Omahas could immediately blend into American society, she still believed that Indians could and should "take their right place" in the larger American society.[85] But the rapid loss of Indian land raised doubts in her mind about the implementation of this final stage of the allotment program. In fact, Susan told the Indian Office that lately she had advised incompetent Indians to wait awhile "till they can show proofs of competency." In closing, she urged the Indian Office to put a hold on all applications from such Indians for at least two years.[86] The new problem for Susan was to find a middle ground where Indians could conduct business with Euro-Americans and still maintain autonomy and control over their own lands and earnings.

In its reply to the Omaha physician's charges, the Indian Office tried to assure her that it had acted in good faith in the matter of fee patents. The Indian Office based this judgment on Superintendent Kneale's report. But a careful reading of the reply reveals that only in one of the four cases she had cited was the contract for sale made after the fee patent had been announced officially. In another of the cases, both Kneale and his superiors took the word of the buyer that his knowledge of the release came from the local newspaper. The Indian Office sidestepped the other two cases and simply insisted that the competency commission had found both of the individuals capable and competent.[87] No doubt Susan's allegations had at least some validity, but unfortunately the Indian Office did little beyond this point about them.

By 1916 close to 90 percent of the Omahas who held fee patents had either sold their lands or taken mortgages they possibly could never repay. By then, the property they had managed to hold onto was deemed taxable. And the only communal tribal land left was a seventy-acre parcel set aside as burial grounds. Their fortunes had taken a turn for the worse after the 1890s because, to borrow the words of a student of Omaha tribal history, "they had been forced to become 'independent' much too soon."[88] The final irony was that what had been perceived as a high degree of acculturation in the Omahas had ultimately led them down the path of dispossession.

But loss of land, and the ensuing poverty, were not unique to the Omahas. Between the passage of the General Allotment, or Dawes, Act of 1887 and the reversal of the allotment policy mandated in the Indian Reorganization Act of 1934, Native American landholdings shrank from 138 to 52 million acres. But the forced assimilation philosophy embodied in the General Allotment Act failed to produce self-supporting Indian citizens, and Indians became even more dependent on the federal government.[89]

Susan never recorded much about her reflections on the Omahas' losses, but she probably wondered why the goal of individual land-ownership—self-support—remained elusive for so many of them. In 1911, fearful that all existing holdings would be lost to subsequent generations of Omahas, she threw her support behind the Gallagher Bill, which proposed to recognize all heirs born under marriages that had been performed according to Indian customs. She argued that the bill would remove legal complications arising from plural unions and numerous heirs and that land jobbers would find it more difficult to manipulate that many landowners.[90]

All this was indeed a rather dramatic turnabout in Susan's personal convictions; as a young woman, she had helped her older sisters to encourage and organize Christian marriages among her people. In backing the Gallagher Bill she displayed a sense of pragmatism that could be traced back to her tribe's practical, self-reliant ethos.[91]

Based on her writings between 1909 and 1910, Susan probably placed the blame for the Indians' failure to attain self-support on the paralytic OIA machinery and on rapacious Euro-Americans. Certainly the former continued to give her trouble, and unfortunately the trouble had to do with an important personal matter: the management of her inherited lands.

Some years ago Susan had inherited portions of land from the estates of her father, her mother, her sister Susette, and a distant relative. The other heirs were mainly her siblings and their children. For years, all of those inherited lands were leased out. But as Susan hinted and as is evident in the family papers, the heirs had disagreed for some time over the management of the lands.[92] In 1910 they finally agreed to sell the lands. But because the trust period for her father's land had yet to expire and minor heirs were involved, the sale ran into complications. Under the law, she and the other heirs could not receive a fee patent to Joseph's land until after the trust period expired. However, they could petition for the partitioning of the land. But the adult heirs would have to prove their competency before they could receive separate fee patents to their small shares of the larger tract. The other option was to sell the entire tract.[93]

Whichever option they pursued would consume a significant amount of time. By now Susan had more than enough first-hand experience with red tape to fully understand the laboriousness of the process, but she knew that time was running out. Given her poor health, Susan feared as early as mid-1911 that her death was imminent, and consequently she urged the Indian Office to draw the procedures to an end so that her children would be well provided for.[94]

Luckily her persistence paid off, and she lived just long enough to see her wish fulfilled. But like so many other heirs of inherited lands, Susan found the process to be fraught with pitfalls. Initially the eleven heirs agreed to partition the land, but they soon set the idea aside since the parcel was too small—about 150 acres—to divide economically. The Indian Office offered the land for sale, but no bids were received. Some of the heirs, including Susan, then offered to buy out the rest, but they could not reach an agreement on the price. By the time they reached a settlement, almost six years had passed. In April 1915 Susan and a few other heirs received the deed to Joseph's land.[95] The Omaha physician had won this personal battle, even though it had taken a long time and had cost her much grief.

Susan's confrontations with government officials had been both personal and political. Her private concerns, particularly the control of her husband's estate, and her daily work for the Omahas almost inevitably brought her into contact with OIA politics. She emerged as a leader who spoke with the unanimous support of her tribe—the factionalism that had been present during the temperance fight receded into the background. No doubt Susan felt honored. To a friend she once confided: "It makes me feel so good to know all the Omahas had so much confidence in me."[96]

Toward the end of her life Susan saw that much of her work had been in vain, as the Omahas lost much of their ancestral land and became even more dependent on the paternalism of the Indian Office. Her struggle to take possession of her share of the family estate, though ending in victory, served as a testament to her own dependence on the Indian Office.

But in the last years of her life, this Omaha physician found other means of expressing her self-worth and asserting her personal independence. As a health reformer, she improved the lives of many. Her work in this arena helped to further augment her personal reputation for perseverance and selflessness.

CHAPTER EIGHT

"Permitted to Serve"

A few years before her death, Susan asserted that she believed "in prevention of disease and hygienic care" more than she did "in giving or prescribing medicine." She said her "constant aim" was "to teach these two things, particularly to young mothers," and her "greatest desire in having the hospital built was to save the little children."[1] At the end of her life, somewhat gaunt and emaciated, she still labored to realize those personal goals. In so doing, she gave credence not only to her legendary fame as a Progressive-Era reformer but also to her position as a leader of the Omahas as they strove to accommodate change in the twentieth-century American West.

Many of her efforts in public health neatly echoed the themes of the public health movement at the turn of the century. By then, both the medical profession and lay public had taken up the banner of prevention. The discovery and acceptance of the theory that germs caused disease gave rise to the cry for an all-out focused attack on bacterial enemies. Sentimentality receded and faith in the efficacy of science to restore social order reached new heights. Fueled by belief in historical progress and a sense of optimism that scientific means were finally available to prevent or control the hazards of infections and diseases, proponents of preventive health saw their cause as part of the larger effort to conserve health, another vital human resource. Through rational social action and pragmatic, empirical methods, proponents rallied the American public to attain a higher level of sanitation and personal hygiene so as to engender well-adjusted healthy bodies.[2]

Susan's thoughts and actions on this subject amply demonstrated the thrust and direction of the voluntary health movement. As a member of the state medical society, she joined six other doctors to form the Thurston County Medical Society in 1907. The intentions of the society included streamlining medical fees, possibly to avoid competition among local physicians. The efforts of these physicians were not unusual. At the turn of the century, medical societies mushroomed at the state and county levels in response to the need for standards and authority.[3]

Until 1911 Susan served several terms on the Walthill health board, her last term as president.[4] By then some Indians had moved into Walthill's white-dominated community, and her work benefited both non-Indians and Indians. Ironically she now found herself in a position to instruct and inculcate higher standards of "civilized living" in Anglo-Americans, the supposed paragons of "civilization."

Some of her health-board duties were recorded in her personal diary; others were duly reported by the local newspaper, the *Walthill Times*. She served notices on owners of unsanitary buildings and imposed fines on repeat offenders. Those who littered public places and streets also came under proscription. The elimination of the sight of foul-smelling garbage became a central goal of the health board. Susan also used her stature to lobby for the erection of a park and children's playground.[5]

She probably proposed the latter in response to the well-known organized-play movement (or small parks and playground movement) of that era. Organized play, according to advocates, was a vital medium for shaping the physical, moral, and cognitive development of adolescents. In addition, they proposed that playgrounds would serve as safe havens for urban youths and slum children would be protected from the deleterious influences of their surroundings. In a larger sense, such organized play facilitated the shaping of future capable workers for American capitalism. Because of her participation in the women's clubs movement, which focused on social reform, she probably knew the rhetoric on the purpose of playgrounds.[6]

As a member of the health board, Susan had an obligation to respond professionally when an epidemic threatened the community. Once, during a diphtheria scare, she supported a quarantine and spent countless hours examining every resident in Walthill and prescribing the necessary treatment. After the scare was over and the quarantine had been lifted, the *Walthill Times* praised "Dr. Picotte" for her preventive work.[7]

Ironically Susan's commitment to prevention landed her in the middle of a controversy in March 1911. According to fragmented evidence, she and the other two physicians who made up the health board disagreed vehemently on the nature of an unidentified contagion that was sweeping through the area. They also parted ways on the need for home quarantine and the closing of public gathering places. Susan apparently agreed to the preventive measures and they were carried out, although enforcement seemed somewhat loose. Some Walthill residents charged that she and the rest of the health board had panicked and taken extreme measures that inconvenienced many and aided few. One board member considered the measures unnecessary, and he ended up in a brawl with the other male member. Much disturbed by this turn of events, Susan telegraphed the state health inspector to come and settle matters. After some investigation, the inspector ruled in favor of those who voted for the quarantine. However, he advised all the current board members to tender their resignations and suggested that in the future the board should be made up of only one physician and two laypersons. The board took the advice, and all, including Susan, resigned.[8]

But her resignation did not significantly damage her professional standing in the Indian or Euro-American communities. Sometime in 1911 the local board of education appointed her health inspector for the schools. In 1906, at the Omahas' request, the reservation boarding school had terminated its operations, and Omaha students subsequently had joined the local public school system. The services Susan rendered as school health inspector reached both Indian and non-Indian school-age youngsters. By the early years of the twentieth century, regular health inspections for children had gained credence in school districts across the country. As health inspector, Susan kept an index-card record—a popular system recommended by government health authorities—on each pupil in the county.[9]

Some years earlier, during one particular smallpox epidemic, she volunteered to vaccinate Indian youngsters against the contagion. Apparently her efforts paid off since only seven died, as compared to more than fifty deaths in the previous year's epidemic.[10] Early detection of illness and infection now became her primary goal. She also made periodic checks on the sanitary conditions of school facilities.[11]

Susan once said: "I feel that what is done for the children is more important than anything else, for what you see in the public life, you must teach in the public school." "The future fathers and mothers of our homes," she continued, "have a right to be educated in health knowledge."[12] At first glance such statements seemed to suggest that her actions were driven by Victorian maternalism, which motivated many Euro-American women reformers of that period.[13] But that would be a facile conclusion, since Susan had always been motivated by her personal search for validation and a desire to aid the struggling Omahas. She hoped that positive attitudes toward public health activities would start with the young people and gradually permeate the adult population. This effort gave her much self-satisfaction and a sense of accomplishment.

Unfortunately, the Indian Office seemed somewhat unreceptive to her advocacy of preventive health care for the young. In 1914, the year before her death, Susan urged Commissioner Cato Sells to initiate monthly examinations of all Indian children attending government schools. Periodic checkups of Indian students had been in place since 1909, but no consistent effort was being made to keep close tabs on them on a regular basis. To drive home her point, Susan related how a young girl who had contracted tuberculosis at her boarding school had returned home and infected both her mother and grandmother; subsequently, all three had lost their lives.[14] No reply has been found in the Indian Office records; presumably none was issued.

Many of the specific health measures—proper disposal of refuse, playgrounds, isolation, and improvement of unsanitary conditions—that she advocated were throwbacks to traditional public health practices of the nineteenth century. Even though turn-of-the-century physicians like Susan had accepted the theory that disease was caused by germs, they realized that dirty environments could foster bacterial growth and diffusion. Basic sanitation campaigns could still aid their efforts to reduce the number of individuals infected with specific communicable diseases. Her advocacy of public health measures also fell in line generally with the growing importance of social science methods such as data collection and the new emphasis on prevention.[15] Susan did her part for the cause, in spite of opposition from some members of the community.

But it was in her role as chair of the state health committee of the Nebraska Federation of Women's Clubs (NFWC) that Susan came to the forefront of public attention. The NFWC was a state branch of the General Federation of Women's Clubs (GFWC), which was committed to the practical improvement of community life. Invoking their domestic, "natural" talents, these largely upper-middle-class white women moved out into the public sphere and subsumed social causes under the wide umbrella of "urban housekeeping." Under the auspices of domesticity, they made a new claim for female influence and expertise in public matters. In the interest of defining themselves as citizens, and not simply wives and mothers, they mobilized to establish an all-female organization that would help them gain sociopolitical leverage. These women reformers of the GFWC (established in 1889) and NFWC (established in 1894) eventually embroiled themselves in a host of activities ranging from the promotion of municipal arts to lobbying for child-labor legislation.[16]

In 1908 the GFWC issued a call for aggressive activism in the field of public health that focused on food sanitation, school hygiene, social hygiene (sex education), and the prevention of tuberculosis. The spirit of the larger voluntary health movement of that era had finally permeated this predominantly female organization. Soon the GFWC's Nebraska auxiliary responded to the call with a campaign against the "white plague," or tuberculosis, and by lobbying for medical inspection.[17]

When Susan received her appointment as chair of the NFWC's health committee, the *Walthill Times* noted that it was "a deserved recognition of her ability in this direction." For three consecutive terms, she continued the work of her predecessor, but her work also branched out into other health-related issues. In her 1911 annual report to the federation, she urged all auxiliaries to end their indifference and suggested that each auxiliary designate a club member to work closely with her on the health agenda. She proposed that the auxiliaries should lobby their local boards of education and health to implement compulsory medical inspection of schools. She also called for the installation of sanitary drinking fountains so as to deal "a blow . . . to all contagious diseases."[18]

According to Susan, the key to the success of the fight against pestilence was "proper education" at the grass-roots level. To that end, auxiliaries should cooperate with local boards to organize Health Days at both school and county levels. All means of relaying life-saving information—including exhibits, booklets, wall cards, and others—should be employed, she asserted. Through such efforts the improved "physical stamina of the race" would in turn increase "mental and moral stamina," she concluded, a common belief of that period.[19]

The Omaha physician tried to practice what she preached to others. She lobbied for the state law requiring medical inspection of schools. Other health-related bills also received her support. In supervising a traveling health exhibit, she found the costs prohibitive, and so she wrote to the Russell Sage Foundation to urge the sale of display materials at lower prices so that the public could be educated.[20]

Susan's major contribution to public health was in the struggle against tuberculosis. By the 1910s this disease had caused more chronic illnesses and deaths than all other acute contagions combined. In the first twenty years of the twentieth century, tuberculosis killed 160,000 persons annually in the United States.[21] Tuberculosis remained the deadliest malady among American Indians, with nearly 17 percent of those examined in 1912 harboring the tubercle bacillus. That year the morbidity rate for Indians was two and a half times higher than that for Euro-Americans. As reported by the agency official in 1910, tuberculosis ranked as the disease with the highest social costs among the Omahas, as lives became disrupted, incapacitated, or destroyed.[22]

As early as 1907 Susan tried to get the Indian Office to pay attention to the malady on the Omaha reservation. In her letter to Commissioner Francis E. Leupp, she related the tragedy: "The spread of tuberculosis among my people is something terrible . . . so many, many of the young children are marked with it in some form. The physical degeneration in 20 years among my people is terrible." She pleaded with Leupp to do something about this "white plague." She was dismayed by Leupp's reply; citing an absence of funds, he turned down her request.[23]

In the interval, the confrontation with government officials over her husband's estate and the Omahas' demand for autonomy in land management probably drew Susan's attention away from the tuberculosis menace. But when she assumed the chair of the health committee, she pledged to place special emphasis on the battle against tuberculosis.[24] In this fight, Susan focused her efforts on public education and prohibitive measures.

Again the malady was as much a personal enemy as it was a public one for Susan. Her husband Henry suffered from tuberculosis and had withered away gradually, and her former beau Thomas Ikinicapi had also died from the disease. As a physician she had treated, often futilely, countless relatives and friends afflicted with the contagion. Now in her public role as educator, she began lecturing on the subject in surrounding towns. On National Tuberculosis Day, she spoke at local churches, and her addresses were published in the newspapers to reach a wider audience.[25]

In her talks the Omaha doctor explained the etiology of the disease and its prevention in terms a layperson could understand. Like most physicians of that period, she increasingly focused her work in public health on the elimination of specific bacteria rather than general environmental concerns. By this time even voluntary organizations, including the GFWC, had switched to promoting tactics to seek out germs responsible for specific diseases. Very much a reformer of her times, Susan had obviously imbued current knowledge on the subject since many of her ideas echoed those dispensed by federal health officials.[26]

By now an accomplished speaker, she structured her talks around a series of questions that were designed to prod her audiences to consider how they too could play a part in the fight against tuberculosis. Her answer, always to the point, was also logical: "The best, surest, and most far reaching [method] is to burn all discharges." She told them that since sputum carried the germ, sickly individuals should spit into paper cups, newspapers, or other disposable receptacles that could be burned easily. Otherwise tuberculosis could be transmitted through the inhalation of such germs. As the disease could be communicated through contaminated hands, food, and utensils, sharing items was inadvisable.[27]

Because specific, effective disease cures were not immediately available, doctors at the turn of the century continued to rely partly on accumulated empirical folklore on the therapeutic value of fresh air, sunshine, a good diet, and rest. So Susan urged her readers—non-Indians and Indians alike—to live in "plenty of fresh air and sunlight" and to be on the look out for accumulated dust, which could harbor germs. "The healthier you are the more difficult it is for the germs to grow," she concluded.[28]

The next year, 1912, she mounted an even more aggressive campaign against the contagion. This time she zeroed in on the housefly, which was considered a major vector of the tubercle bacillus and other contagious germs. To educate the public about this danger, she designed a dramatic, almost lurid, poster entitled "War Declared on the Fly." Around the edge she showed flies engaged in life-threatening activities such as infesting food, hovering above an invalid, and even eating a dead dog. The poster explained the dangers that flies pose to human health and offered ways to eliminate them. She hoped to convince both Indians and non-Indians that flies bred filth and that filth led in turn to diseases, tuberculosis only one of them. To get rid of flies, Susan offered simple, practical suggestions: cover all foodstuff; screen windows and doors; and use common poisons, such as kerosene and chloride of lime, on privy vaults and garbage cans. More than 150 womens' clubs in the region received the poster, and it was also widely reprinted in Nebraska newspapers.[29] Besides the poster, Susan also wrote a long article on the habits of the housefly and on how to combat the pest through the use of flyswatters and flytraps. Such devices could be homemade, and so Susan provided the necessary directions. Later, at the 1913 annual state convention of the NFWC, the Omaha physician demonstrated the use of these homemade contraptions, and eventually she succeeded in persuading representatives to use them in their own talks to club members and local groups.[30]

In the campaign against tuberculosis, the "evils of the [common] drinking cup" also came under her scrutiny. According to one account, she once persuaded Walthill's town council to have the tin cup that hung from a faucet on the main street removed. Apparently the cup helped spread the malady. Later she wrote an article for the local newspaper and inveighed against such cups elsewhere. The proper substitute was drinking fountains which dispensed with the mouthing of contaminated utensils, she urged. Her health committee crusaded against common cups and helped to secure state legislation banning their use. Disposable cups, and even ice-cream dishes and spoons, were soon made available in stores, and sanitary drinking fountains were erected in local schools. Her campaigns against both houseflies and common drinking cups were hardly unique. By then various government agencies, including the Indian Office, had identified these as health hazards and launched vigorous efforts to combat them. The role she and her committee played complemented and augmented those efforts.[31]

Much of what Susan did as a health reformer was done for the benefit of both Omahas and non-Omahas. But her most well-known legacy served to better the lives of her people, the Omaha Indians. This was the building of the reservation hospital.

Susan had promoted the idea since her college days. In the late 1880s when the Women's National Indian Association (WNIA) announced plans to help build a "home [hospital] for the sick and care-worn women and children," the young medical student enthusiastically endorsed it.[32] But the plans went awry. Though more than half the money had been raised by mid-1890, the WNIA simply gave up on the project after a few false starts. No explanation was offered for the project's abandonment, though the delays were credited to the lack of cost estimates and to unavoidable "local conditions."[33]

As the years passed, Susan became more involved with the local white population. Her practice in Walthill served a number of white patients, and she moved with ease into the local social circle. But she never criticized or abandoned her Indian roots. Late in life, she proudly recounted Omaha stories and legends in writing, and she published some of them in the local newspapers. "These ceremonies," she wrote in an article on rituals associated with the sacred corn, "were beautiful and symbolic . . . tending to preserve integrity and unity as a people." In speeches and interviews, she also willingly shared her knowledge of the Omahas' historical past. A review she wrote on John G. Neihardt's collection of Indian stories, *The Lonesome Trail* (1907), was particularly revealing. She said she was relieved to read of Indians with believable characteristics, but she went on to lament the passing of traditional traits, as her people went through "so-called civilization," which resulted in their having neither an Indian nor Caucasian identity.[34] Perhaps she was also reflecting on her own predicament; after all, her ambivalent bicultural identity had at times trapped her in the middle on Indian-white issues.

Susan never neglected her people. Her work on temperance and allotment-related issues maintained her ties to the tribal community. In fact from late 1910 on, she began to refuse calls for medical aid from Euro-Americans in order to "save" herself for "Indian work."[35] The memories of her long, hard drives across the prairies to offer succor to dying patients lingered on and sustained her emotional bond with the tribespeople.

When the Connecticut Indian Association chose to revive the hospital project in 1908, the Omaha physician wrote to offer her support. A ten-acre portion of land was secured from the government and some money was collected. But again, and probably much to Susan's dismay, the proposal was scuttled. The CIA cited the high costs, the "malarious conditions" of the proposed site, and the possibility of raising "factional fights" (although it is unclear what the

CIA meant by this) as the main reasons for the second failure.[36]

This botched attempt may have strengthened her growing misgivings about the so-called "maternalism" of these Euro-American women. Certainly any semblance of common sisterhood, even one tempered by a racial hierarchy, seemed to have disappeared. That disappointment, coupled with her concomitant frustrations with the federal government over land management, forced her to reevaluate her relationship with the Euro-American world during her middle-age years.[37] The experience also marked another turning point in Susan's life; her ties to her white female sponsors became attenuated and apparently she never sought their aid to help build the hospital.

But she never gave up her dream. When the CIA failed, her lifelong wish became a personal crusade. However, she could not turn to the Indian Office. Obsessed with the goal of ending Indians' dependency on the government, Commissioner Francis E. Leupp objected to the idea of establishing government hospitals for Indians since he believed that they would only serve to preserve that unhealthy relationship. He felt that only private organizations should establish and maintain hospitals among the Indians. Leupp's successor, Commissioner Robert G. Valentine, secured appropriations to build facilities to treat trachoma and sanatoriums for tuberculosis patients, but kept his silence on general hospitals for reservations.[38]

With little hope of receiving federal aid, in late 1910 Susan turned to the Presbyterian Home Mission Board, the missionary organization of her denomination. "We need a hospital more than anything else," she pleaded in her letter. The death of so many babies "for want of care," and the manifold cases of tuberculosis made her request an imperative one, she argued. To assuage fears that the hospital would turn into a burden for the organization, she assured the authorities that "it would be pretty nearly if not entirely self-supporting."[39]

Even before she received a reply from the Home Mission Board, Susan had already begun drumming up support. She spoke in churches about the need for such a facility and sent morbidity and fatality data to eastern women reformers, imploring their assistance. When a few officials of the Home Mission Board visited the reservation in January 1911, she presented her case for the reservation hospital and called it a "crying need." Susan clearly understood the mind-set of privileged, white, middle-class Americans and used that to devise the best possible rhetoric and strategy for her fund-raising campaign. Like other cultural brokers, she constantly recast knowledge of the "Other" as a tool for tribal autonomy.[40]

Her arguments did not initially convince the Home Mission Board, but she persevered and resubmitted her appeal. Also, she persuaded Susan Pingry, who sat on the board and had been one of her teachers at Elizabeth Institute (her finishing school in New Jersey), to lobby on her behalf. Once again, her eastern connections came in handy. Her persistence yielded results. In early fall of 1911 the board voted to appropriate a little over $7,000 for the hospital project. The Omaha doctor considered the sum a little inadequate and soon filed another request. In response, the board earmarked an additional $1,300. Susan's letter-writing efforts to her eastern friends also brought in a gift of $500 from the Massachusetts Society for the Propagation of the Gospel Among the Indians, a Presbyterian-related organization. In all, her denomination underwrote 90 percent of the $10,000 proposed budget.[41]

But the appropriated funds fell short of the actual costs. The planning committee, which included Susan, wanted to keep the size of the hospital forty-two feet by seventy-eight feet, as originally planned, and the space allocated for staff quarters. But it scrapped the proposal for the building to be mission style with tiled floors and cement plastered walls, and it accepted the construction of a functional, bungalow-like structure. Even with these changes, little money was left for landscaping, sanitation improvement, and, most importantly, for furnishings and equipment.[42]

Susan decided to write to friends and organizations, both in the East and in the West, for support. Her old friend from college days Marian B. Heritage pledged the money to furnish the nurses' rooms, and two concerned Euro-American individuals in Pittsburgh held a benefit concert and donated the proceeds to equip the kitchen and office. Various missionary organizations and churches in the region also offered to underwrite the costs of certain sections of the hospital, including the nursery and two of the five private rooms.[43]

Susan also approached local townspeople and Omahas. Various Walthill residents offered to furnish the maternity room and the two general wards. She and her sister Marguerite pooled their resources to dedicate the operating theatre in their father's memory. Marguerite's husband, Walter T. Diddock, donated a one-acre elevated site overlooking the town. Some tribal members also pledged a total of two hundred dollars.[44]

Though the building was completed on schedule, the opening had to be delayed because Susan was ill for more than half of 1912. She underwent surgery, probably for the pain in her ears, but was left with a paralysis of facial muscles and a "nervous condition." By late fall she had recovered sufficiently to oversee the furnishing of the hospital. On January 10, 1913, the Omaha physician finally witnessed the dedication—complete with speeches, a lavish banquet, and prayers in the Omaha language—of her long-awaited hospital.[45]

Without federal aid or that of her eastern "mothers," the members of the CIA, she had gotten the project off the ground with money raised in part by playing benevolent groups off against each other. In getting both Indians and non-Indians to contribute to the project, she had again demonstrated the cross-cultural agility successful mediators must possess. "To Dr. Picotte, more than any other person is due the credit for the erection of the hospital," the *Walthill Times* commended.[46]

At first, because of her health, there was some uncertainty as to whether Susan could serve as physician-in-charge of the new hospital, though the *Walthill Times* announced in its coverage of the dedication that she would serve in that capacity. But later the same newspaper and her family correspondence hinted that the plan had run aground. Susan did not assume the position until the spring of the following year, and even then her professional obligations were limited because of her frail health.[47]

As in many other instances, her poor physical condition stood in the way of Susan's personal fulfillment. Still, the hospital was a success. Indians flocked to it, and shortly after it opened the hospital administration reversed its Indians-only policy so that non-Indians could also use its services. In accordance with Susan's wish, classes on dietary and preventive health were also offered at the hospital.[48] She probably felt satisfied that her life-long aspiration had become a reality.

The hospital was completed just two years before her death. By early March 1915 she was in critical condition. By then, doctors in Omaha had diagnosed her as suffering from "a . . . malady of the bones of the head and face," probably cancer. She went through a series of operations to remove the "infected bones," and by late summer of that year she had made "decided improvement," according to the *Walthill Times*.[49]

But her doctors had already surmised that her illness was terminal and that they could do little else for her. Susan went home and spent the last few months of that summer in the company of her youngest son, Pierre, by then a student at the Nebraska Military Academy, a private institution in Lincoln (her other son, Caryl, was attending Bellevue College). Her niece Marguerite also took care of Susan. Together, they kept her spirits up. But her malady was too far along, and death claimed her in the early morning on September 18, 1916.[50]

The funeral services for this remarkable woman symbolically captured the direction of her short but productive life and her movement between two worlds—that of the Omahas and that of the Euro-Americans. At her home in Walthill an overflow crowd of Indians and whites surrounded the three Presbyterian clergymen who performed the simple but dignified service. Following that, an Omaha tribal leader offered the closing prayer in the Omaha language. In the afternoon Susan was borne to the Bancroft cemetery, where she was finally laid to rest beside her Indian husband, Henry Picotte.[51]

Though her life was cut short at the age of fifty, Susan La Flesche Picotte, M.D., had undoubtedly left her mark in both the Indian and non-Indian communities. The outpouring of affection and the tributes from all parts of the country following her death attested to the impact she had made as a progressive reformer and tribal leader. "Her life was dedicated to their [Indians'] needs . . . to the furtherance of . . . their personal and collective welfare . . . as she gave willingly to her people," the *Walthill Times* editor wrote in an extended issue covering the funeral. One Indian reform periodical praised her efforts against "reservation evils," an obvious reference to her work in the areas of temperance and public health. *The Southern Workman*, the voice of her alma mater in Virginia, characterized her adulthood as "one of unselfish usefulness."[52]

Laudatory remarks also came from friends who had kept abreast of the twists and turns in Susan's life. In a letter to Marguerite, Alice Fletcher, Susan's old mentor, asserted that she had left a "worth[sic] record of service to God and to man and that is much to bequest." In a pointed reference to her ties with two cultures, Harry L. Keefe, the longtime attorney for the tribe, wrote: "In her death the Indians lose their best and surest friend [while] the community and state sustains an irreparable loss." Her Hampton teacher Josephine E. Richards described the Omaha physician as an exemplar of womanhood to Hampton female students and also praised her work on behalf of "her own people."[53]

Richards's comments succinctly captured the essence of Susan La Fleshe Picotte's persona. Born into a fairly acculturated Omaha family and surrounded by many tribal members who embraced the spirit of accommodation to white ways, she grew up fully acquainted with the government's mission of Americanization. She attended western schools, where teachers augmented her growing faith in Christianity and supported her desire to pursue a career in medicine. The lessons of those teachers also gave credence to her father's belief in the role of historical change—that the Omahas would have to adopt at least some of the Euro-American's ways or else they would perish.

However, her father and many Omahas parted ways with Euro-American reformers on the issue of cultural identity. Joseph La Flesche and other acculturated Omahas, the so-called "make-believe white men," willingly accepted various aspects of white culture, but they kept enough distance from it to avoid disappearing into the Euro-American society. Like her father, Susan understood the Omahas' need to "climb higher," to borrow the phrase she used during her salutatory address in 1886.[54]

To that end, she initially saw her role—one partly shaped by ties to her sponsor, the Connecticut Indian Association—as that of an educator of selective aspects of Euro-American, middle-class culture. The CIA expected Susan, in her capacity as a physician and through her position as an educated, refined daughter of an Indian chief, to channel knowledge of the white world to Omaha families, particularly to women, who would in turn parlay their honed skills and values for the benefit of the tribal nation. Seemingly she gave the association the impression that she would fulfill that particular mediatory role.

But Susan never forgot the value of her tribal identity; frequently she spoke in defense of it. In her early days as a medical student and OIA physician, she exhibited a hint of white-like superiority. She disparaged the "backwardness" of the Omahas and their lack of appreciation for sanitation and western medicine. But though she identified with the Euro-American order, her cultural brokerage was never simply a one-way promotion of Christian civilization. She did not experience a total cultural transformation or cross permanently to the other side of the Indian-white dividing line. Later in life she even sought to educate non-Indians on the richness of her Omaha heritage. Always she tried to identify common ground across the supposed cultural divide.

After completing her medical studies and returning to the reservation, the Indian physician quickly expanded her sphere of influence beyond the home and into the surrounding landscape. The prescriptive role of a Victorian "true" woman simply never mirrored Susan's multifaceted persona.

She was motivated by her Christian faith and the legacy of her father's activism, but just as important was her fervent desire for personal empowerment, which developed in part from her family's tenuous claim to Omaha identity. Susan probably longed for a sense of belonging. Her father's controversial role as tribal leader and, later, her siblings' unwitting instigation of factionalism on the reservation sullied the family's reputation. Perhaps she thought that mediation on behalf of the Omahas could restore the integrity of the La Flesche name and stabilize her own claim to tribal honors. Of course, Susan could have chosen to embrace "whiteness"; after all, she purposely interacted with Euro-Americans and they in turn welcomed her. The fact that she did not choose this path suggests that, despite her acceptance of the Euro-American message of historical change, she had retained her sense of tribal patriotism. In not necessarily attributing her achievements to part-white "blood," Susan distanced herself somewhat from "white civilization" and linked her fortunes to the convoluted ones of other Omahas.

And the observations she made as a youth about the general dissipation and loss of autonomy that enveloped neighboring tribes and the chaos unleashed on the Omahas by the demands of reservation life also affected Susan's mind-set about her role in shaping the future of the tribal nation. She was hardly enchanted by everything that western civilization had to offer, and her progression into a sociopolitical role seemed inevitable. The Omahas' needs were obvious, and the time was right.

By the turn of the century the Omahas suffered from an even larger host of serious socioeconomic problems, ranging from alcoholism to mismanagement of land resources. Led by "paper chiefs" who often did the bidding of paternalistic OIA field officials, the Omahas were left defenseless. Unguided and unprotected, Omahas fell victim to predatory whites bent on robbing the Indians of their land, their identity. No less devastating to their pride was the fact that some of the best-educated Omahas at times chose to align with predatory Euro-Americans.

Susan stepped into that leadership vacuum. In the fight against intemperance, she delivered fiery lectures, wrote passionate letters to reformers and the Indian Office, and lobbied for the passage of prohibitive measures. When her efforts produced half-hearted results, she abandoned that direction, and returned to religion. She revived a dispirited congregation and brought Omahas into the fold of Christianity. Even then, she fought a losing battle against another alliance—that of the peyote religion.

Soon she had to accept the efficacy of peyotism. In so doing, she paralleled the attitudes of many other acculturated Omahas, who saw nothing wrong in endorsing a native religion that superficially incorporated some Christian elements. This blend artfully kept them in two worlds, those of the Indians and of the Euro-Americans. In endorsing peyotism, Susan recognized that this indigenous religion kept its followers on the road to progress and yet still allowed them to preserve native traits. Such a recognition suggests that she wanted to embrace acculturation but not total amalgamation into white society. In that way her life was no different from that of many other people of color or immigrants; for all of them linear, straightforward assimilation into American ways was a rarity.[55]

Susan's claim to personal power was very much rooted in her somewhat contested Omaha heritage. Her father had been a tribal chief and her family had produced fairly well-known professionals and leaders. Her siblings assumed public roles that provided an entrée for cultural brokerage: Francis, an ethnologist, researched and wrote on Indian lore and customs; Marguerite, a teacher (and later an OIA field matron), promoted Victorian domesticity; and the well-known Susette, or "Bright Eyes," lectured on Indian rights. Many members of the family played mediatory roles either throughout or during some part of their adult lives.

Although Omaha women traditionally held no political offices within the tribe, they were never excluded from the orbit of influence.[56] As a result, Susan was readily accepted as a leader by most tribal members. Apparently her gender did not set hard and fast limits on her rise to sociopolitical power. The fact that she used her gender and its concomitant image of Victorian womanhood to further personal and tribal ends was evident in her earlier attempts to secure medical succor for and destroy alcoholism among her people. As she further solidified her stature within the tribal society, her gender became less important, although Euro-Americans continued to try to apply the strictures of Euro-American womanhood to her. Racial identity stood out as the trait Susan cleaved to in order to further her goals.

Helpless against the sway of alcoholism within her family and tribe and fed up with the drawn-out legal battle to gain control of her husband's estate, Susan became disenchanted with white ways and gradually distanced herself from the ineffective Indian Office. In her role as interpreter for Omahas, she witnessed enough inertia and injustice to convince her of the unreliability of the Indian department. To some extent, Susan probably saw the OIA's ineptitude as a betrayal of the Euro-Americans' promise to help Omahas "climb higher." By turning her focus away from white society, she opened a door to enter into tribal politics and assume a leadership role. Her mediation efforts became increasingly centered on promoting the needs of her people and less on extolling the value of the non-Indian world.

With the antagonism arising from the fight over intemperance seemingly erased, the Omahas drew toward Susan and other astute leaders, and together they fought for fiscal and political autonomy and freedom from the reins of government control. Ironically the autonomy they sought and gained was followed by the dissolution of more Indian landholdings and an even heavier dependence on the Indian Office.

Susan was hardly a naive person. She knew that some Indians simply could not handle the awesome responsibilities associated with a capitalist, money-oriented economy. Unprepared for the challenges of the white world, some Indians engaged in debauchery and squandered away their earnings, as she had witnessed time and again.

To reconcile that knowledge of her people's limitations with the demand for Omaha autonomy, Susan adamantly blamed the troublesome past on the incompetence of the Indian Office. She implied that its failure to guide and protect the Omahas had left them helpless against rapacious non-Indians. But here lies the contradiction the Omaha doctor never resolved: she never found, or at least never expressed, a way for Indians to receive protection and yet maintain their sense of independence. Because Susan never resolved the conflict between the needs for protection and autonomy, she wavered between the two; she certainly was not a very systematic thinker when it came to reform of Indian policy. To strike a balance between the two needs—an act that required walking a tightrope between paternalism and unsupervised freedom—was clearly difficult. In an era when the cry for efficiency and economy took precedence, the Indian Office chose to offer the Indians independence (via fee patents on their allotments) but refused to offer adequate assistance during the transition, and thus created a situation that led to the Indian tragedy.

No doubt Susan was just as mired in the restraints of the historical ward-guardian relationship as any other turn-of-the-century Indian. Her protracted fight to gain her share of the family estate offers proof of that. But her work in the field of public health gave her the opportunity to move out of the dictates of the Indian Office. On her own, she carved a niche for herself in the town of Walthill and the state of Nebraska. Though her efforts echoed many of the government's campaigns, she rarely approached the Indian Office for assistance. This was evident in her fight for the reservation hospital. Having long given up on the government, Susan turned to her racially mixed circle of friends and acquaintances. The realization of this life-long dream gave her much self-satisfaction and the independence she had sought ever since she had witnessed, as a young girl, the tragic removal of the Poncas and their attempted flight back to Nebraska.

As a cultural broker, Susan showed not only receptiveness to the other side of the cultural divide, but also dogged determination. Without that characteristic, she would have failed in medical school. Without her persistence, the lobbying efforts for prohibitive laws against drinking would have amounted to nothing. Admittedly the laws were ineffective, but that was hardly within her realm of control. Without perseverance she certainly would have ended her quest for personal and tribal autonomy in land management.

She sometimes ran up against difficulties on both sides of the cultural divide in her brokerage efforts. Indeed, to borrow the words of historian Margaret Connell Szasz, "the nature of mediation was that of a juggling act" for Susan.[57] When the juggling fails, either one side or the other, or the juggler, will suffer the consequences.

The fear of antagonizing either the Indians or white Americans always loomed in her mind. When she fought against alcoholism, she intimated that she had stirred up hostile feelings against her within the tribe. Although she publicly brushed such factionalism aside, the fact that she brought this up suggests some concern on her part. The moral uprighteousness she displayed during the crusade must have also irritated many Omahas. Certainly in her confrontation with the Indian Office over the consolidation plan and land-related issues, Susan had to come to grips with the fact that she was parting ways with a bureaucracy—and certain aspects of a lifeway—that she had always supported. The strife and foraying back and forth between cultures must have created a personal identity crisis of sorts at times as she struggled to locate her ethnic identity.

Toward the end of her life Susan attenuated her association with official paternalism to some degree. The protracted fight against the negative effects of white presence in and around the reservation gave her insights into the unequal ward-guardian relationship that under-girded Indian–Euro-American affairs. No doubt she continued to lobby the Indian Office for help on specific health issues, but she also forged her own path of selective adaptation. Undoubtedly she embraced Progressive-Era reforms and pursued the Euro-American route to financial stability through investments; according to one report she willed altogether approximately $50,000 to her sons.[58]

Yet clearly Susan never rejected her tribal roots. Though three of her sisters—Susette, Rosalie, and Marguerite—married Euro-American men, she chose an Indian man whose social background was incomparable to hers. She took pride in Omaha values: courage, love for the home and family, respect for traditions, and adaptability to dynamic change. And though the demands of the modern world may have forced the Omahas to give up most aspects of their material culture, such as lodge homes, traditional clothing, and subsistence farming, it is evident in Susan's published and unpublished writings that she was proud of that cultural milieu and certainly never severed her link to the traditional past. Like her father, she viewed that past in a teleological way; past actions constituted events that shaped her evolving sense of self.

In the final tally, the measure of Susan's personal achievements lay in the legacy she left behind. Neither of her sons ever became doctors, though they went on to lead productive lives. Caryl, the older son, made the army his career and served with distinction during World War II. Apparently he later moved to Detroit, Michigan. The other son, Pierre lived in Walthill for most of his life and raised a family of three children. Information on his profession or work is scant; one writer reported that Pierre worked in the post office.[59]

Shortly after the Omaha doctor's death, the facility she had helped build was renamed Dr. Susan Picotte Memorial Hospital. It continued to serve both Indians and non-Indians until 1947, when competition from a nearby government hospital drove it out of business. Used over the years for various purposes, ranging from a nursing home to a bakery, in 1988 the building became the Susan La Flesche Picotte Center, which serves as a multipurpose facility dedicated to the principles that guided her life: "education, service, stewardship, and justice." In 1989 the building became a historical landmark on the national register of historic places and a permanent exhibition was unveiled in commemoration of her legacy.[60]

On the occasion of that celebration, Congressman Doug Bereuter of Nebraska offered a tribute in the U.S. House of Representatives to Susan's life. In his address, Representative Bereuter extolled her as one whose "own accomplishments were the means to bridge the cultural and economic gulf that threatened to divide" the Indians and non-Indians. "Her public accomplishments is [sic] a reminder that color and culture are no barriers to success and respect," he concluded.[61] Finally, in remembrance of Dr. Picotte's respect for "cultural diversity and devotion to community service," in 1993 a new elementary school in the city of Omaha was named after her.[62]

Near the end of her life, in response to some commendation, Susan said: "I cannot see how any credit is due me. I am only thankful that I have been called and permitted to serve. I feel blessed for that privilege."[63] Despite this public display of humility, she was indeed a proud woman. Undoubtedly she cared for her people, but occasionally she also exhibited personal pride in her accomplishments to the non-Indian world. She claimed credit for her work in temperance and evangelism. Even her defiance of the OIA on the issue of land autonomy offered a hint of arrogance. But such pride never set her apart from Omahas who were less fortunate. To the end of her life, she remained wedded to the Indian community and never hesitated to identify herself as part of that ethnic group.

Susan successfully found a place for herself in the larger American society, but she never lost her Indianness. Her linguistic proficiency, multicultural expertise, ambition, and sincerity helped her get along with all kinds of people on both sides of the Indian-white dividing line. Her life provided testimony to how cultural mediation could serve to better all Americans, regardless of race or creed. Moving between two seemingly disparate worlds, Susan La Flesche Picotte inspired her contemporaries. And her faith in the value of "education, service, stewardship, and justice" continues to inspire Americans today.

Abbreviations

AIC	American Indian Correspondence, Presbyterian Historical Society, Philadelphia, Pennsylvania
AR	*Annual Report of the Commissioner of Indian Affairs to the Secretary of the Interior*
BIA	Bureau of Indian Affairs
CCF	Central Consolidated Files, 1907–1939. Record Group 75, Bureau of Indian Affairs, National Archives and Record Service, Washington, D.C.
CIA	Commissioner of Indian Affairs
FLP-NAA	Fletcher–La Flesche Papers, National Anthropological Archives, Smithsonian Institution, Washington, D.C.
HUA	Hampton University Archives, Hampton, Virginia
IB	*The Indian Bulletin*
LFP-NSHS	La Flesche Family Papers, Nebraska State Historical Society, Lincoln, Nebraska
LR-OA	*Letters Received by the Indian Office, 1824–1881*, Omaha Agency, 1864–1870, Record Group 75, Bureau of Indian Affairs, M234, reel 605, National Archives and Records Service, Washington, D.C.
NA	National Archives and Records Service, Washington, D.C.
NSHS	Nebraska State Historical Society, Lincoln, Nebraska
PHS	Presbyterian Historical Society, Philadelphia, Pennsylvania

RF	Rosalie Farly
RIFJ	*Reports of Inspection of the Field Jurisdictions of the Office of Indian Affairs, 1873–1900*, RG 75, BIA, M1016, reel 32, NA
SAF-HUA	Susan La Flesche Alumni File, Hampton University Archives, Hampton, Virginia
SLF	Susan La Flesche Picotte
SNSR	*Superintendents' Annual Narrative and Statistical Reports from Field Jurisdictions of the Bureau of Indian Affairs, 1907–1938*, RG 75, BIA, M1011, reel 169, NA
STK-CSL	Sara Thomson Kinney Papers, Connecticut State Library, Hartford, Connecticut
SW	*Southern Workman*
WT	*Walthill Times*

Notes

INTRODUCTION

1. For a theoretical discussion of cultural brokerage, see Margaret Connell Szasz, "Introduction," in *Between Indian and White Worlds: The Cultural Broker*, ed. Margaret Connell Szasz (Norman: University of Oklahoma Press, 1994), 3–20; Szasz, "Conclusion," in Szasz, *Between Indian and White Worlds*, 294–300; James A. Clifton, "Alternate Identities and Cultural Frontiers," in *Being and Becoming Indian: Biographical Studies of North American Frontiers*, ed. James A. Clifton (Chicago: Dorsey Press, 1989), 1–37; L. G. Moses and Raymond Wilson, "Introduction," in *Indian Lives: Essays on Nineteenth- and Twentieth-Century Native American Leaders*, 2d ed., ed. L. G. Moses and Raymond Wilson (Albuquerque: University of New Mexico Press, 1993), 1–18.

2. Daniel K. Ritcher, "Cultural Brokers and Intercultural Politics: New York–Iroquois Relations, 1664–1701," *Journal of American History* 75 (June 1988): 40–41.

3. Stuart Hall, "Ethnicity: Identity and Difference," *Radical America* 23, no. 4 (1989): 15; Stuart Hall, "Cultural Identity and Diaspora," in *Identity: Community, Culture, Difference*, ed. Jonathan Rutherford (London: Lawrence & Wishart, 1990), 222, 225.

4. For a critique of the concept of separate spheres, see Linda K. Kerber, "Separate Spheres, Female Worlds, Woman's Place: The Rhetoric of

Women's History," *Journal of American History* 75 (June 1988): 9–39. See also Janet D. Spector, *What This Awl Means: Feminist Archaeology at a Wahpeton Dakota Village* (St. Paul: Minnesota Historical Society Press, 1993), 33.

5. Theodore Stern, *The Klamath Tribe: A People and Their Reservation* (Seattle: University of Washington Press, 1965), 229–30; Malcolm McFee, "The 150% Man, A Product of Blackfeet Acculturation," *American Anthropologist* 70 (1968): 1100–101. Clifton, "Alternate Identities," 29. For sociological discussion on biculturalism see Antonio Darder, "The Politics of Biculturalism: Culture and Difference in the Formation of Warriors for *Gringostroika* and The New Mestizas," in *Culture and Difference: Critical Perspectives on the Bicultural Experience in the United States*, ed. Antonio Darder (Westport, Conn.: Bergin & Garvey, 1995), 1–20.

6. Quoted in *Indian Voices: The First Convocation of American Indian Scholars* (San Francisco: Indian Historian Press, 1970), 49; Moses and Wilson, "Introduction," 10.

7. Kathleen Barry, "The New Historical Syntheses: Women's Biography," *Journal of Women's History* 1 (Spring 1989): 101. For a multifaceted discussion on the usefulness of historical biographies, see Stephen B. Oates, ed., *Biography as High Adventure: Life-Writers Speak on Their Art* (Amherst: University of Massachusetts Press, 1986). See also Stephen B. Oates, *Biography as History* (Waco: Markham Press Fund, 1991).

8. Szasz, "Introduction," 20.

CHAPTER 1. "I NEVER SAW A BATTLE"

1. "Glimpses of a Woman's Work among the Omahas," *Omaha World-Herald*, March 22, 1908.

2. Roger L. Welsch, *Omaha Tribal Myths and Trickster Tales* (Athens, Ohio: Sage/Swallow Press Books, 1981), 242; Paul A. Olson, ed., *The Book of the Omaha: Literature of the Omaha People* (Lincoln: Nebraska Curriculum Development Center, 1979), 1.

3. James Owen Dorsey, *Omaha Sociology*, Bureau of American Ethnology Third Annual Report (Washington, D.C.: Government Printing Office, 1884): 211; Alice C. Fletcher and Francis La Flesche, *The Omaha Tribe*, Bureau of American Ethnology Twenty-Seventh Annual Report, 1905–1906 (Washington, D.C.: Government Printing Office, 1911), 73–74.

4. Dorsey, *Omaha Sociology*, 21; Fletcher and La Flesche, *Omaha Tribe*, 85–86.

5. John M. O'Shea and John Ludwickson, *Archaeology and Ethnohistory of the Omaha Indians: The Big Village Site* (Lincoln: University of Nebraska Press, 1992), 1.

6. Olson, *Book of the Omaha*, 4; Lawrence J. Evers, "The Literature of the Omahas" (Ph.D. diss., University of Nebraska, Lincoln, 1972), 19, 54–56.

7. John Ernest Weaver, *Native Vegetation of Nebraska* (Lincoln: University of Nebraska Press, 1965), 3, 13, 33, 113; Richard White, *The Roots of Dependency: Subsistence, Environment, and Social Change among the Choctaws, Pawnees, and Navajos* (Lincoln: University of Nebraska Press, 1983), 167.

8. Susan La Flesche [hereafter SLF], "The Origin of the Corn," *Walthill Times* [hereafter *WT*], March 8, 1912.

9. Edwin James, *Account of an Expedition from Pittsburgh to the Rocky Mountains*, 2 vols. (Philadelphia: H. C. Carey & I. Lea, 1823; reprint, Ann Arbor: University Microfilms, 1966), 1:201, 212–13; Paul Wilhelm, Duke of Wurttemberg, *Travels in North America, 1822–1824*, ed. Savoie Lottinville (Norman: University of Oklahoma Press, 1973), 335; John Bradbury, *Travels in the Interior of America, in the Years 1809, 1810, and 1811* (London: Sherwood, Neely, & Jones, 1817; reprint, Ann Arbor: University Microfilms, 1966), 69; Fletcher and La Flesche, *Omaha Tribe*, 261–70, 339; Rebecca Tsosie, "Changing Women: The Cross-Currents of American Indian Feminine Identity," *American Indian Culture and Research Journal* 12, no. 1 (1988): 5; Margot Liberty, "Hell Came with Horses: Plains Indian Women in the Equestrian Era," *Montana, The Magazine of Western History* 32 (Summer 1982): 14.

10. David J. Wishart, *An Unspeakable Sadness: The Dispossession of the Nebraska Indians* (Lincoln: University of Nebraska Press, 1994), 25–27; Fletcher and La Flesche, *Omaha Tribe*, 274, 342–45; "Letterbox," *St. Nicholas Magazine* 7 (September 1880): 918; Bradbury, *Travels*, 69.

11. James, *Account*, 1:201–12, 217, 220–21; SLF to Rosalie Farley [hereafter RF], March 2, 1887, LFP-NSHS.

12. Laura F. Klein and Lillian A. Ackerman, "Introduction," in *Women and Power in Native North America*, ed. Laura F. Klein and Lillian A. Ackerman (Norman: University of Oklahoma Press, 1995), 14; Carol Devens, *Countering Civilization: Native American Women and Great Lakes Missions, 1630–1900* (Berkeley: University of California Press, 1992), 13; Nancy Shoemaker, "Introduction," in *Negotiators of Change: Historical Perspectives on Native American Women*, ed. Nancy Shoemaker (New York: Routledge, 1995), 7–9; Karen Anderson, *Changing Woman: A History of*

Racial Ethnic Women in Modern America (New York: Oxford University Press, 1996), 22, 24; Fletcher and La Flesche, *Omaha Tribe*, 313–14, 325–27, 337, 362–63.

13. Nancy Shoemaker, "Rise or Fall of Iroquois Women," *Journal of Women's History* 2 (Winter 1991): 40, 52; Marla N. Powers, *Oglala Women: Myth, Ritual, and Reality* (Chicago: University of Chicago Press, 1986), 2–3; Mona Etienne and Eleanor Leacock, "Introduction," in *Women and Colonization: Anthropological Perspectives*, ed. Mona Etienne and Eleanor Leacock (New York: Praeger Publishers, 1980), 20–21; Patricia C. Albers, "Autonomy and Dependency in the Lives of Dakota Women: A Study in Historical Change," *Review of Radical Political Economics* 17, no. 3 (1985): 119–20; Ted C. Hinckley, "Glimpses of Societal Change Among Nineteenth-Century Tlingit Women," *Journal of the West* 32 (July 1993): 15; Fletcher and La Flesche, *Omaha Tribe*, 325–33, 337, 340–48.

14. W. Raymond Wood, "Plains Trade in Prehistoric and Protohistorical Intertribal Relations," in *Anthropology on the Great Plains*, ed. W. Raymond Wood and Margot Liberty (Lincoln: University of Nebraska Press, 1980), 100, 106; Fletcher and La Flesche, *Omaha Tribe*, 76–401.

15. G. Hubert Smith, "Notes on Omaha Ethnohistory, 1763–1820," *Plains Anthropologist* 18 (November 1973): 259; Preston Holder, *The Hoe and the Horse on the Plains: A Study of Cultural Development among North American Indians* (Lincoln: University of Nebraska Press, 1970), 16–17, 66.

16. Fletcher and La Flesche, *Omaha Tribe*, 35–36.

17. Gary E. Moulton, ed., *The Journals of the Lewis and Clark Expedition*, 8 vols. (Lincoln: University of Nebraska Press, 1983–), 3:398–99; James MacKay, "Journal," in *Before Lewis and Clark: Documents Illustrating the History of the Missouri, 1783–1804*, ed. Abraham P. Nasatir, 2 vols. (St. Louis: St. Louis Historical Documents Foundation, 1952), 1:358; Bradbury, *Travels*, 69; Prince of Wied-Neuwied Maximilian, *Travels in the Interior of North America, 1832–1834*, 3 vols, ed. Reuben Gold Thwaites (Cleveland: Arthur H. Clark, 1906), 1:474.

18. Barbara R. Marsh, "Intertribal Conflicts of the Omaha Indians: Traditional and Contemporary Accounts, 1673–1837" (master's thesis, Wichita State University, 1956), 57–58; George E. Hyde, *The Pawnee Indians* (Norman: University of Oklahoma Press, 1951), 129–32; Reuben Gold Thwaites, ed., *Original Journals of the Lewis and Clark Expedition, 1804–1806*, 8 vols. (New York: Dodd, Mead, 1904–1905; reprint, New York: Arno Press, 1969), 1:98, 102, 112, 167–68, 7:64, 315; Richard White, "The Winning of the West: The Expansion of the Western Sioux in the Eighteenth and Nineteenth Centuries," *Journal of American History* 65 (September

1978): 321, 323; Pierre-Jean De Smet, *Life, Letters, and Travels of Father Pierre-Jean De Smet, S.J. 1801–1873*, 4 vols., ed. Hiram M. Chittenden and Alfred Talbot Richardson (New York: Francis P. Harper, 1905; reprint, New York: Arno Press, 1969), 2:628; Rudolph Friederich Kurz, *Journal of Rudolph Friederich Kurz*, ed. J. N. B. Hewitt, Bureau of American Ethnology, Bulletin 115 (Washington, D.C.: Government Printing Office, 1937; reprint, Lincoln: University of Nebraska Press, 1970), 66; G. Hubert Smith, *Omaha Indians: Ethnohistorical Report on the Omaha People*, Indian Claims Commission docket no. 225A (Washington, D.C.: Government Printing Office, 1957; reprint, New York: Garland Publishing, 1974), 79, 129, 181.

19. Alan Klein, "The Political-Economy of Gender: A 19th Century Plains Indian Case Study," in *The Hidden Half: Studies of Plains Indian Women*, ed. Patricia Albers and Beatrice Medicine (Washington, D.C.: University Press of America, 1983), 154–56; Nancy C. Wright, "Economic Development and Native American Women in the Early Nineteenth Century," *American Quarterly* 33 (Fall 1981): 525–26.

20. John M. O'Shea and John Ludwickson, "Omaha Chieftainship in the Nineteenth Century," *Ethnohistory* 39 (Summer 1992): 319–23.

21. SLF, "Origin"; Fletcher and La Flesche, *Omaha Tribe*, 6, 597–99, 608–609.

22. Michael C. Coleman, "The Mission Education of Francis La Flesche: An American Indian Response to the Presbyterian Boarding School in the 1860s," *American Studies in Scandinavia*, 18 (1986): 68; Fletcher and La Flesche, *Omaha Tribe*, 201; O'Shea and Ludwickson, *Archaeology*, 23. See also Nasatir, *Before Lewis and Clark*, 1:264, 282–86, 298, 358, 2:608; Abraham Nasatir, "John Evans, Explorer and Surveyor," *Missouri Historical Review* 25 (April 1931): 455–56.

23. James, *Account*, 1:225–26, 228–29.

24. Thomas F. Schilz and Jodye L. D. Schilz, "Beads, Bangles, and Buffalo Robes: The Rise and Fall of the Indian Fur Trade Along the Missouri and Des Moines Rivers, 1700–1820," *Annals of Iowa* 49 (Summer/ Fall 1987): 11–12; Preston Holder, "The Fur Trade as Seen from the Indian Point of View," in *The Frontier Re-examined*, ed. John Francis McDermott (Urbana: University of Illinois Press, 1967), 133. For an overview of the fur trade, see David J. Wishart, *The Fur Trade of the American West, 1807–1840: A Geographical Synthesis* (Lincoln: University of Nebraska Press, 1979).

25. Henry Fontenelle, letter, January 20, 1891, in J. A. MacMurphy, "Some Frenchmen of Early Days on the Missouri River," in *Transactions and Reports of the Nebraska State Historical Society* 5 (1893): 54; Maximilian, *Travels*, 266.

26. Norma Kidd Green, *Iron Eye's Family: The Children of Joseph La Flesche* (Lincoln: Nebraska State Historical Society, 1969), 2–4; Dorsey, *Omaha Sociology*, 255–56; Fontenelle, letter in MacMurphy, "Some Frenchmen," 54; R. H. Barnes, "A Legacy of Misperception and Invention: The Omaha Indians in Anthropology," in *The Invented Indian: Cultural Fictions and Government Policies*, ed. James A. Clifton (New Brunswick: Transaction Publishers, 1990), 219–20.

27. "Joseph La Flesche," *Talks and Thoughts* (October 1889): 3, SAF-HUA; "Joseph La Flesche," *The Bulletin* 1 (January 1889): 3; Fletcher and La Flesche, *Omaha Tribe*, 63.

28. John Ewers, "Intertribal Warfare as the Precursor of Indian-White Warfare on the Northern Great Plains," *Western Historical Quarterly* 6 (October 1975): 407; Paul Wilhelm, *Travels*, 337.

29. Bert Anson, "Variations of the Indian Conflict: The Effects of the Emigrant Indian Removal Policy, 1830–1854," *Missouri Historical Review* 59 (October 1964): 72–75; Schilz and Schilz, "Beads, Bangles," 18–19.

30. Quote in Wishart, *Unspeakable Sadness*, 77; Wishart, *Fur Trade*, 66–67.

31. White, *Roots of Dependency*, 192; Ray H. Mattison, "The Indian Frontier on the Upper Missouri to 1865," *Nebraska History* 39 (September 1958): 248; John Dougherty, "A Description of the Fur Trade in 1831 by John Dougherty," ed. Richard E. Jensen, *Nebraska History* 56 (Spring 1975): 114, 117.

32. Fletcher and La Flesche, *Omaha Tribe*, 631–32.

33. Roger L. Nichols, ed., *The Missouri Expedition, 1818–1820: The Journal of Surgeon John Gale with Related Documents* (Norman: University of Oklahoma Press, 1969), x–xi; H. Winnett Orr, *Selected Pages from the History of Medicine in Nebraska* (Lincoln: n.p., 1952), 11.

34. Nichols, *Missouri Expedition*, x–xi; Green, *Iron Eye's Family*, 5.

35. Green, *Iron Eye's Family*, 5; David D. Smits, "'Squaw Men,' 'Half-Breeds,' and Amalgamators: Late Nineteenth-Century Anglo-American Attitudes Toward Indian-White Race-Mixing," *American Indian Culture and Research Journal* 15, no. 3 (1991): 56; Sherry L. Smith, *The View from Officers' Row* (Tucson: University of Arizona Press, 1990), 58–64, 87, 90.

36. Irving S. Cutter, *Dr. John Gale, A Pioneer Army Surgeon* (Springfield, Ill.: Schnepp & Barnes, 1931), 11.

37. S. D. Bangs, "History of Sarpy County," in *Transactions and Reports of the Nebraska State Historical Society* (Lincoln: State Journal, 1887), 2: 300.

38. Green, *Iron Eye's Family*, 5; "Mary Gale La Flesche," *WT*, March 5, 1909; MacMurphy, "Some Frenchmen," 52–53; Joan Mark, *A Stranger in*

Her Native Land: Alice Fletcher and the American Indians (Lincoln: University of Nebraska Press, 1984), 125; John Ewers, "Mothers of Mixed Bloods: The Marginal Women in the History of the Upper Missouri," in *Probing the American West: Papers from the Santa Fe Conference*, ed. K. Ross Toole (Santa Fe: Museum of New Mexico Press, 1962), 69.

39. "Glimpses of a Woman's Work"; Janis Chapman Thorne, "People of the River: Mixed Blood Families on the Lower Missouri" (Ph.D. diss., University of California, Los Angeles, 1987), 302.

40. Thorne, "People of the River," 387–92; Alice C. Fletcher, "Obituary Notice," *Journal of American Folklore* 2 (January/March 1889): 11; Fletcher and La Flesche, *Omaha Tribe*, 632. For an overview of the Métis people, see Jacqueline Peterson and Jennifer S. H. Brown, ed., *The New Peoples: Being and Becoming Métis in North America*, (Lincoln: University of Nebraska Press, 1985).

41. O'Shea and Ludwickson, "Omaha Chieftainship," 330, 338–39.

42. Fletcher and La Flesche, *Omaha Tribe*, 622–23; Smith, *Omaha Indians*, 116–19; Charles J. Kappler, *Indian Affairs: Laws and Treaties*, 2 vols. (Washington, D.C.: Government Printing Office, 1904), 2:611–14; De Smet, *Life, Letters*, 1:200.

43. Joseph Jablow, *Ethnohistory of the Ponca* (New York: Garland Publishing, 1974), 261; Robert A. Trennert, Jr., *Alternative to Extinction: Federal Indian Policy and the Beginnings of the Reservation System, 1846–51* (Philadelphia: Temple University Press, 1975), 138; De Smet, *Life, Letters*, 3:1188; Wishart, *Unspeakable Sadness*, 87.

44. 0'Shea and Ludwickson, "Omaha Chieftainship," 338–39; Wishart, *Unspeakable Sadness*, 78; Fletcher and La Flesche, *Omaha Tribe*, 83–84; U.S. Commissioner of Indian Affairs, *Annual Report of the Commissioner of Indian Affairs to the Secretary of the Interior* [hereafter CIA, *AR*], 1845, 12–13.

45. "Joseph La Flesche"; Fletcher and La Flesche, *Omaha Tribe*, 638.

46. See Trennert, *Alternative to Extinction*. For the "Great American Desert" myth, see Henry Nash Smith, *Virgin Land: The American West as Symbol and Myth* (New York: Vintage Books, 1950), 201–26.

47. Jeri Ferris, *Native American Doctor: The Story of Susan La Flesche Picotte* (Minneapolis: Carolrhoda Books, 1991), 45.

48. CIA, *AR*, 1856, 103–105; see also, CIA, *AR*, 1857, 149–50. Initially the Omahas harbored serious trepidations about moving to this new land because it was so exposed to Sioux attacks. They accepted the terms of the treaty of 1854 only when the federal government promised to offer military protection from the Sioux. But the government never delivered on the promise.

49. Norma Kidd Green, "The Make-Believe White Man's Village," *Nebraska History* 56 (Summer 1975): 243–44.

50. Senate, *Memorial of the Members of the Omaha Tribe of Indians for a Grant of Land in Severalty*, S. Misc. Doc. 31, 47th Cong., 1st sess., 1882, serial 1993, 7; Green, "Make-Believe," 243–44; Rebecca Hancock Welch, "Alice Cunningham Fletcher, Anthropologist and Indian Rights Reformer" (Ph.D. diss, George Washington University, 1980), 61.

51. Norma Kidd Green, "The Presbyterian Mission to the Omaha Indian Tribe," *Nebraska History* 48 (Autumn 1967): 269; "Presbyterian Mission to the Omahas," Melvin R. Gilmore Papers, NSHS.

52. For discussion of these accounts, see Gary C. Stein, "A Fearful Drunkenness: The Liquor Trade to the Western Indians as Seen by European Travelers in America, 1800–1860," *Red River Valley Historical Review* 1 (Summer 1974): 109–21; Allan M. Winkler, "Drinking on the American Frontier," *Quarterly Journal of Studies on Alcohol* 29, no. 6 (1968): 413–45.

53. Green, *Iron Eye's Family*, 24; Fletcher and La Flesche, *Omaha Tribe*, 618–19.

54. "An Indian Chief's Crusade for Temperance," *The Indian School Journal* 9 (March 1909): 35.

55. CIA, *AR*, 1855, 86–87; Burtt to Walter Lowrie, June 6, 1860 and July 18, 1861, "Presbyterian Missionary Letters Relating to the American Indians in Nebraska Country," PHS; William T. Hagan, *Indian Police and Judges: Experiments in Acculturation and Control* (New Haven: Yale University Press, 1966), 14; Melvin R. Gilmore, "First Prohibition Law in America," *Journal of American History* 4 (July/September 1910): 397.

56. Clyde A. Milner II, *With Good Intentions: Quaker Work among the Pawnees, Otos, and Omahas in the 1870s* (Lincoln: University of Nebraska Press, 1982), 182.

57. Wishart, *Unspeakable Sadness*, 124; Fletcher and La Flesche, *Omaha Tribe*, 633.

58. Burt to Lowrie, July 18, 1861, "Presbyterian Missionary Letters"; CIA, *AR*, 1861, 62–65; CIA, *AR*, 1863, 236.

59. Robert C. Farb, "Robert C. Furnas as Omaha Indian Agent, 1864–1866," *Nebraska History* 32 (September 1951): 189–90.

60. CIA, *AR*, 1881, 188.

61. Robert S. Gardner to CIA, June 28, 1884, *Reports of Inspection of the Field Jurisdictions of the Office of Indian Affairs, 1873–1900*, [hereafter *RIFJ*] Record Group 75, Bureau of Indian Affairs, M1016, reel 32, Report 2910, National Archives and Records Service, Washington, D.C. [hereafter

RG 75, BIA, NA]. See also Samuel S. Benedict to CIA, March 5, 1883, *RIFJ*; Matthew R. Barr to CIA, January 10, 1884, *RIFJ*; CIA, *AR*, 1889, 239.

62. Szasz, "Conclusion," 294–300; Clifton, "Alternate Identities," 24.

CHAPTER 2. "FOR THE DELIGHT OF THOSE DAYS"

1. "Letterbox," 918.

2. Ibid.

3. See Francis Paul Prucha, *American Indian Policy in Crisis: Christian Reformers and the Indian, 1865–1900* (Norman: University of Oklahoma Press, 1976); Margaret Connell Szasz, *Education and the American Indian: The Road to Self-Determination since 1928* (Albuquerque: University of New Mexico Press, 1977).

4. SLF, "The Home Life of the Indian," *The Indian's Friend* 4 (June 1892): 40.

5. Fletcher and La Flesche, *Omaha Tribe*, 327.

6. Questionnaire, November, 1888, SAF-HUA; Cuming County, "Nebraska Marriages, Book V, 1894–1898," 2, NSHS.

7. CIA, *AR*, 1864, 349–52; Robert W. Furnas to CIA, December 3, 1865, *Letters Received by the Indian Office, 1824–1881*, Omaha Agency, 1864–1870 [hereafter *LR*-OA], Record Group 75, Bureau of Indian Affairs, M234, reel 605, RG 75, BIA, NA; William Callon to Superintendent Denman, June 30, 1868, *LR*-OA; see also CIA, *AR*, 1868, 697, 700; CIA, *AR*, 1869, 187.

8. Fletcher and La Flesche, *Omaha Tribe*, 635; Milner, *With Good Intentions*, 158–59.

9. Addison E. Sheldon, *Land Systems and Land Policies in Nebraska*, Publications of the Nebraska State Historical Society, vol. 22 (Lincoln: Nebraska State Historical Society, 1936), 75–93.

10. Kappler, *Indian Affairs*, 2:872.

11. Robin Ridington, "Omaha Survival: A Vanishing Indian Tribe that Would Not Vanish," *The American Indian Quarterly* 11 (Winter 1987): 38.

12. Furnas to CIA, February 28, 1866, December 30, 1865, *LR*-OA; Furnas to Walter Lowrie, May 5, 1866, American Indian Correspondence, 1833–1893 [hereafter AIC], PHS, Box A, vol. 1, letter 371.

13. Farb, "Robert W. Furnas," 186–96; CIA to Furnas, June 18, 1864, Robert W. Furnas Papers, NSHS.

14. CIA to Dennis N. Conley, March 27, 1866, *LR*-OA; S. Orlando Lee to Walter Lowrie, April 18, 1866, AIC, Box A, vol. 1, letter 64; Green, *Iron Eye's Family*, 36; Milner, *With Good Intentions*, 159.

15. Fletcher and La Flesche, *Omaha Tribe*, 634; Kristin Herzog, "The La Flesche Family: Native American Spirituality, Calvinism, and Presbyterian Missions," *American Presbyterians* 65 (Fall 1987): 224–25.

16. Alice C. Fletcher, "Glimpses of Child-Life among the Omaha Tribe of Indians," *Journal of American Folklore* 1 (July/September 1888): 115–16; Olson, *Book of the Omaha*, 5.

17. Fletcher and La Flesche, *Omaha Tribe*, 634; Ridington, "Omaha Survival," 40–41; Robin Ridington, "Images of Cosmic Union: Omaha Ceremonies of Renewal," *History of Religions* 28 (November 1978): 145.

18. Fletcher and La Flesche, *Omaha Tribe*, 226, 404–6; "Glimpses of a Woman's Work."

19. Margaret Connell Szasz, "Native American Children," in *American Childhood: A Research Guide and Historical Handbook*, ed. Joseph M. Hawes and N. Ray Hiner (Westport, Conn.: Greenwood Press, 1985), 314, 323; David H. DeJong, *Promises of the Past: A History of Indian Education in the United States* (Golden, Colo.: North American Press, 1993), 5, 10.

20. Fletcher and La Flesche, *Omaha Tribe*, 330; SLF, "My Childhood and Womanhood," *Southern Workman* [hereafter SW] 15 (July 1886): 78; Fletcher and La Flesche, *Omaha Tribe*, 330; Dorsey, *Omaha Sociology*, 265; Marguerite La Flesche, "Some Indian Customs: Commencement Address of Marguerite La Flesche," *SW* 16 (August 1887): 88; for an early nineteenth-century eyewitness account of Omaha children's work see James, *Account*, 1:239. For more on the centrality of work in defining Indian self-identity, see Klein and Ackerman, "Introduction," 3–16; Anderson, *Changing Woman*, 22.

21. SLF, "My Childhood," 78.

22. Fletcher and La Flesche, *Omaha Tribe*, 326; Alice C. Fletcher, "The Indian Woman and Her Problems," *SW*, 28 (May 1899): 174; Dorsey, *Omaha Sociology*, 266–67. For examples of other tribes exhibiting the same pattern, see Devens, *Countering Civilization*; Laura F. Klein, "'She's One of Us, You Know,' The Public Life of Tlingit Women: Traditional, Historical, and Contemporary Perspectives," *The Western Canadian Journal of Anthropology* 6, no. 3 (1976): 164–183; Victoria D. Patterson, "Evolving Gender Roles in Pomo Society," in *Women and Power in Native North America*, ed. Laura F. Klein and Lillian A. Ackerman (Norman: University of Oklahoma Press, 1995), 126–45.

23. Alice C. Fletcher, "Glimpses of Indian Child Life," *The Outlook*, May 16, 1896, 892.

24. Fannie Reed Giffen, *Oo-Ma-Ha-Ta-Wa-Tha (Omaha City)* (Lincoln: n.p., 1898), 32; Ferris, *Native American Doctor*, 18.

25. Dorsey, *Omaha Sociology*, 1266.

26. SLF, "My Childhood," 78; Susette La Flesche, "Nedawi," *St. Nicholas Magazine* 8 (January 1881): 228; Fletcher, "Glimpses of Indian Child Life," 892.

27. Fletcher, "Glimpses of Child-Life," 119, 123.

28. SLF, "The Dance of the Turkey," LFP-NSHS; Fletcher, "Glimpses of Child-Life," 123.

29. SLF, "My Childhood," 78; Fletcher, "Glimpses of Indian Child-Life," 890.

30. SLF, "An Indian Mud Lodge: A Peculiar Home," *The Indian Helper*, June 17, 1892, 4.

31. Fletcher, "Glimpses of Indian Child Life," 892.

32. SLF, "Home Life of the Indian," 39.

33. James Owen Dorsey, *Omaha and Ponka Letters*, Bureau of American Ethnology Bulletin 11, Smithsonian Institution (Washington, D.C.: Government Printing Office, 1891), 65–69; Fletcher and La Flesche, *Omaha Tribe*, 70–71, 608–10; Evers, "Literature of the Omahas," 19, 54, 56.

34. Dorsey, *Omaha and Ponka Letters*, 65–69.

35. "Mary La Flesche," *WT*, March 5, 1909; "Joseph La Flesche," *SW* 17 (December 1888): 127; SLF, "My Childhood," 78.

36. Norma Kidd Green, "Four Sisters: Daughters of Joseph La Flesche," *Nebraska History* 45 (June 1964): 173; CIA, *AR*, 1868, 702.

37. Kappler, *Indian Affairs*, 614; Hamilton to Walter Lowrie, December 9, 1856, "Presbyterian Missionary Letters," PHS. See also *Historical Sketch of the Missions* (Philadelphia: Women's Board of Home Missions, 1891), 178.

38. Michael C. Coleman, *Presbyterian Missionary Attitudes toward American Indians, 1837–1893* (Jackson: University Press of Mississippi, 1985), 43–45, 147; Robert F. Berkhofer, Jr., *Salvation and Savage: An Analysis of Protestant Missions and American Indian Response, 1787–1862* (Lexington: University Press of Kentucky, 1965), 4–7, 34.

39. Coleman, *Presbyterian Missionary Attitudes*, 17.

40. Michael C. Coleman, "Not Race, but Grace: Presbyterian Missionaries and American Indians, 1837–1893," *Journal of American History* 67 (June 1980): 42, 57, 59; Hamilton to John C. Lowrie, February 1, 1868, typescript, PHS.

41. I. R. Rolph to Walter Lowrie, October 21, 1857, AIC, Box 4, vol. 2.

42. Coleman, *Presbyterian Missionary Attitudes*, 94–96.

43. Barbara Welter, "The Cult of True Womanhood, 1820–1860," *American Quarterly* 18 (Summer 1966): 151–74; Nancy Cott, *The Bonds of Womanhood: "Woman's Sphere" in New England, 1780–1835* (New Haven: Yale University Press, 1987), 69, 71, 195; Kathryn Kish Sklar, *Catharine Beecher: A Study in American Domesticity* (New York: W. W. Norton, 1973), 156, 161, 163–64. For critiques on the prescriptive nature of domestic ideology see Elizabeth Jameson, "Women as Workers, Women as Civilizers: True Womanhood in the American West," in *The Women's West*, ed. Susan Armitage and Elizabeth Jameson (Norman: University of Oklahoma Press, 1987), 145–64; Nancy A. Hewitt, "Beyond the Search for Sisterhood: American Women's History in the 1980s," in *Unequal Sisters: A Multicultural Reader in U.S. Women's History*, 2d ed., ed. Vicki L. Ruiz and Ellen Carol Dubois (New York: Routledge, 1994), 1–19; Robert L. Griswold, "Anglo Women and Domestic Ideology in the American West in the Nineteenth and Early Twentieth Centuries," in *Western Women: Their Land, Their Lives*, ed. Lillian Schlissel, Vicki L. Ruiz, and Janice Monk (Albuquerque: University of New Mexico Press, 1988), 15–34; Kerber, "Separate Spheres," 9–39; Susan M. Reverby and Dorothy O. Helly, "Introduction: Converging on History," in *Gendered Domains: Rethinking Public and Private in Women's History*, ed. Dorothy O. Helly and Susan M. Reverby (Ithaca, N.Y.: Cornell University Press, 1992), 1–26.

44. Reverby and Helly, "Introduction," 1–26.

45. Ray H. Mattison, "Indian Missions and Missionaries on the Upper Missouri to 1900," *Nebraska History* 38 (June 1957): 136; Phillips G. Davies, "Davis Jones and Gwen Davies, Missionaries in Nebraska Territory, 1853–1860," *Nebraska History* 60 (Spring 1979): 83.

46. "Quaker Report on Indian Agencies in Nebraska, 1869," *Nebraska History* 54 (Summer 1973): 182; Hamilton to E.S. Painter, October 17, 1869, AIC, Box B, vol. 1, letter 220; Hamilton to John C. Lowrie, February 3, 1869, AIC, Box B, vol. 1, letter 153; Davies, "Davis Jones," 83.

47. Hamilton to John C. Lowrie, February 1, 1868, typescript.

48. Hamilton to John C. Lowrie, August 20, 1869, AIC, Box B, vol. 1, letter 204; "Quaker Report," 182.

49. Hamilton to Edward Painter, September 7, 1869, AIC, Box B, vol. 1, letter 175; CIA, *AR*, 1888, 702.

50. Hamilton to Painter, October 17, 1869, AIC, Box B, vol. 1, letter 229.

51. CIA, *AR*, 1868, 503.

52. Francis Paul Prucha, *The Great Father: The United States Government and the American Indians*, 2 vols. (Lincoln: University of Nebraska Press, 1984), 2:490–500.

53. Ibid.

54. For more on Grant's Peace Policy, see Robert M. Utley, "The Celebrated Peace Policy of General Grant," *North Dakota History* 20 (1953): 121–42; Henry E. Fritz, *The Movement for Indian Assimilation, 1860–1890* (Philadelphia: University of Pennsylvania Press, 1963), 72–86; Robert H. Keller, Jr., *American Protestantism and United States Indian Policy, 1869–82* (Lincoln: University of Nebraska Press, 1983), 26, 28.

55. Fritz, *Movement for Indian Assimilation*, 72.

56. Milner, *With Good Intentions*, 15–16.

57. Prucha, *Great Father*, 2:523–24; James L. Sellers, ed., "Diary of Dr. Joseph A. Paxson, Physician to the Winnebago Indians, 1869–1870," *Nebraska History* 27 (July/September 1946): 180, 182; Hamilton to John C. Lowrie, February 24, 1869, AIC, Box B, vol. 1, letter 161; Hamilton to Painter, October 17, 1869, AIC, Box B, vol. 1, letter 220.

58. Hamilton to John C. Lowrie, February 3, 1869, AIC, Box B, vol. 1, letter 153; CIA, *AR*, 1869, 472; CIA, *AR*, 1868, 687–88; Hamilton to John C. Lowrie, February 24, 1869, AIC, Box B, vol. 1, letter 161; Hamilton to John C. Lowrie, February 16, 1869, AIC, Box B, vol. 1, letter 158.

59. Hamilton to Painter, September 7, 1869, AIC, Box B, vol. 1, letter 175; Hamilton to John C. Lowrie, September 28, 1869, AIC, Box B, vol. 1, letter 184; Keller, *American Protestantism*, 48.

60. Norma Kidd Green, "The Presbyterian Mission," 280; Board of Foreign Missions of the Presbyterian Church in the U.S.A., *Thirty-Third Annual Report of the Board of Foreign Missions of the Presbyterian Church in the United States of America* (New York: Board of Foreign Missions, 1870), 13.

61. Orrin C. Painter, *William Painter and His Father, Dr. Edward Painter: Sketches and Reminiscences* (Baltimore: Arundel Press, 1914), 138; SLF, "My Childhood," 78.

62. "Letterbox," 918; CIA, *AR*, 1871, 863; SLF, "My Childhood," 78; CIA, *AR*, 1870, 252; E.C. Kemble to CIA, November 4, 1874, *RIFJ*.

63. "Glimpses of a Woman's Work"; SLF, "My Childhood," 79.

64. Milner, *With Good Intentions*, 8–9, 21; Hamilton to John C. Lowrie, February 5, 1878, AIC, Box E, vol. 1, letter 12.

65. For parallels between the Presbyterian faith and Omaha religion, see Herzog, "La Flesche Family," 230.

66. CIA, *AR*, 1877, 540; Joseph La Flesche to John C. Lowrie, September 16, 1879, AIC, Box E, vol. 1, letter 212; Dorsey, *Omaha and Ponka Letters*, 36.

67. Hamilton to John C. Lowrie, September 10, 1879, AIC, Box E, vol. 1, letter 210; Fritz, *Movement for Indian Assimilation*, 136.

68. Margaret Crary, *Susette La Flesche: Voice of the Omaha Indians* (New York: Hawthorn Books, 1973), 140–41; Milner, *With Good Intentions*, 174.

69. James T. King, "A Better Way: General George Crook and the Ponca Indians," *Nebraska History* 50 (Fall 1969): 239–55; see also Thomas H. Tibbles, *Buckskin and Blanket Days: Memoirs of a Friend of the Indians*, ed. Theodora Bates Cogswell (Garden City, N.Y.: Doubleday, 1957), 193–235.

70. Green, *Iron Eye's Family*, 62, 76; Rayna Green, "The Pocahontas Perplex: The Image of the Indian Woman in American Culture," *Massachusetts Review* 16 (1975): 698–714; see also Glenda Riley, "Some European (Mis)perceptions of American Indian Women," *New Mexico Historical Review* 59 (July 1984): 237–66.

71. *The City of Elizabeth, New Jersey Illustrated* (Elizabeth, N.J.: Elizabeth Daily Journal, 1889), 107; Elias D. Smith, *The School Interests of Elizabeth, A City of New Jersey, U.S.A.* (Elizabeth, N.J.: n.p., 1911), 71–72; Green, *Iron Eye's Family*, 122–23.

72. Milner, *With Good Intentions*, 159–61; Mark, *Stranger*, 69–70; Jacob Vore to CIA, January 16, 1878, *Letters Received by the Indian Office, 1824–1881*, Nebraska Agencies, 1876–1880, RG 75, BIA, microfilm 234, reel 524, NA; CIA, *AR*, 1873.

73. Wilcomb E. Washburn, *The Assault on Indian Tribalism: The General Allotment Law (Dawes Act) of 1887*, ed. Harold H. Hyman (Philadelphia: Lippincott, 1975), 11.

74. Mark, *Stranger*, 74–75; Nancy Oestreich Lurie, "The Lady from Boston and the Omaha Indians," *American West* 3 (Fall 1966), 31–33, 80–85; Alice C. Fletcher, "Preparation of Indians for Citizenship," *SW* 34 (August 1905): 425–28; Welch, "Alice Cunningham Fletcher, 82, 126–27.

75. Alice C. Fletcher, "Lands in Severalty to Indians; Illustrated by Experiences with the Omaha Tribe," *Proceedings of the American Association for the Advancement of Science* 33 (1884): 665; Francis La Flesche, "Protection of Indian Lands," in *Report of the Annual Mohonk Conference on the Indian and Other Dependent Peoples* (Mohonk Lake, N.Y.: The Conference, 1914–1916), 70; CIA, *AR*, 1882, 172–73; see U.S. Senate Miscellaneous Document, *Memorial of the Members of the Omaha Tribe*, 1, 14 for another similar petition.

76. CIA, *AR*, 1882, 4; Delos Socket Otis, *The Dawes Act and the Allotment of Indian Lands*, ed. Francis Paul Prucha (Norman: University of Oklahoma Press, 1973), 8; Janet A. McDonnell, *The Dispossession of the American Indian, 1887–1934* (Bloomington: Indiana University Press, 1991), 42.

77. Mark, *Stranger*, 88–90.

78. *Historical Sketch of the Missions*, 179; Questionnaire, SAF-HUA; Robert S. Gardner to CIA, June 28, 1884, *RIFJ*, Report 2910; Charles Howard to Secretary of Interior, October 14, 1881, *RIFJ*, Report 2681; James A. Haworth to Secretary of Interior, December 29, 1882, *RIFJ*, Report 144; CIA, *AR*, 1882, 173; CIA, *AR*, 1883, 164.

79. Mark, *Stranger*, 90, 125; Welch, "Alice Cunningham Fletcher," 123; Alice C. Fletcher, "The Preparation of the Indian for Citizenship," *Lend a Hand* 9 (September 1892): 197.

80. Philip Gleason, "American Identity and Americanization," in *Harvard Encyclopedia of American Ethnic Groups*, ed. Stephen Thernstrom (Cambridge, Mass.: Belknap Press, 1980), 31–58.

81. Richard Hofstatder, *Social Darwinism in American Thought*, rev. ed. (New York: George Braziller, 1959), 51–66; Brian W. Dippie, *The Vanishing American: White Attitudes and U.S. Indian Policy* (Lawrence: University Press of Kansas, 1982), 102–106, 170–71.

82. "Glimpses of a Woman's Work."

CHAPTER 3. "HOME IS THE FOUNDATION"

1. SLF to RF, undated, LFP-NSHS; SLF to "My Dear Girls," undated, LFP-NSHS.

2. The first American Indian to be admitted into Hampton Institute was Peter Johnson, a Ute Indian who arrived in the fall of 1877 but only stayed for about twelve months. See Donal F. Lindsey, *Indians at Hampton Institute, 1877–1923* (Urbana: University of Illinois Press, 1995). Samuel Chapman Armstrong, *Indian Education in the East: At Hampton, Va. and Carlisle, Penn.* (Hampton, Va.: Normal School Steam Press, 1880), 1; Prucha, *Great Father*, 2:687–700.

3. Richard H. Pratt, *Battlefield and Classroom: Four Decades with the American Indian, 1867–1904*, ed. Robert M. Utley (New Haven, Conn.: Yale University Press, 1964), 215; William N. Hailmann, *Education of the Indian*, Monographs on Education in the U.S., no. 19 (St. Louis: Division of Exhibits, Department of Education, Universal Exposition, 1904), 9; Hampton Institute, *Ten Years' Work for Indians at Hampton, Virginia, 1878–1888* (Hampton, Va.: Hampton Institute Press, 1888), 12; Hampton Institute, *Twenty-Two Years' Work of the Hampton Normal and Agricultural Institute at Hampton, Virginia, Record of Negro and Indian Graduates and Ex-Students* (Hampton, Va.: Normal School Press, 1893), 241; *SW* 15 (March 1886): 25.

4. *SW* 13 (September 1884): 99; Armstrong, "Annual Report," in CIA, *AR,* 1884, 237; Armstrong, "Annual Report," in CIA, *AR,* 1885, 463.

5. SLF to Miss Richards, August 7, 1885, SAF-HUA; *SW* 15 (March 1886): 32; Armstrong, "Annual Report," in CIA, *AR,* 1885, 472; SLF, letter, December 19, 1887, in Hampton Institute, *Ten Years' Work,* 56; Armstrong, "Annual Report," *SW* 14 (June 1885): 75; Hampton Institute, *Concerning Indians* (Hampton, Va.: Normal School Steam Press, 1883), 21; K. Tsianina Lomawaima, *They Called it Prairie Light: The Story of Chilocco Indian School* (Lincoln: University of Nebraska Press, 1994), xiv, 131.

6. Armstrong, "Annual Report," *SW* 13 (October 1884): 111; SLF, letter, December 19, 1887, in Hampton Institute, *Ten Year's Work,* 56; Samuel Chapman Armstrong, *The Ideas on Education Expressed by Samuel C. Armstrong* (Hampton: For the Armstrong League of Hampton Workers by the Hampton Institute Press, 1909), 3, 5, 34; Edith Armstrong Talbot, *Samuel Chapman Armstrong: A Biographical Study* (New York: Doubleday, Page, 1904), 211, 213–14, 277; *SW* 9 (February 1880): 38; Francis Greenwood Peabody, *Education for Life: The Story of Hampton Institute* (Garden City, N.Y.: Doubleday, 1919), 154.

7. Armstrong, *Ideas,* 30; Hampton Institute, *Twenty-Two Years' Work,* 314. For an analysis of gender-based acculturation in Indian schools, see K. Tsianina Lomawaima, "Domesticity in the Federal Indian Schools: The Power of Authority over Mind and Body," *American Ethnologist* 20 (May 1993): 227–40 and also Robert A. Trennert, "Educating Indian Girls at Non-reservation Boarding Schools, 1878–1920," *Western Historical Quarterly* 13 (July 1982), 271–90.

8. Samuel Chapman Armstrong, "Education of the Indian," *The Journal of Proceedings and Addresses of the National Education Association* (1884): 177; Samuel Chapman Armstrong, *Annual Report of the Principal to the Board of Trustees, 1891* (Hampton, Va.: Hampton Institute Press, 1891): 6; Armstrong, *Indian Education,* 2, 4; Armstrong, "Annual Report," *SW* 20 (1891): 195; Samuel Chapman Armstrong, *The Indian Question* (Hampton, Va.: Normal School Steam Press, 1883), 15.

9. Carolyn L. Attneave and Agnes Dill, "Indian Boarding Schools and Indian Women: Blessing or Curse?," in *Proceedings of the Conference on the Educational and Occupational Needs of American Indian Women* (Washington, D.C.: Government Printing Office, 1976), 213; David Wallace Adams, "The Federal Indian Boarding School: A Study of Environment and Response" (Ph.D. diss., Indiana University, 1975), 46–47; Lindsey, *Indians at Hampton,* 9, 182; Lomawaima, "Domesticity in the Federal Indian Schools," 228–29.

10. Prucha, *Great Father*, 2:690; Armstrong, "Annual Report," in CIA, *AR*, 1885, 465; Lindsey, *Indians at Hampton*, 183–84; Dippie, *Vanishing American*, 115–16.

11. *SW* 14 (January 1885): 8; *SW* 14 (July 1885): 82; *SW* 14 (May 1885): 56; *SW* 15 (April 1886): 44.

12. Armstrong, "Annual Report," *SW* 14 (June 1885): 66; SLF, letter, December 19, 1887, in Hampton Institute, *Ten Year's Work*, 56; Chapman, "Annual Report," *SW* 14 (June 1885): 75; *SW* 14 (April 1885): 44; Lindsey, *Indians at Hampton*, 134; SLF, diary, January 17, 1911, LFP-NSHS.

13. SLF, letter, December 19, 1887, in Hampton Institute, *Ten Year's Work*, 56; SLF to Miss Richards, August 7, 1885, SAF-HUA.

14. The full name of Susan's classmate Sam is unknown. SLF to RF, undated, LFP-NSHS.

15. SLF, letter, December 19, 1887, in Hampton Institute, *Ten Years' Work*, 56.

16. Ibid.

17. For other examples, see David Wallace Adams, *Education for Extinction: American Indians and the Boarding School Experience, 1875–1928* (Lawrence: University Press of Kansas, 1995), 240, 256; Michael C. Coleman, "American Indian School Pupils as Cultural Brokers: Cherokee Girls at Brainerd Mission, 1828–1829," in *Between Indian and White Worlds: The Cultural Broker*, ed. Margaret Connell Szasz (Norman: University of Oklahoma Press, 1994), 127, 130–31. For more on the concept of cognitive dissonance or acculturation stress, see George D. Spindler, "Psychocultural Adaption," in *The Study of Personality: An Interdisciplinary Appraisal*, ed. Edward Norbeck, Douglas Price-Willams, and William M. McCord (New York: Holt, Rinehart, and Winston, 1968), 337–43; John Ogbu, "Cultural Discontinuities and Schooling," *Anthropology and Education Quarterly* 8 (December 1982): 290–307; Harry F. Wolcott, "The Teacher as an Enemy," in *Education and Cultural Process: Toward an Anthropology of Education*, ed. George D. Spindler (New York: Holt, Rinehart, and Winston, 1974), 411–25.

18. Ake Hultkranz, *Native Religions of North America: The Power of Visions and Fertility* (San Francisco: Harper & Row, 1987), 32; Adams, "Federal Indian Boarding School," 140.

19. Joseph Willard Tingey, "Blacks and Indians Together: An Experiment in Biracial Education at Hampton Institute (1878–1923)" (Ph.D. diss., Columbia Teacher's College, 1978), 157; Armstrong, "Annual Report," *SW* 15 (June 1886): 65; *SW* 14 (June 1885): 65, 67–68, 71.

20. *SW* 14 (June 1885): 65, 67–68, 71; SLF to Miss Richards, August 7, 1885, SAF-HUA; Tingey, "Blacks and Indians Together," 157.

21. Armstrong, "Annual Report," in CIA, *AR*, 1884, 236–37; Armstrong, "Annual Report," *SW* 15 (June 1885): 69; SLF to "My Dear Girls," undated, LFP-NSHS; *SW* 14 (November 1885): 109; Helen W. Ludlow, *Hampton Normal and Agricultural Institute: Its Work for Indians* (Springfield, Mass.: n.p., n.d.), 4; Armstrong, "Annual Report," *SW* 15 (June 1886): 65.

22. Armstrong, "Annual Report," in CIA, *AR*, 1885, 462; Hampton Institute, *The Hampton Normal and Agricultural Institute and its Work for Negro and Indian Youth* (Hampton, Va.: n.p., 1894), 4; Hampton Institute, *Concerning Indians*, 12–13; SLF to Miss Richards, August 7, 1885, SAF-HUA.

23. Josephine E. Richards to Alice C. Fletcher, March 3, 1886, Fletcher–La Flesche Papers, National Anthropological Archives, Smithsonian Institution, Washington, D.C. [hereafter FLP-NAA].

24. "Dr. Susan Picot, Indian Physician, Dead at Walthill," *WT*, September 18, 1915.

25. "Glimpses of a Woman's Work"; SLF to J. M. Gould, September 2, 1887, reprinted in "The Indian," Scrapbook 1, Sara Thomson Kinney Papers, Connecticut State Library, Hartford, Connecticut [hereafter STK-CSL].

26. "Glimpses of a Woman's Work"; SLF to J. M. Gould, September 2, 1887, reprinted in "The Indian," Scrapbook 1, STK-CSL.

27. "Connecticut Indian Association," *Hartford Courant*, June 25, 1886.

28. Senate, *Notes on the Returned Students of the Hampton Normal and Agricultural Institute*, S. Rept. Exec. Doc. 31, 52d Cong., 1st sess., 1892, serial 2892, 3–12; Trennert, "Educating Indian Girls," 289.

29. Trennert, "Educating Indian Girls," 287–88.

30. Valerie Sherer Mathes, "Native American Women in Medicine and the Military," *American Indian Quarterly* 2, no. 2 (1975): 42–43.

31. Alice C. Fletcher to SLF, April 24, 1886, SAF-HUA; Alice C. Fletcher, quote, in Valerie Mathes, "Portrait for a Western Album," *American West* 16 (May/June 1979): 39; Welch, "Alice Cunningham Fletcher," 52.

32. For more on Charles Eastman, see Raymond Wilson, *Ohiyesa: Charles Eastman, Santee Sioux* (Urbana: University of Illinois Press, 1983); for more on Carlos Montezuma, see Peter Iverson, *Carlos Montezuma and the Changing World of American Indians* (Albuquerque: University of New Mexico Press, 1982); John Duffy, *From Humors to Medical Science: A History of American Medicine* (Urbana: University of Illinois Press, 1993), 294.

33. Mary Roth Walsh, *"Doctors Wanted: No Women Need Apply": Sexual Barriers in the Medical Profession, 1835–1975* (New Haven: Yale University Press, 1977), xii, 1–9; Duffy, *From Humors to Medical Science*, 46; for the early history of the Woman's Medical College of Pennsylvania,

see Clara Marshall, *The Woman's Medical College of Pennsylvania: An Historical Outline* (Philadelphia: P. Blakiston, Son, 1897).

34. Walsh, *"Doctors Wanted,"* 72; Virginia G. Drachman, "Women Doctors and the Women's Medical Movement: Feminism and Medicine, 1850–1895" (Ph.D. diss., State University of New York at Buffalo, 1976), 30, 32; Richard H. Shyrock, *Medicine in America: Historical Essays* (Baltimore: Johns Hopkins University Press, 1966), 176.

35. Shyrock, Medicine in America, 183; Regina M. Morantz-Sanchez, *Sympathy and Science: Women Physicians in American Medicine* (New York: Oxford University Press, 1985), 51, 54; Walsh, *"Doctors Wanted,"* 8–9, 133–34; Regina Morantz-Sanchez, "The Female Student Has Arrived: The Rise of the Women's Medical Movement," in *"Send Us a Lady Physician": Women Doctors in America, 1835–1920,* ed. Ruth J. Abram (New York: W. W. Norton, 1985), 63–64.

36. Morantz-Sanchez, "The Female Student Has Arrived," 63–64; Morantz-Sanchez, *Sympathy and Science,* 54; Rosalind Rosenberg, *Beyond Separate Spheres: Intellectual Roots of Modern Feminism* (New Haven: University of Yale Press, 1982), xv, 5–7, 11; Ruth J. Abram, "Will There Be a Monument?: Six Pioneer Women Doctors Tell Their Own Stories," in *"Send Us a Lady Physician,"* 100; Duffy, *From Humors to Medical Science,* 289; Walsh, *"Doctors Wanted,"* 133–34.

37. Walsh, *"Doctors Wanted,"* xvi.

38. Marshall, *Woman's Medical College,* 46–47.

39. Morantz-Sanchez, "The Female Student Has Arrived," 60–61.

40. Rosenberg, *Beyond Separate Spheres,* 14–17.

41. Biographical sketch, Martha M. Waldron Papers, HUA; Martha M. Waldron, "The Indian Health Question," *Lend a Hand* 5 (November 1890): 773.

42. Alfred Jones to Martha M. Waldron, March 26, 1886, FLP-NAA. See also *Thirty-Seventh Annual Announcement of the Woman's Medical College of Pennsylvania* (Philadelphia: n.p., 1886), 17.

43. Fletcher to SLF, April 24, 1886.

44. For the history of the Women's National Indian Association, see Helen M. Wanken, "Woman's Sphere and Indian Reform: The Women's National Indian Association, 1875–1901" (Ph.D. diss., Marquette University, 1981); for the early years of the Connecticut Indian Association, see Ellen Terry Johnson, *Historical Sketch of the Connecticut Indian Association from 1881 to 1888* (Hartford: Fowler & Miller, 1888); see also "Fifteen Years of Work," *The Indian Bulletin* [hereafter *IB*] 10 (December 1896): 5–6; "Wisdom from Hartford," *SW* 17 (March 1888): 33.

45. For a definition of "maternalism," see Linda Gordon, "Putting Children First: Women, Maternalism, and Welfare in the Early Twentieth Century," in *U.S. History as Women's History: New Feminist Essays*, ed. Linda K. Kerber, Alice Kessler-Harris, and Kathryn Kish Sklar (Chapel Hill: University of North Carolina Press, 1995), 65.

46. Wanken, "Woman's Sphere," 65, 74–75; Laurence M. Hauptman, "Medicine Woman: Susan La Flesche, 1865–1915," *New York State Journal of Medicine* 78 (September 1978): 1784; *IB*, December 1891, 2.

47. Fletcher to SLF, April 24, 1886, SLF-HUA.

48. "Eighteenth Anniversary of Hampton Institute," *SW* 15 (June 1886): 73; Alice C. Fletcher to RF, May 21, 1886, LFP-NSHS.

49. "Connecticut Indian Association," *Hartford Courant*, June 25, 1886; Samuel Chapman Armstrong to CIA, August 20, 1886, Letters Received by the Indian Office, 1881–1907, [hereafter Letters Received] RG 75, BIA, File 2250, Fletcher to RF, May 21, 1886, LFP-NSHS.

50. SLF, "My Childhood," 78.

51. Ibid.; *SW* 15 (April 1886): 37; U.S. House, *Congressional Record* 17, part 4 (March 10, 1886), 2264–66 and (March 17, 1886), 2464; see also Armstrong, *Indian Question*, 17.

52. SLF, "My Childhood," 78.

53. Ibid., 79.

54. Ibid.

55. Ibid.

56. Fletcher to RF, May 21, 1886, LFP-NSHS; "Eighteenth Anniversary," *SW* 15 (June 1886): 73.

57. "Report of Meeting of May 21st, 1886, Minute Book 1, Box 3, STK-CSL; Sara Thomson Kinney to Miss Richards, May 14, 1886, SAF-HUA; *Thirty-Seventh Annual Announcement*, 17.

58. "Connecticut Indian Association," *Hartford Courant*, June 25, 1886.

59. Ibid.

60. Ibid.; Maxine Van de Wetering, "The Popular Concept of 'Home' in Nineteenth-Century America," *Journal of American Studies* 18 (April 1984): 23–25; Glenna Matthews, *"Just a Housewife": The Rise and Fall of Domesticity in America* (New York: Oxford University Press, 1987), 90.

61. Anne F. Scott, "On Seeing and Not Seeing: A Case of Historical Invisibility," *Journal of American History* 71 (June 1984): 16–17; Dolores Janiewski, "Learning to Live 'Just Like White Folks': Gender, Ethnicity, and the State in the Inland Northwest," in *Gendered Domains: Rethinking Public and Private in Women's History*, ed. Dorothy O. Helly and Susan M.

Reverby (Ithaca, N.Y.: Cornell University Press, 1992), 172–73; Matthews, *"Just a Housewife,"* 92–93, 115. For some examples of women who diverged from the rigid male-female division of public versus private spheres, see Alice Kessler-Harris, *Out to Work: A History of Wage-Earning Women in the United States* (New York: Oxford University Press, 1982); Martha Verbrugge, *Able-Bodied Womanhood: Personal Health and Social Change in Nineteenth-Century Boston* (New York: Oxford University Press, 1988); Polly Welts Kaufman, *National Parks and the Woman's Voice: A History* (Albuquerque: University of New Mexico Press, 1996).

62. "Report from the Omahas," *SW* 15 (September 1886): 99.

63. Sara Thomson Kinney to CIA, September 6, 1886, Letters Received, File 23847.

64. Sara Thomson Kinney to CIA, September 10, 1886, Letters Received, File 24280.

65. Francis La Flesche to Ed Farley, September 27, 1886, LFP-NSHS.

65. SLF, "My Childhood," 79.

CHAPTER 4. "KIND OF GETTING THERE"

1. Sara Thomson Kinney to RF, undated, LFP-NSHS; Johnson, *Historical Sketch*, 13; "Report of Meeting of October 9th," Minute Book No. 1, 1881–1887, Box 3, STK-CSL; see also "Connecticut Indian Association," *Hartford Courant*, October 8, 1886, Scrapbook 1, Box 3, STK-CSL.

2. SLF to RF, October 27, 1886, Wednesday, probably December, 1886, LFP-NSHS.

3. Marshall, *Woman's Medical College*, 68–69; *Pioneer-Pacesetter-Innovator: The Story of the Medical College of Pennsylvania* (New York: Newcomen Society in North America, 1971), 9, 16; Mary Putnam Jacobi, "Woman in Medicine," in *Woman's Work in America*, ed. Annie Nathan Meyer (New York: Henry Holt, 1891), 170.

4. SLF to RF, October 24, 1886, LFP-NSHS; Gulielma Fell Alsop, *History of the Woman's Medical College, Philadelphia, Pennsylvania, 1850–1950* (Philadelphia: J. B. Lippincott, n.d.), 135, 142.

5. Alsop, *History of the Woman's Medical College*, 124; SLF to RF, October 24, 1886, LFP-NSHS; SLF to RF, October 27, 1886, LFP-NSHS.

6. SLF to RF, October 24, 1886, LFP-NSHS; Carol Lopate, *Women in Medicine* (Baltimore: Johns Hopkins University Press, 1968), 9.

7. Sara Thomson Kinney to CIA, October 2, 1886, Letters Received, File 26206; Kinney to CIA, October 5, 1886, Letters Received, File 26690;

Acting Secretary of Interior to CIA, October 14, 1886, Letters Received, File 5784, enclosure; CIA, *AR*, 1886, 160.

8. See agreements and vouchers for 1887 and 1888 in STK-CSL. See also Johnson, *Historical Sketch*, 23; Sara Thomson Kinney to Herbert Welsh, February 12, 1889, *Indian Rights Association Papers, 1868–1968*, 136 microfilm reels (Glen Rock, N.J.: Microfilming Corporation of America, 1974), reel 4.

9. Shyrock, *Medicine in America*, 193.

10. Morantz-Sanchez, *Sympathy and Science*, 77; *Pioneer-Pacesetter-Innovator*, 12, 15; Marshall, *Woman's Medical College*, 69; Ruth J. Abram, "Give Her Knowledge: The Class of 1879 in Training," in *"Send Us a Lady Physician": Women Doctors in America, 1835–1920*, ed. Ruth J. Abram (New York: W. W. Norton, 1985), 140.

11. "Report of the Committee on Examinations, 1887," in Rachel L. Bodley Papers, Folder 3, Box 2, Archives and Special Collections on Women in Medicine, The Medical College of Pennsylvania and Hospital, Philadelphia, Pennsylvania; *Fortieth Annual Announcement of the Woman's Medical College of Pennsylvania* (Philadelphia: n.p., 1889), 8; Marshall, *Woman's Medical College*, 36–38; Alsop, *History of the Woman's Medical College*, 72; *Pioneer-Pacesetter-Innovator*, 14; Ruth J. Abram, "Soon the Baby Died: Medical Training in Nineteenth-Century America," in *"Send Us a Lady Physician,"* 18.

12. *Thirty-Seventh Annual Announcement of the Woman's Medical College of Pennsylvania* (Philadelphia: n.p., 1886), 1; see also *Thirty-Eighth Annual Announcement of the Woman's Medical College of Pennsylvania* (Philadelphia: n.p., 1887), 6.

13. *Thirty-Eighth Announcement*, 6.

14. *Thirty-Nineth Annual Announcement of the Woman's Medical College of Pennsylvania* (Philadelphia: n.p., 1888), 7.

15. SLF to RF, October 27, 1886, LFP-NSHS; *Thirty-Eighth Annual Announcement*, 9; SLF to RF, December 24, 1887, LFP-NSHS.

16. SLF, letter, December 19, 1887, in Hampton Institute, *Ten Years' Work* , 56; SLF to RF, October 24, 1886, October 29, 1886, October 27, 1886, LFP-NSHS; *Thirty-Seventh Annual Announcement*, 15; "Report of the Committee on Examinations, 1887," in Bodley Papers.

17. SLF to RF, November 17, 1886, LFP-NSHS.

18. SLF to RF, undated, Wednesday, probably December 1886, LFP-NSHS.

19. SLF to RF, December 24, 1887, undated fragment of a letter after letter dated January 4, 1888, LFP-NSHS.

20. Ibid.
21. Ibid.
22. SLF to RF, March 2, March 9, 1887, LFP-NSHS.
23. SLF to Sara Thomson Kinney, April 2, 1888, reprinted in *The Bulletin* 1 (April 1888): 1; "Hartford Indian Association," *Hartford Courant*, March 21, 1888, Scrapbook 1, Box 3, STK-CSL; *SW* 17 (May 1888), clipping, SAF-HUA.
24. SLF to RF, March 9, 1887, undated, Wednesday, probably December, 1886, LFP-NSHS; Frances B. Cogan, *All-American Girl: The Ideal of Real Womanhood in Mid-Nineteenth-Century America* (Athens: University of Georgia Press, 1989), 29–31; Stephanie L. Twin, "Women and Sport," in *Sport in America: New Historical Perspectives*, ed. Donald Spivey (Westport, Conn.: Greenwood Press, 1985), 204. See also Allen Guttmann, *Women's Sports: A History* (New York: Columbia University Press, 1991), 85–105.
25. SLF, letter, December 17, 1887, LFP-NSHS; SLF to RF, April 4, 1887, October 24, 1886, January 19, 1887, LFP-NSHS; Sara Thomson Kinney to CIA, June 29, 1887, Letters Received, File 16996; SLF to RF, January 12, 1887, LFP-NSHS.
26. SLF to RF, October 24, 1886, January 19, 1887, undated, Wednesday, probably December 1886, LFP-NSHS; SLF to RF, April 5, 1887, LFP-NSHS; Mrs. Heritage to Joseph La Flesche, December 23, 1887, LFP-NSHS; SLF to RF, undated fragment of a letter after letter dated January 4, 1888, LFP-NSHS.
27. "Speaking for the Indians," 1888, "The Indian Association," 1889, newspaper clippings, SAF-HUA; SLF to RF, undated fragment of letter, April 4, 1887, April 5, 1887, January 4, 1888, December 15, 1886, LFP-NSHS.
28. SLF to RF, January 19, 1887, October 24, 1886, November 5, 1886, April 4, 1887, March 9, 1887, LFP-NSHS; for the history of the Lincoln Institute and the Educational Home, see John Thomas Scharf and Thompson Westcott, *History of Philadelphia, 1609–1884*, 3 vols. (Philadelphia: L. H. Everts, 1884), 2:1457, 1487.
29. SLF to RF, February 9, 1887, February 2, 1887, January 26, 1887, LFP-NSHS.
30. SLF to RF, February 9, 1887, February 2, 1887, LFP-NSHS.
31. *Talks and Thoughts*, August, 1889, Scrapbook 1, Box 3, STK-CSL; SLF to RF, February 2, 1887, February 9, 1887, LFP-NSHS.
32. SLF to RF, November 17, 1886, LFP-NSHS; SLF to RF, December 1, 1886, LFP-NSHS.
33. SLF to RF, probably January 1–4, 1888, LFP-NSHS; SLF to RF, April 5, 1887, LFP-NSHS.

34. SLF to RF, March 2, 1887, February 2, 1887, undated fragment of letter, October 29, 1886, LFP-NSHS.
35. *Twenty-Two Years' Work*, 66; SLF to RF, October 24, 1886, LFP-NSHS.
36. SLF to RF, December 1, 1886, LFP-NSHS.
37. Ibid.; SLF to RF, March 2, 1887; "Report of Meeting of June 22d, 1886," Minute Book No. 1, 1881–1887, Box 3, STK-CSL; Kessler-Harris, *Out to Work*, 98–100, 128.
38. SLF to RF, January 26, 1887, December 1, 1886, February 2, 1887, April 4, 1887, December 24, 1887, LFP-NSHS; Cogan, *All-American Girl*, 138, 141–43.
39. SLF to RF, January 26, 1887, December 1, 1886, February 2, 1887, April 4, 1887, December 24, 1887, LFP-NSHS.
40. SLF to RF, November 17, 1886, December 1, 1886, April 4, 1887, January 19, 1887, LFP-NSHS.
41. SLF to RF, March 9, 1887, January 19, 1887, April 4, 1887, LFP-NSHS.
42. SLF to RF, January 4, 1888, LFP-NSHS.
43. Ibid.; SLF to RF, undated, Wednesday, probably, December, 1886, LFP-NSHS.
44. SLF to RF, undated, Wednesday, probably December, 1886, January 26, 1887, March 2, 1887, LFP-NSHS; *SW* 16 (July 1887), SAF-HUA.
45. SLF to Sara Thomson Kinney, November 19, 1888, Box 3, STK-CSL; see also *The Bulletin* 1 (December 1888): 3.
46. SLF to Sara Thomson Kinney, November 19, 1888, Box 3, STK-CSL; see also *The Bulletin* 1 (December 1888): 3.
47. Giffen, *Oo-Ma-Ha-Ta-Wa-Tha (Omaha City)*, 40; *SW* 17 (December 1888): 127.
48. Ibid.
49. SLF to RF, December 15, 1886, February 2, 1887, March 2, 1887, LFP-NSHS.
50. SLF to RF, undated, Wednesday, probably December, 1886, December 24, 1887, LFP-NSHS; La Flesche to Kinney, November 19, 1888; *Hartford Courant*, October 1, 1887, Scrapbook 1, Box 3, STK-CSL.
51. *Hartford Courant*, October 1, 1887; "Indian Association and the Lawn Party," *Hartford Courant*, October 3, 1887, October 4, 1887, Scrapbook 1, Box 3, STK-CSL.
52. "Aiding Indian Civilization: A Delightful Lawn Festival and Fair," *Hartford Courant*, October 5, 1887, Scrapbook 1, Box 3, STK-CSL. For

home building see Johnson, *Historical Sketch*, 11–12, 22; Wanken, "Woman's Sphere," 63–64; *SW* 18 (September 1889): 97; SLF, "An Indian on Home Building," *The Indian's Friend* 1 (July 1889): 1.

53. "Aiding Indian Civilization," *Hartford Courant*, STK-CSL.

54. Sara Thomson Kinney to Mrs. Bull, undated, Saturday, p.m., Box 5, STK-CSL; SLF to Mrs. Bull, March 4, 1889, Box 5, STK-CSL.

55. *Fortieth Annual Announcement*, 4; Alsop, *History of the Woman's Medical College*, 154; "Dr. Susan La Flesche," *The Bulletin* 1 (March 1889): 1; *SW* 18 (April 1889): 37.

56. SLF to CIA, June 13, 1889, Letters Received, File 15736; *The Bulletin* 1 (March 1889): 1; *Fortieth Annual Announcement*, 15.

57. *The Bulletin* 1 (June 1889): 1; "Reception to Dr. Susan La Flesche," *Hartford Times*, April 5, 1889, Scrapbook 1, Box 3, STK-CSL.

58. "Indian Association," *Waterbury American*, April 3, 1889, *Waterbury Republican*, April 3, 1889, *Norwich Courier*, April 7, 1889, "For the Indians," *Hartford Courant*, April 9, 1889, *Winsted Citizen*, April 10, 1889, Scrapbook 1, Box 3, STK-CSL; *The Bulletin* 1 (December 1889): 2; "Eight Annual Report, Connecticut Indian Association, November 5, 1889," Minute Book 2, 1887–1892, Box, STK-CSL; see also "State Indian Associations," *Lend a Hand* 4 (December 1889): 877.

59. *The Bulletin* 1 (June 1889): 1; *SW* 18 (May 1889), SAF-HUA; Putnam-Jacobi, "Woman in Medicine," 190; Duffy, *From Humors to Medical Science*, 209.

60. SLF to CIA, June 13, 1889, Letters Received, File 15736.

61. Ibid.

62. CIA, *AR*, 1890, xxii; see also Francis Paul Prucha, "Thomas Jefferson Morgan (1889–93)," in *The Commissioners of Indian Affairs, 1824–1977*, ed. Robert M. Kvasnicka and Herman J. Viola (Lincoln: University of Nebraska Press, 1979), 197; see also *Worcester Spy*, September 10, 1889, Scrapbook 1, Book 3, STK-CSL.

63. SLF to CIA, August 5, 1889, Letters Received, File 21752.

64. *SW* 14 (November 1885), SAF-HUA.

CHAPTER 5. "MY WORK AS A PHYSICIAN AMONG MY PEOPLE"

1. SLF, "My Work as Physician Among My People," *SW* 21 (August 1892): 133.

2. Ibid.; SLF to Miss Burbanks, November 6, 1891, reprinted in "A Letter from Dr. La Flesche," *IB* 3 (December 1891): 4.

3. Eastman and Montezuma supported the pan-Indianism movement through the Society of American Indians, which was established in 1911 to promote the betterment and mutual concerns of all Native American peoples. Hazel W. Hertzberg, *The Search for an American Identity: Modern Pan-Indian Movements* (Syracuse, N.Y.: Syracuse University Press, 1971), 19.

4. "Rules for Indian Schools," in CIA, *AR*, 1890, cxlix.

5. Frank C. Armstrong to CIA, November 7, 1889, *RIFJ*.

6. SLF to Members of the Connecticut Indian Association, January 13, 1890, reprinted in "Some Interesting Letters," *The Bulletin* 1 (April 1890): 3; "Christmas for the Indians," *Hartford Post*, November 26, 1889, Scrapbook 1, Box 3, STK-CSL; "Work of the Indian Association," *Hartford Times*, November 26, 1889, Scrapbook 1, Box 3, STK-CSL.

7. Diane Theresa Putney, "Fighting the Scourge: American Indian Morbidity and Federal Policy, 1897-1928" (Ph.D. diss., Marquette University, 1980), 1-22.

8. SLF to CIA, January 29, 1890, Letters Received, File 3161; William W. Junkin to CIA, September 17, 1892, *RIFJ*, Report 7215; SLF to Members of the Connecticut Indian Association, January 13, 1890, 3; "From Indian Trained Nurse," *SW* 19 (December 1890): 131; Joseph Barnaby, "Letter," *SW* 20 (February 1891): 155.

9. SLF to Mrs. Quinton, undated, reprinted in "From Dr. Susan La Flesche," *The Indian's Friend* 2 (December 1889): 2; SLF to CIA, January 29, 1890, Letters Received; SLF to Members of the Connecticut Indian Association, January 13, 1890, 3.

10. SLF to Mrs. Quinton, undated, 2; SLF to Members of the Connecticut Indian Association, January 13, 1890, 3.

11. CIA, *AR*, 1890, 140; CIA, *AR*, 1891, 290.

12. CIA, *AR*, 1893, 197; CIA, *AR*, 1892, 308; William W. Junkin to CIA, May 29, 1890, *RIFJ*, Report 3645.

13. Edmund Mallet to CIA, July 3, 1889, *RIFJ*, Report 4058.

14. Mary L. Barnes to Mr. W. Rankin, February 18, 1887, AIC.

15. Barnes to John C. Lowrie, July 6, 1888, Box J, vol. 1, AIC.

16. Lawrence M. Hensel, *Report of Our Omaha Mission* (n.p., 1888), 1-8; *SW* 17 (May 1888): 55; CIA, *AR*, 1890, 240.

17. SLF to Members of the Connecticut Indian Association, January 13, 1890, 3; SLF to Mrs. Quinton, undated, 2.

18. "Glimpses of a Woman's Work."

19. SLF to Mrs. Quinton, undated, 2.

20. Fletcher and La Flesche, *Omaha Tribe*, 326; Alice C. Fletcher, "The Indian Woman and Her Problems," 174; Dorsey, *Omaha Sociology*, 266–67.

21. SLF, "My Work as Physician among My People," 133; "From Dr. Susan La Flesche," in *The Hampton Normal and Agricultural Institute and Its Work for the Education of the Indian*, clipping, SAF-HUA; Sara Thomson Kinney, *Indians as I Have Seen Them* (n.p., n.d.), 4, STK-CSL.

22. "Connecticut Indian Association," *Hartford Courant*, June 25, 1886; *WNIA*, November, 1890, clipping, SAF-HUA; Amelia Stone Quinton, *Missionary Work of the Women's National Indian Association* (n.p., 188–?), 1; Valerie Sherer Mathes, "Nineteenth Century Women and Reform: The Women's National Indian Association," *American Indian Quarterly* 14 (Winter 1990): 7–9.

23. "From Dr. Susan La Flesche," in *The Hampton Normal and Agricultural Institute*; SLF, *Report of Susan La Flesche, M.D., Medical Missionary of The Women's National Indian Association Among the Omaha Indians*, Women's National Indian Association, October 24, 1891, 6–7, Sophia Smith Collection, Smith College, Northampton, Massachusetts; SLF to Mrs. Quinton, undated, 2.

24. Gloria Moldow, *Women Doctors in Gilded-Age Washington: Race, Gender, and Professionalization* (Urbana: University of Illinois Press, 1987), 127; Ruth J. Abram, "Private Practice: Taking Every Case to Heart," in *"Send Us a Lady Physician,"* 154–55.

25. Robert H. Ashley to CIA, December 10, 1889, Letters Received, File 5955; SLF to CIA, January 29, 1890, Letters Received, File 3161; CIA, *AR*, 1892, 308.

26. Kinney, *Indians as I Have Seen Them*, 8; Robert H. Ashley to CIA, March 3, 1891, Letters Received, File 8906; Arthur M. Tinker to CIA, December 21, 1891, *RIFJ*, Report 106.

27. Robert S. Gardner, October 27, 1891, *RIFJ*, Report 8012, Exhibit 1; CIA, *AR*, 1890, 140; Kinney, *Indians as I Have Seen Them*, 8; "In the Indian Country," *Hartford Courant*, October 10, 1891; "Well Done," *IB* 3 (April 1891): 2; SLF, *Report of Susan La Flesche, M.D.*, 6.

28. Wilson, *Ohiyesa*, 43.

29. "From Dr. Susan La Flesche," in *Hampton Normal and Agricultural Institute*; see also SLF to Miss Burbanks, November 6, 1891, 4; CIA, *AR*, 1891, 609.

30. SLF to Miss Burbanks, November 6, 1891, 4; Kinney, *Indians as I Have Seen Them*, 4–5.

31. CIA, *AR*, 1889, 13.

32. SLF, "My Work as Physician Among My People," 133.

33. Arthur M. Tinker to CIA, November 4, 1899, *RIFJ*, Report 7499; "Annual Report, Winnebago and Omaha Agencies, July 1, 1910," *Superintendents' Annual Narrative and Statistical Reports from Field Jurisdictions of the Bureau of Indian Affairs, 1907–1938* [hereafter SNSR], RG 75, BIA, M1011, reel 169, NA; SLF, *Report of Susan La Flesche, M.D.*, 5; SLF, "My Work as Physician Among My People," 133.

34. Putney, "Fighting the Scourge," 70–71; Ashley to CIA, March 3, 1891, *RIFJ*; Julius F. Schwarz, *History of the Presbyterian Church in Nebraska* (n.p., 1924), 35; "Our Medical Mission," *The Indian's Friend* 4 (May 1892): 37.

35. Ashley to CIA, March 3, 1889, Letters Received, File 8906; Junkin to CIA, May 29, 1890, *RIFJ*, Report 3645; Junkin to CIA, September 17, 1892, *RIFJ*, Report 7215; Ruth M. Raup, *The Indian Health Program from 1800 to 1955* (Washington, D.C.: U.S. Public Health Service, Division of Indian Health, 1955), 6; Virginia R. Allen, "Agency Physicians to the Southern Plains Indians, 1868–1900," *Bulletin of the History of Medicine* 49 (Fall 1975): 319; *WNIA*, November, 1890, clipping, SAF-HUA.

36. CIA, *AR*, 1889, 12–13; CIA, *AR*, 1890, xii; CIA, *AR*, 1892, 101; William T. Hagan, "Daniel M. Browning (1893–1897)," in *The Commissioners of Indian Affairs, 1824–1977*, ed. Robert M. Kvasnicka and Herman J. Viola (Lincoln: University of Nebraska, 1979), 205–10; Putney, "Fighting the Scourge," 22, 44–47.

37. Putney, "Fighting the Scourge," 69–71.

38. Charles Eastman, "The Indians' Health Problem," *American Indian Magazine* 4 (April/June 1916): 141–42.

39. SLF, *Report of Susan La Flesche, M.D.*, 5.

40. L. Webster Fox, "Trachoma Problem among North American Indians," *Journal of the American Medical Association* 86 (February 1926): 405; CIA, *AR*, 1911, 10; CIA, *AR*, 1912, 17; Joseph A. Murphy, "Health Problems of the Indians," *Annals of the American Academy of Political and Social Science* 37 (March 1911): 349.

41. SLF, "My Work as Physician Among My People," 133.

42. Tinsley Randolph Harrison, *Principles of Internal Medicine*, 7th ed. (New York: McGraw Hill, 1974), 980; Putney, "Fighting the Scourge," 143–44.

43. SLF, "Report of Physician for Omahas," in CIA, *AR*, 1893, 197.

44. See William N. Hailmann, *Circular Letter of Instruction* (Washington, D.C.: Government Printing Office, 1895); Putney, "Fighting the Scourge," 165–66.

45. Putney, "Fighting the Scourge"; CIA, *AR*, 1914, 16.

46. "Our Medical Mission," 37; SLF, "My Work as Physician among My People," 133.

47. SLF, *Report of Susan La Flesche, M.D.*, 4; SLF, "My Work as Physician Among My People," 1–33.

48. "Our Medical Mission," 37.

49. Women's National Indian Association, *Sketches of Delightful Work* (n.p., 1893), 50–51.

50. Putney, "Fighting the Scourge," 23, 44–44; CIA, *AR*, 1909, 2; see William Osler, *Principles and Practice of Medicine*, 2d ed. (New York: Appleton, 1895), 203–77 for information on the etiology of tuberculosis; Charles E. Rosenberg, "American Medicine in 1879," in *"Send Us a Lady Physician": Women Doctors in America, 1835–1920*, ed. Ruth J. Abram (New York: W. W. Norton, 1985), 28.

51. Ales Hrdlicka, *Tuberculosis among Certain Indian Tribes of the United States* (Washington, D.C.: Government Printing Office, 1909), 3–4; CIA, *AR*, 1904, 34; CIA, *AR*, 1912, 40; Putney, "Fighting the Scourge," 79, 92, 140.

52. SLF, "Report of Physician for Omahas," 197; "Glimpses of a Woman's Work."

53. See Hrdlicka, *Tuberculosis among Certain Indian Tribes*, 30, 32, for arguments that parallel those of Susan La Flesche; Harrison, *Principles of Internal Medicine*, 858–59; Osler, *Principles and Practice of Medicine*, 272–74.

54. SLF, "Report of Physician for Omahas," 197; "Letterbox," 918; SLF, "Home Life of the Indian," 1; SLF, "Indian Mud Lodge," 1, 4.

55. SLF to Robert H. Ashley, April 16, 1892, Letters Received, File 15077, enclosure 1; SLF to RF, ca. 1887, LFP-NSHS.

56. RF to Francis La Flesche, January 1, 1893, LFP-NSHS.

57. SLF, "From Dr. Susan La Flesche," *The Indian's Friend* 5 (June 1893): 3; *IB* 6 (December 1894): 3; RF to Francis La Flesche, August 17, 1893, LFP-NSHS.

58. SLF to William H. Beck, October, 1863, Letters Received, File 38476, enclosure 3; William H. Beck to CIA, October 9, 1893, Letters Received, File 38476.

59. Beck to CIA, October 9, 1893, Letters Received.

60. RF to Francis La Flesche, November 20, 1893, LFP-NSHS.

61. Ibid.

62. William H. Beck to CIA, October 29, 1893, Letters Received, File 40940; *Talks and Thoughts*, December 1893, clipping, SAF-HUA.

63. *IB* 6 (December 1894): 3; Marian B. Heritage to RF, June 22, 1894, LFP-NSHS.

64. Cuming County, "Nebraska Marriages Book V, 1894–1898," 2, NSHS; John G. Neihardt, *Patterns and Coincidences: A Sequel to All is But a Beginning* (Columbia: University of Missouri Press, 1978), 40–41; First Assistant Secretary to CIA, February 20, 1907, Letters Received, File 18063, "Findings of Fact," March 3, 1906, enclosure 1; Lisa E. Emmerich, "Marguerite La Flesche Diddock: Office of Indian Affairs Field Matron," *Great Plains Quarterly* 13 (Summer 1993): 166; *SW* 23 (August 1894): 195.

65. SLF to Dear friend, October 12, 1905, SAF-HUA; Neihardt, *Patterns and Coincidences*, 40.

66. Patricia C. Albers, "From Illusion to Illumination: Anthropological Studies of American Indian Women," in *Gender and Anthropology: Critical Reviews for Research and Teaching*, ed. Sandra Morgen (Washington, D.C.: American Anthropological Association, 1989), 137; Barbara J. Berg, *The Remembered Gate: Origins of American Feminism: The Woman and the City, 1800–1860* (New York: Oxford University Press, 1978), 92–93.

67. SLF to RF, Wednesday, December 1886, December 1, 1886, LFP-NSHS.

68. SLF to RF, December 24, 1887, LFP-NSHS; Cuming County, "Nebraska Marriages Book V," 2.

69. Marguerite La Flesche Picotte, "Letter," *SW* 24 (January 1895): 10; Ellen J. Smith, "Medical Societies: Lifted from the Ranks of Mere Pretenders," in *"Send Us a Lady Physician,"* 216; RF to Francis La Flesche, July 29, 1895, LFP-NSHS; for more on self-employment see Lucy Eldersveld Murphy, "Business Ladies: Midwestern Women and Enterprise, 1850–1880," *Journal of Women's History* 3 (Spring 1991): 70, 83.

70. "A New Role," *IB* 10 (February 1896): 1.

71. SLF, letter, undated, reprinted in *IB* 10 (March 1896): 1.

72. SLF to Mrs. Kinney, November 14, 1896, reprinted in "News from Dr. Picotte," *IB* 11 (February 1897): 2.

73. "Report of the Educational Committee," *IB* 12 (December 1898): 3; Green, *Iron Eye's Family*, 147; Moldow, *Women Doctors in Gilded-Age Washington*, 124–25.

74. SLF, letter, undated, reprinted in *IB* 10 (March 1896): 1; SLF to Mrs. Kinney, November 14, 1896, 2; Mrs. Gould to RF, October 13, 1898, LFP-NSHS.

75. SLF, letter, undated, reprinted in *IB* 10 (March 1896): 1; SLF to Mrs. Kinney, November 14, 1896, 2; Mrs. Gould to RF, October 13, 1898, LFP-NSHS; Alice C. Fletcher to RF, June 1, 1896, LFP-NSHS; Raup, *Indian*

Health Program, 5; Laurence F. Schmeckebier, *The Office of Indian Affairs: Its History, Activities and Organization* (Baltimore: Johns Hopkins Press, 1927), 228.

76. SLF to CIA, June 13, 1896, Letters Received, File 23011, enclosure 2.

77. Councilmen to CIA, March 11, 1896, Letters Received, File 23011, enclosure 1; William Beck to CIA, June 15, 1896, Letters Received, File 23011.

78. SLF to Mrs. Kinney, November 14, 1896, 2.

79. Green, *Iron Eye's Family*, 148.

80. SLF to Miss Richards, December 9, 1897, SAF-HUA.

CHAPTER 6. "THIS CURSE OF DRINK"

1. SLF to Thomas [sic] W. Jones, January 27, 1900, Letters Received, File 6049.

2. For the differences between evangelical Protestantism and the social gospel movement, see Martin E. Marty, *Righteous Empire: The Protestant Experience in America* (New York: Dial Press, 1970), 179, 185; J. Christopher Soper, *Evangelical Christianity in the United States and Great Britain: Religious Beliefs, Political Choices* (New York: New York University Press, 1994), 63–64; Ian Tyrrell, *Woman's World/Woman's Empire: The Woman's Christian Temperance Union in International Perspective, 1880–1930* (Chapel Hill: University of North Carolina Press, 1991), 66.

3. "Indian Chief's Crusade," 35; SLF to RF, January 19, 1887, LFP-NSHS; Paula Baker, "The Domestication of Politics: Women and American Political Society, 1780–1920," in *Unequal Sisters: A Multicultural Reader in U.S. Women's History*, 2d ed., ed. Vicki L. Ruiz and Ellen Carol Dubois (New York: Routledge, 1994), 95.

4. Jean V. Matthews, "'Woman's Place' and the Search for Identity in Ante-Bellum America," *The Canadian Review of American Studies* 10 (Winter 1979): 301; Barbara Leslie Epstein, *The Politics of Domesticity: Women, Evangelism, and Temperance in Nineteenth-Century America* (Middletown, Conn.: Wesleyan University Press, 1981), 1–2, 103; *Annual Report of the Women's National Indian Association, December 1892* (Philadelphia: n.p., 1892), 21; see also Janet Zollinger Giele, *Two Paths to Women's Equality: Temperance, Suffrage, and the Origins of Modern Feminism* (New York: Twayne Publishers, 1995), x, xii, 76–80; Ruth Bordin, *Woman and Temperance: The Quest for Power and Liberty, 1873–1900* (Philadelphia: Temple University Press, 1981), xiv–xviii, 3–14; for a

summary of other theories on the motivation of the temperance movement see Soper, *Evangelical Christianity*, 89-93.

5. McDonnell, *Dispossession of the American Indian*, 43-44.

6. James McLaughlin to CIA, June 19, 1895, *RIFJ*.

7. CIA, *AR*, 306.

8. William A. Junkin to CIA, September 14, 1892, *RIFJ*, Report 7152.

9. Quoted in Francis La Flesche, "An Indian Allotment," *The Independent* 52 (November 8, 1900): 2688.

10. SLF to Jones, January 27, 1900, Letters Received.

11. Junkin to CIA, September 14, 1892, *RIFJ*, Report 7152, Exhibit E; McLaughlin to CIA, June 19, 1895, *RIFJ*, Report 4883; CIA, *AR*, 1895, 200.

12. McDonnell, *Dispossession of the American Indian*, 56-57.

13. SLF to CIA, July 7, 1909, *Indian Rights Association Papers*, reel 21.

14. Francis La Flesche, "Protection of Indian Lands," in *Report of the Annual Lake Mohonk Conference*, 72; Orr, *Selected Pages from the History of Medicine in Nebraska*, 12. See also *WT*, January 7, 21, 1910.

15. "Testimony of Susan La Flesche Picotte, investigating the death of Henry Warner," May 22, 1914, LFP-NSHS.

16. Robert K. Thomas, "History of North American Indian Alcohol Use as a Community-Based Phenomenon," *Journal of Studies on Alcohol* 42, no. 9 (1981): 29-39; Welsch, *Omaha Tribal Myths and Trickster Tales*, 4.

17. Thomas W. Hill, "Peyotism and the Control of Heavy Drinking: The Nebraska Winnebago in the Early 1900s," *Human Organization* 49 (Fall 1990): 256; E. P. Dozier, "Problem Drinking Among American Indians: The Role of Sociocultural Deprivation," *Quarterly Journal of Studies on Alcohol* 27, no. 1 (1966): 74, 85; Nancy O. Lurie, "The World's Oldest On-Going Protest Demonstration: North American Indian Drinking Patterns," *Pacific Historical Review* 40 (August 1971): 315-16.

18. Francis La Flesche to Caryl Farley, February 3, 1901, LFP-NSHS.

19. Sara T. Kinney to Lake Mohonk Conference, undated, in CIA, *AR*, 1891, 1191.

20. SLF to Jones, January 27, 1900, Letters Received.

21. "Testimony of Susan La Flesche Picotte," May 22, 1914, LFP-NSHS.

22. Sara Thomson Kinney, *Indians as I Have Seen Them*, 9, STK-CSL.

23. Epstein, *Politics of Domesticity*, 1, 89; Tyrrell, *Woman's World*, 2, 256; SLF, letter, undated, reprinted in *The Indian's Friend* 6 (November 1890): 2; SLF, letter, undated, reprinted in "From Dr. La Flesche," *The*

Indian's Friend 3 (February 1891): 3; Kinney, *Indians as I Have Seen Them*, 10, STK-CSL.

24. SLF, letter, undated, 3; Jack S. Blocker, Jr., *American Temperance Movements: Cycles of Reform* (Boston: Twayne, 1989), 104; James H. Timberlake, *Prohibition and the Progressive Movement, 1900–1920* (Cambridge: Harvard University Press, 1963), 145–46; K. Austin Kerr, *Organized for Prohibition: A New History of the Anti-Saloon League* (New Haven: Yale University Press, 1985), 2–3; John J. Rumbarger, *Profits, Power, and Prohibition: Alcohol Reform and the Industrializing of America, 1800–1930* (Albany: State University of New York, 1989), 159, 162.

25. SLF, letter, undated, 3.

26. Ibid.; SLF, "The Omahas and Citizenship," *SW* 20 (April 1891): 177; Judith A. Boughter, "Betraying Their Trust: The Dispossession of the Omaha Nation, 1790–1916" (master's thesis, University of Nebraska at Omaha, 1995), 201; for liquor laws, see *Federal Indian Law* (Washington, D.C.: Government Printing Office, 1958; reprint, New York: Association on American Indian Affairs, 1966), 381–93. See also Francis Paul Prucha, *American Indian Policy in the Formative Years: The Indian Trade and Intercourse Acts, 1790–1834* (Cambridge: Harvard University Press, 1962), 269.

27. SLF, letter, undated, 3.

28. CIA, *AR*, 1892, 186–87.

29. "Omahas Drinking," *The Word Carrier* 21 (August 1892): 21; CIA, *AR*, 1905, 27.

30. SLF, letter, probably spring, 1893, reprinted in "From Dr. Susan La Flesche," *The Indian's Friend* 5 (June 1893): 3.

31. Ibid.; CIA, *AR*, 1894, 63, 189; CIA, *AR*, 1892, 62; *Federal Indian Law*, 287; *U.S. Statutes at Large* 27 (1892): 260; SLF to Dear Friends, probably April, 1894, reprinted in "Letter from Dr. Susan La Flesche," *IB* 8 (May 1894): 3.

32. Boughter, "Betraying Their Trust," 201–202; Arthur M. Tinker to CIA, December 22, 1891, *RIFJ*, Report 105; Prucha, *American Indian Policy in Crisis*, 321.

33. SLF, letter, probably spring, 1893, 3; "From Dr. Susan La Flesche," *Talks and Thoughts*, July 1893, clipping, SAF-HUA.

34. SLF to Dear Friends, probably April 1894, 3.

35. Ibid.

36. Ibid.

37. Ibid.

38. CIA, *AR*, 1894, 189.

39. McLaughlin to CIA, June 19, 1895, *RIFJ*.

40. Senate, *Sale of Intoxicating Liquors to Indians*, Sen. Rept. Doc. 1294, 54th Cong., 2d sess., 1897, serial 3474, 13; U.S. Statutes at Large 29 (1897): 506–507.

41. Senate, *Sale of Intoxicating Liquors to Indians*, Sen. Rept. Doc. 1294, 7–8.

42. CIA, *AR*, 1895, 51; CIA, *AR*, 1897, 56.

43. CIA, *AR*, 1894, 62; CIA, *AR*, 1895, 57.

44. CIA, *AR*, 1899, 36.

45. *Bancroft Blade*, December 21, 1899; William J. McConnell to CIA, May 18, 1900, Report 3710, enclosure 9, *RIFJ*.

46. SLF to Jones, January 27, 1900, Letters Received; see also SLF, "Another Appeal," *The Indian's Friend* 12 (March 1900): 8.

47. SLF to R. G. Valentine, July 2, 1909, SAF-HUA.

48. Peggy Pascoe, *Relations of Rescue: The Search for Female Moral Authority in the American West, 1874–1939* (New York: Oxford University Press, 1990), 135; SLF, Diary, September 26, 27, 1910, January 19, 1911, LFP-NSHS.

49. Emmerich, "Marguerite La Flesche Diddock," 168–69.

50. SLF to Jones, January 27, 1900, Letters Received.

51. Harry L. Keefe to Thomas[sic] W. Jones, January 30, 1900, Letters Received, File 6097; William J. McConnell to CIA, May 11, 1900, Report 3484, *RIFJ*.

52. Harry L. Keefe to George D. Meiklejohn, January 30, 1900, Letters Received, File 7368, enclosure 1.

53. SLF, "Another Appeal," 8–9; SLF to Herbert Welsh, January 30, 1900, *Indian Rights Association Papers*, reel 15; CIA, *AR*, 1902, 52.

54. CIA, *AR*, 1902, 241; CIA, *AR*, 1904, 56; CIA, *AR*, 1905, 24, 249; *In The Matter of Heff*, 25 Sup. Ct. 605 (1905).

55. SLF to Wilbur F. Crafts, D.D., October 16, 1905, Letters Received, File 84470.

56. Ibid.

57. CIA, *AR*, 1903, 203.

58. John G. Neihardt, quoted in Donald Schnier, "A History of Bancroft, Nebraska" (master's thesis, University of Nebraska at Omaha, 1967), 41.

59. Anne P. Diffendel, "The La Flesche Sisters: Susette, Rosalie, Marguerite, Lucy, Susan," in *Perspectives: Women in Nebraska History*, ed. Susan Pierce (Lincoln: Nebraska Department of Education and the Nebraska

State Council for the Social Studies, 1984), 223; *Bancroft Blade*, April 3, 1908; "Dr. Picotte at Bancroft," *WT*, April 10, 1908.

60. "Testimony of Susan La Flesche Picotte," May 22, 1914, LFP-NSHS; John M. Commons to CIA, January 14, 1908, Central Consolidated Files, 1907–1939, RG 75, BIA, File 43395 (126) Omaha, NA [hereafter CCF].

61. SLF to CIA, July 2, 1909, SAF-HUA.

62. Commons to CIA, January 14, 1908, CCF.

63. RF to Francis La Flesche, January 28, 1894, May 14, 1893, January 2, 1894, May 14, 1898, LFP-NSHS; Green, *Iron Eye's Family*, 111.

64. Neihardt, *Patterns and Coincidences*, 40; Green, *Iron Eye's Family*, 149; SLF to My dear friend, October 12, 1905, SAF-HUA; for characteristics of temperance advocates, see Giele, *Two Paths to Women's Equality*, 76–80, 84.

65. William Johnson to CIA, August 28, 1907, CCF, File 73132-07 (126) Omaha.

66. SLF to Francis E. Leupp, November 15, 1907, CCF, File 90863 (162) Omaha.

67. For more on the field matron program, see Helen M. Bannan, *"True Womanhood" on the Reservation: Field Matrons in the United States Indian Service* (Tucson: University of Arizona Southwest Institute for Research on Women, 1984) and Lisa E. Emmerich, "'Right in the Midst of My Own People': Native American Women and the Field Matron Program," *American Indian Quarterly* 15 (Spring 1991): 201–16; Francis E. Leupp to SLF, November 20, 1907, CCF, File 90863 (162) Omaha.

68. SLF to Leupp, November 15, 1907, CCF.

69. Ibid.

70. Johnson to CIA, August 28, 1907, CCF.

71. SLF, "The Varied Work of an Indian Missionary," *Home Mission Monthly* 22 (August 1908): 246; "Indian Association," *Litchfield Enquirer*, October 15, 1908, Scrapbook 1, Box 3, STK-CSL; Presbyterian Church in the U.S., "Niobrara Presbytery, Minutes 1885–1950," 4 vols., 1: April 18–19, 1905, 21st Stated Spring Meeting, September 19–20, 1905, Stated Fall Meeting, 2: April 16, 18, 1907, Stated Spring Meeting, PHS; Green, *Iron Eye's Family*, 149–50; Lake Mohonk Conference of Friends of the Indian and Other Dependent Peoples, *Annual Report of Proceedings*, 1906, 112–13.

72. Jacqueline Peterson and Mary Drake, "American Indian Women and Religion," in *Women and Religion in America: The Colonial and Revolutionary Periods*, vol. 2 of *Women and Religion in America*, ed. Rosemary Radford Ruether and Rosemary Skinner Keller (San Francisco: Harper & Row, 1983), 3, 5; Kay Parker, "American Indian Women and Religion on the Southern

Plains," in *Women and Religion in America: The Nineteenth Century*, vol. 1 of *Women and Religion in America*, ed. Rosemary Radford Ruether and Rosemary Skinner Keller (San Francisco: Harper & Row, 1983), 53.

73. Barbara Welter, "She Hath Done What She Could: Protestant Women's Missionary Careers in Nineteenth-Century America," *American Quarterly* 30 (Winter 1978): 637; Green, *Iron Eye's Family*, 150.

74. SLF to Francis E. Leupp, May 21, 1907, Letters Received, File 48623; Blocker, *American Temperance Movements*, xiv–xv.

75. SLF, "Varied Work of an Indian Missionary," 246; Blocker, *American Temperance Movements*, 86–87; Prucha, *Great Father*, 2:625.

76. SLF, "Varied Work of an Indian Missionary," 246–47; SLF to Leupp, May 21, 1907, Letters Received; Green, *Iron Eye's Family*, 150.

77. SLF, "Varied Work of an Indian Missionary," 246–47; SLF to Leupp, May 21, 1907, Letters Received; Green, *Iron Eye's Family*, 150.

78. SLF, "Varied Work of an Indian Missionary," 247.

79. "Omaha Indians Unite with Church," *WT*, December 6, 1907; SLF, "Varied Work of an Indian Missionary," 247; *The Indian's Friend* 21 (September 1908): 1; "Dr. Picotte at Kansas City," *WT*, May 29, 1908.

80. SLF, "From the Omahas," *The Word Carrier* 39 (July/August 1910): 16; Herzog, "La Flesche Family,: 230.

81. "Glimpses of a Woman's Work."

82. SLF to Francis E. Leupp, July 8, 1909, Letters Received, File 61405; Green, *Iron Eye's Family*, 152.

83. *Arrow*, September 24, 1909, clipping, SAF-HUA; SLF to Miss Andrus, June 24, 1909, SAF-HUA; *WT*, May 22, 1908, March 29, April 2, 5, May 24, 1912; *Winnebago Chieftain*, May 29, 1908, clipping, SAF-HUA.

84. SLF to Valentine, July 2, July 13, 1909, SAF-HUA; Robert C. Ogden to Dr. Frissell, June 27, 1900, SAF-HUA; Boughter, "Betraying Their Trust," 240.

85. SLF to Valentine, July 2, 1909, SAF-HUA; Fletcher and La Flesche, *Omaha Tribe*, 625; *WT*, May, 17, 1907; "Walthill was One Year Old Wednesday," *WT*, May 24, 1907; "Winnebago and Omaha Agencies, Annual Report, July 1, 1910," *SNSR*.

86. SLF to Valentine, July 2, 1909, SAF-HUA.

87. Boughter, "Betraying Their Trust," 233.

88. Ibid., 205; *Bancroft Blade*, May 1, 8, 1908; William Johnson to CIA, August 28, 1907, CCF, File 73132-07 (126) Omaha; *WT*, November 20, December 11, December 25, 1908; "Winnebago and Omaha Agencies, Annual Report, July 1, 1910," *SNSR*.

89. Johnson to CIA, August 28, 1907, CCF, 73132-07 (126) Omaha; "Annual Report of the Omaha Indian School, 1916," *SNSR*; Green, *Iron*

Eye's Family, 152. CIA, *AR*, 1903, 203; Boughter, "Betraying Their Trust," 204.

90. T. Kue Young, *The Health of Native Americans: Toward a Biocultural Epidemiology* (New York: Oxford University Press, 1994), 208.

91. Ake Hultkrantz, *Shamanic Healing and Ritual Drama: Health and Medicine in Native American Religious Traditions* (New York: Crossroads Publishing, 1992), 79–80.

92. "Mescal Society," 4–5, Melvin R. Gilmore Papers, NSHS; Weston La Barre, *The Peyote Cult*, 5th ed. (Norman: University of Oklahoma Press, 1989), 45, 82–83, 91–92, 165–66; James H. Howard, "Omaha Peyotism," *Hobbies—The Magazine for Collectors* 56 (September 1951): 142.

93. "Testimony of Susan La Flesche Picotte," LFP-NSHS; La Barre, *Peyote Cult*, 116.

94. La Barre, *Peyote Cult*, 109–11, 116; see also Thomas R. Roddy, "The Winnebago Mescal-Eaters," in *The Indian Tribes of the Upper Mississippi Valley and Region of the Great Lakes*, ed. Emma Helen Blair (Cleveland: Arthur H. Clark, 1912), 2:282.

95. SLF, "Varied Work of an Indian Missionary," 247; "Glimpses of a Woman's Work."

96. CIA, *AR*, 1909, 14; F. H. Abbott to Omaha delegation, 25 March 1912, CCF, File 2989-1908 (126), pt. 1c: Liquor Traffic. OIA officials even held that peyote, like alcohol, was addictive, but according to contemporary research, peyote is neither a narcotic nor habit forming. J. S. Slotkin, *The Peyote Religion* (Glencoe, Ill.: Free Press, 1956), 50; Weston La Barre, "Twenty Years of Peyote Studies," *Current Anthropology* 1 (January 1960): 45.

97. Malcom J. Arth, "A Functional View of Peyotism in Omaha Culture," *Plains Anthropologist* 2 (October 1956): 25; "Omaha Indian School, Annual Report 1914," 3, *SNSR*; "Mescal Society," 4–5; W. H. Kearns, "The New Presbyterian Hospital for the Omaha Indians," in *American Indian Missions, Reprint of Assembly Herald Articles*, 1913 (n.p., n.d.), 5.

98. "Testimony of Susan La Felsche Picotte," LFP-NSHS; SLF, Diary, November 3, November 19, 1910, LFP-NSHS; Omaha Mescal Society to CIA, 25 March 1912, CCF, File 2989-08, pt. 3a: Liquor Traffic.

99. La Barre, *Peyote Cult*, 21, 207, 301.

100. Arth, "Functional View," 25–26.

101. SLF to Francis La Flesche, undated, reprinted in Omer C. Stewart, *Peyote Religion: A History* (Norman: University of Oklahoma Press, 1987), 221; "Mescal Meetings," *WT*, December 24, 31, 1909; La Barre, *Peyote Cult*, 7; Slotkin, *Peyote Religion*, 76.

102. "Omaha Indian School, Annual Report, 1914," 1, *SNSR*; "Testimony of Susan La Flesche Picotte," LFP-NSHS; SLF to Cato Sells, April 29, 1914, LFP-NSHS.

103. "Testimony of Susan La Flesche Picotte," LFP-NSHS.

104. Ibid.

CHAPTER 7. "A MORE LIBERAL POLICY"

1. SLF to Francis E. Leupp, July 8, 1907, Letters Received, File 61405; First Assistant Secretary to U.S. CIA, February 20, 1907, Letters Received, File 18063, "Findings of Fact," March 3, 1906, enclosure 1; McDonnell, *Dispossession of the American Indian*, 55; Frederick E. Hoxie, *A Final Promise: The Campaign to Assimilate the Indians, 1880–1920* (Lincoln: University of Nebraska Press, 1984), 159–60.

2. *Federal Indian Law*, 811; McDonnell, *Dispossession of the American Indian*, 55; Hoxie, *Final Promise*, 160.

3. SLF to Leupp, July 8, 1907, Letters Received.

4. R. J. Taylor to CIA, November 2, 1906, Letters Received, File 98043; Thos. Ryan to CIA, February 20, 1907, Letters Received, File 18063.

5. SLF to Francis E. Leupp, May 21, 1907, Letters Received, File 48628; Prucha, *Great Father*, 2:876; Hoxie, *Final Promise*, 160.

6. SLF to Leupp, May 21, 1907, Letters Received; Anderson, *Changing Woman*, 40–41; for information on the impact of OIA gendered policies on individual tribes, see Janiewski, "Learning to Live," 174–75; Carolyn Garrett Pool, "Reservation Policy and the Economic Position of Wichita Women," *Great Plains Quarterly* 8 (Summer 1988): 164, 166; Patterson, "Evolving Gender Roles in Pomo Society," 136, 144.

7. SLF to Leupp, May 21, 1907, Letters Received.

8. R. J. Taylor to SLF, May 16, 1907, Letters Received, File 48628; see also R. J. Taylor to CIA, May 29, 1907, Letters Received, File 51403.

9. SLF to Leupp, May 21, 1907, Letters Received.

10. Taylor to CIA, May 29, 1907, Letters Received.

11. SLF to CIA, July 1, 1907, Letters Received, File 60157.

12. R. J. Taylor to SLF, July 1, 1907, Letters Received, File 61405.

13. SLF to Leupp, July 8, 1907, Letters Received, File 61405.

14. Ibid.

15. Ibid.

16. Ibid.; Questionnaire, November, 1888, SAF-HUA.

17. F. M. Conser to SLF, July 1, 1907, Letters Received, File 61405, enclosure 1; R. J. Taylor to CIA, March 24, 1909, CCF.

18. SLF to Mr. Commons, July 27, 1907, Letters Received, File 66499; John M. Commons to CIA, July 30, 1907, Letters Received, File 66499-2; Acting Commissioner to Superintendent in Charge, August 6, 1907, Letters Received, File 61405, enclosure 2.

19. SLF to Acting Commissioner, July 1908, CCF, File 46224/108 (223) Omaha; Acting Commissioner to Superintendent, Omaha Indian School, July 23, 1908, CCF, File 46224/108 (223) Omaha; Murphy, "Business Ladies," 67–68; Glenda Riley, *The Female Frontier: A Comparative View of Women on the Prairie and the Plains* (Lawrence: University Press of Kansas, 1988), 108–11, 128–30; *WT*, August 17, 28, 1908.

20. SLF to Mr. Conser, February 18, 1909, CCF, File 23479 (354) Yankton; R. J. Taylor to CIA, March 24, 1909, CCF, File 23479 (354) Yankton; SLF to CIA, February 9, 1910, CCF, File 11308-10 (225) Yankton. The outcome of this attempt remains unknown, since evidence on the subject beyond early 1910 is non-existent.

21. SLF, Diary, September 20, 24, 26, 27, 30, October 10, November 1, 1910, LFP-NSHS.

22. SLF, Diary, September 29, October 1, 10, 17, November 7, 8, 15, December 9, 10, 1910, LFP-NSHS; McDonnell, *Dispossession of the American Indian*, 56–57, 89–90.

23. SLF, Diary, September 24, 26, October 3, 1910, LFP-NSHS; CIA, *AR*, 1898, 329.

24. SLF, Diary, October 4, 7, September 30, November 28, December 5, 19, 1910, LFP-NSHS.

25. SLF, Diary, November 5, 10, 1910, LFP-NSHS.

26. SLF, Diary, September 24, October 3, September 30, November 21, 26, 1910, LFP-NSHS.

27. Prucha, *Great Father*, 2:875–76; McDonnell, *Dispossession of the American Indian*, 56; SLF, Diary, September 24, October 1, 4, 10, November 11, 15, 17, December 12, 1910, LFP-NSHS; SLF to Francis E. Leupp, January 29, 1906, Letters Received, File 10324.

28. SLF, Diary, September 27, 28, October 2, 4, November 1, 2, 3, 7, 8, 15, 29, 1910, January 6, 1911, LFP-NSHS; Prucha, *Great Father*, 2: 870–72.

29. Samuel E. Brosius to SLF, January 24, 1909, *Indian Rights Association Papers*, reel 21; H. B. Frissell to Dear Doctor, March 17, 1909, SAF-HUA.

30. SLF to Robert G. Valentine, July 2, 1909, SAF-HUA; Boughter, "Betraying Their Trust," 239–40; SLF to Secretary of the Interior, July 7, 1909, *Indian Rights Association Papers*, reel 21.

31. Robert G. Ogden to Mr. Frissell, June 30, 1909, SAF-HUA; SLF to M. K. Sniffen, July 7, 1909, telegram, *Indian Rights Association Papers*, reel 21; Boughter, "Betraying Their Trust," 243–44.

32. SLF to Secretary of the Interior, July 7, 1909, *Indian Rights Association Papers*.

33. Ibid.

34. Ibid.

35. Ibid.

36. Ibid.

37. SLF to Robert G. Valentine, July 13, 1909, SAF-HUA.

38. Ibid.; see also Boughter, "Betraying Their Trust," 239, and Janet A. McDonnell, "Land Policy on the Omaha Reservation: Competency Commissions and Forced Fee Patents," *Nebraska History* 63 (Fall 1982): 401–402.

39. Boughter, "Betraying Their Trust," 240; McDonnell, "Land Policy," 402.

40. McDonnell, "Land Policy," 402.

41. Ibid., 402–407; see also "250 Omahas Get Patent," *WT*, March 4, 1910.

42. SLF, testimony, "Omaha Indian Conference, Indian Office, Washington," January 28, 1910, CCF, File 13212-10 (056) Omaha.

43. Ibid.; SLF, "Dr. Picotte's Appeal," *WT*, March 4, 1910; SLF, "Omaha-Winnebago Merger," *WT*, January 7, 1910.

44. SLF to F. H. Abbott, December 2, 1909, CCF, File 97680-09 (133) Omaha Part 1.

45. Ibid.; Prucha, *Great Father*, 2:780–81; F. H. Abbott to SLF, December 7, 1909, CCF, File 97680-09 (133) Omaha Part 1; SLF, "Omaha-Winnebago Merger," *WT*, January 7, 1910.

46. SLF to Alice Fletcher, n.d., December 2, 1909, FLP-NAA.

47. SLF to Abbott, December 2, 1909, CCF; see also SLF to Robert G. Valentine, December 22, 1909, CCF, File 97680-09 (133) Omaha Part 1.

48. SLF to Abbott, December 2, 1909, CCF.

49. Ibid.

50. Abbott to SLF, December 7, 1909, CCF.

51. Andrew G. Pollock to F. H. Abbott, December 3, 1909, CCF, File 97680-09 (133) Omaha Part I.

52. Ibid.

53. SLF to Mr. Abbott, December 11, 1909, CCF, File 97680-09 (133) Omaha Part 1.

54. Ibid.
55. SLF to Valentine, December 22, 1909, CCF.
56. Ibid.
57. Ibid.
58. bid.
59. CIA to Dr. Susan and Mr. Hiram Chase, December 28, 29, 1909, CCF, File 97680-09 (133) Omaha Part 1.
60. SLF, "Omaha-Winnebago Merger," *WT*, January 7, 1910; "Those Washington Dispatches to the Omaha Bee," *WT*, February 4, 1910.
61. SLF, "Dr. Picotte Discusses the New Policy," *WT*, December 31, 1909; see also SLF, "Omaha-Winnebago Merger," *WT*, January 7, 1910; SLF, "Dr. Picotte's Appeal," *WT*, March 4, 1910.
62. SLF, "Dr. Picotte's Appeal."
63. SLF, "Dr. Picotte Discusses the New Policy," *WT*, December 31, 1909.
64. Ibid.
65. Ibid.; SLF, "Omaha-Winnebago Merger," *WT*, January 7, 1910; "Omahas Will Seek Liberty in the Courts," *Omaha Sunday World-Herald*, January 23, 1910, 6-M; SLF, "An Indian on Home-Building," *Indian's Friend* 1 (July 1889): 1.
66. SLF, "Omaha-Winnebago Merger," *WT*, January 7, 1910; "Big Council Meeting," *WT*, January 7, 1910; Milner, *With Good Intentions*, 184.
67. SLF, "Omaha-Winnebago Merger," *WT*, January 7, 1910.
68. Ibid.; SLF, "Dr. Picotte Discusses the New Policy," *WT*, December 31, 1909.
69. "Omahas Will Stand Pat," *WT*, December 1, 1909; "The Parting of the Ways," *WT*, January 21, 1910.
70. SLF to Miss Folsom, February 15, 1910, SAF-HUA. For an explanation of neurasthenia, see Barbara Sicherman, "The Uses of a Diagnosis: Doctors, Patients, and Neurasthenia," *Journal of the History of Medicine* 32 (January 1977): 33, 36; also see Lorna Duffin, "The Conspicuous Consumptive: Woman as an Invalid," in *The Nineteenth-Century Woman: Her Cultural and Physical World*, ed. Sara Delamont and Lorna Duffin (New York: Barnes & Noble Books, 1978), 36–38.
71. "Those Washington Dispatches to the Omaha Bee," *WT*, February 4, 1910; SLF, testimony, "Omaha Indian Conference," CCF; SLF, "Dr. Picotte's Appeal," *WT*, March 4, 1910; SLF to Miss Folsom, February 15, 1910, SAF-HUA.
72. SLF to Miss Folsom, February 15, 1910, SAF-HUA.
73. SLF, testimony, "Omaha Indian Conference," CCF; SLF, "Dr. Picotte's Appeal," *WT*, March 4, 1909.

74. SLF, testimony, "Omaha Indian Conference," CCF.
75. Ibid.
76. Ibid.
77. Ibid.
78. "Those Washington Dispatches to the Omaha Bee," *WT*, February 4, 1910.
79. "250 Omahas Get Patent," *WT*, March 4, 1910; *Fremont Tribune*, March 11, 1910, quoted in Green, *Iron Eye's Family*, 157.
80. SLF to F. H. Abbott, October 3, 1910, telegram, CCF, File 79461-10 (312) Omaha.
81. Ibid.; SLF to CIA, October 13, 1910, CCF, File 79461-10 (312) Omaha.
82. SLF to CIA, October 13, 1910, CCF, File 79461-10 (312) Omaha.
83. Ibid.
84. McDonnell, "Land Policy," 404–5; SLF to CIA, October 13, 1910, CCF.
85. SLF, "Dr. Picotte's Appeal," *WT*, March 4, 1910.
86. SLF to CIA, October 13, 1910, CCF.
87. C. F. Hanke to SLF, December 29, 1910, CCF, File 79461-10 (312) Omaha.
88. McDonnell, *Dispossession of the American Indian,* vii–viii; Boughter, "Betraying Their Trust," 255, 263–64.
89. "Committee Conducts Strange Hearings," *WT*, March 8, 1911.
90. SLF to CIA, June 16, 1911, CCF, File 60679-10 (12) Omaha; Francis La Flesche to RF, July 14, 1899, LFP-NSHS; Francis La Flesche to Edward Farley, December 4, 1899, LFP-NSHS.
91. Green, *Iron Eye's Family*, 142.
92. SLF to CIA, June 16, 1911, CCF.
93. C. F. Hanke to SLF, November 17, 1910, CCF, File 60679-10 (312) Omaha; C. F. Hanke to SLF, June 24, 1911, CCF, File 60679-10 (312) Omaha.
94. Charles Monroe to Secretary of the Interior, September 5, 1914, CCF, File 34547-13 (310) Omaha; Apel Johnson to CIA, May 17, 1916, CCF, File 34547-13 (310) Omaha.
95. SLF to Miss Folsom, February 15, 1910, SAF-HUA.

CHAPTER 8. "PERMITTED TO SERVE"

1. "Pioneer Medical Women: Dr. Susan La Flesche Picotte," *The Medical Woman's Journal* 37 (1930): 20.

2. George A. Rosen, *Preventive Medicine in the United States, 1900–1975: Trends and Interpretations* (New York: Science History Publications, 1975), 6, 151; John Whiteclay Chambers, II, *The Tyranny of Change: America in the Progressive Era, 1900–1917* (New York: St. Martin's Press, 1980), 74; William Leach, *True Love and Perfect Union: The Feminist Reform of Sex and Society*, 2d ed. (Middletown, Conn.: Wesleyan University Press, 1989), 156–57, 328–29, 344, 346.

3. *Nebraska State Medical Society Proceedings* (Lincoln: n.p., 1890–1899); "Thurston County Medical Society," *WT*, September 20, 1907; Duffy, *From Humors to Medical Science*, 215, 217. Little else is known about Susan La Flesche Picotte's involvement in the Thurston County Medical Society; a close reading of local newspapers uncovered no other coverage of the society's activities.

4. *WT*, January 13, 1911.

5. SLF, Diary, November 5, 10, 17, 1910, LFP-NSHS; *WT*, January 13, 1911; "Clean Up," *WT*, October 22, 1909; "Pioneer Women," 21.

6. Dominick Cavallo, *Muscles and Morals: Organized Playgrounds and Urban Reform, 1880–1920* (Philadelphia: University of Pennsylvania Press, 1981), 1–8; Alan G. Ingham, "Games, Structures, and Agency: Historians on the American Play Movement," *Journal of Social History* 17 (Winter 1983): 289; for a radical, "social control" interpretation see Cary Goodman, *Choosing Sides: Playground and Street Life on the Lower East Side* (New York: Schocken Books, 1979).

7. "Diptheria Scare is Over," *WT*, September 17, 1909.

8. "Appoint a New Board of Health," *WT*, March 17, 1911.

9. "Medical Inspection for Pupils," *WT*, April 24, 1911; Duffy, *From Humors to Medical Science*, 227; Putney, "Fighting the Scourge," 90, 104. See also John Duffy, "School Buildings and the Health of American School Children in the Nineteenth Century," in *Healing and History: Essays for George Rosen*, ed. Charles E. Rosenberg (New York: Science History Publications, 1979), 161–78.

10. CIA, AR, 1899, 233; John Farley to Caryl Farley, November 20, 1900, LFP-NSHS.

11. "Medical Inspection of Pupils."

12. Albert F. Tyler, ed., *History of Medicine in Nebraska* (Omaha: Magic City Printing, 1977), 28.

13. For more on the intersection of maternalism and social activism, see Gordon, "Putting Children First," 64–70. See also Estelle Freedman, "Separatism as Strategy: Female Institution Building and American Feminism, 1870–1930," in *Women and Power in American History: A Reader, vol. II*

from 1870, ed. Kathryn Kish Sklar and Thomas Dublin (Englewood Cliffs, New Jersey: Prentice Hall, 1991), 15–17; Nancy S. Dye, "Introduction," in *Gender, Class, Race, and Reform in the Progressive Era*, ed. Noralee Frankel and Nancy S. Dye (Lexington: University Press of Kentucky, 1991), 1, 5.

14. SLF to Cato Sells, April 29, 1914, LFP-NSHS; Putney, "Fighting the Scourge," 90, 107–8; Hrdlicka, *Tuberculosis among Certain Indian Tribes*, 35.

15. Judith Walker Leavitt, *The Healthiest City: Milwaukee and the Politics of Health Reform* (Princeton, N.J.: Princeton University Press, 1982), 70–71; Baker, "The Domestication of Politics," 94.

16. Karen J. Blair, *Clubwoman as Feminist: True Womanhood Redefined, 1868–1914* (New York: Holmes & Meier, 1980), 98, 104, 115, 142, 144; Anne Firor Scott, *Natural Allies: Women's Associations in American History* (Urbana: University of Illinois Press, 1991), 111, 142, 155–57; Mildred W. Wells, *Unity in Diversity: The History of the General Federation of Women's Clubs* (n.p.: General Federation of Women's Clubs, 1953), vii, 29, 168; *Sixty Years of Nebraska Federation of Women's Clubs, Inc., 1894–1954* (Lincoln: n.p., 1954), 1; Freedman, "Separatism as Strategy," 12, 15.

17. Mary I. Wood, *The History of the General Federation of Women's Clubs* (New York: The History Department, General Federation of Women's Clubs, n.d.), 227, 282; Blair, *Clubwoman as Feminist*, 103–4; Wells, *Unity in Diversity*, 226; George A. Rosen, *A History of Public Health* (New York: MD Publications, 1957), 383–84; Inez C. Philbrick, "Health Committee," in *Nebraska Federation of Women's Clubs Yearbook, 1909–1910* (Lincoln: n.p., 1910), 28–29.

18. *WT*, January 13, 1911; SLF, "Health Department," in *Nebraska Federation of Women's Clubs Yearbook, 1910–1911* (Lincoln: n.p., 1911), 36–37; *Nebraska Federation of Women's Clubs Yearbook, 1911–1912* (Lincoln: n.p., 1912), 8.

19. SLF, "Health Department," 36–37.

20. Tyler, *History of Medicine in Nebraska*, 28.

21. Stuart Galishoff, *Safeguarding the Public Health: Newark, 1895–1918* (Westport, Conn.: Greenwood Press, 1975), 120, 122.

22. CIA, *AR*, 1912, 17, 40; "Annual Report, Winnebago and Omaha Agencies, July 1, 1910," *SNSR*.

23. SLF to Francis E. Leupp, November 15, 1907, CCF, File 90863 (162) Omaha; Leupp to SLF, November 20, 1907, CCF, File 90863 (162) Omaha.

24. *WT*, January 13, 1911.

25. "How to Protect Yourself Against Tuberculosis," *WT*, May 12, 1911; "White Plague," *WT*, March 10, 1911.

26. "White Plague," *WT*, March 10, 1911; Blair, *Clubwoman as Feminist*, 103–104; Hrdlicka, *Tuberculosis among Certain Indian Tribes*, 30–33; see also Murphy, "Health Problems of the Indians," 347–53.

27. "How to Protect Yourself Against Tuberculosis" *WT*, May 12, 1911; "White Plague," *WT*, March 10, 1911.

28. "White Plague," *WT*, March 10, 1911.

29. "War Declared on the Fly," *WT*, May 31, 1912.

30. "The Fly Our Most Dangerous Foe," *WT*, May 31, 1912; *WT*, October 17, 1913.

31. S. James Rowland, Jr., "Susan La Flesche: Princess, Physician, Prairie Preacher," *A.D.* 4 (November 1975): 40; SLF, Diary, January 11, 1911, LFP-NSHS; Tyler, *History of Medicine in Nebraska*, 28; Valerie Sherer Mathes, "Dr. Susan La Flesche Picotte: The Reformed and the Reformer," in *Indian Lives: Essays on Nineteenth- and Twentieth-Century Native American Leaders*, 2d ed., ed. L. G. Moses and Raymond Wilson (Albuquerque: University of New Mexico Press, 1993), 80; Putney, "Fighting the Scourge," 107–108, 183; CIA, *AR*, 1912, 65, 68; Ales Hrdlicka, "Contribution to the Knowledge of Tuberculosis," *SW* 35 (November 1908): 632.

32. Sara T. Kinney, "Indian Home Building," *The Indian's Friend* 2 (April 1889): 3; "Speaking for the Indians," 1889, clipping, SAF-HUA; CIA, *AR*, 1889, 910.

33. *The Indian's Friend* 2 (March 1890): 1; *IB* 1 (November 1890): 2; *The Indian's Friend* 2 (November 1890): 3.

34. SLF, "How the Silver Fox Taught the Coyote to Fish," "When and How Fire Came to be First Cured," "Primitive Farming among the Omaha Indians," "Folklore Tales of the American Indians," LFP-NSHS; "Indian Woman Feature of Farmers' Institute," *Western Paper*, February, 1912, clipping, SAF-HUA; SLF, "The Origin of the Corn," *WT*, March 8, 1912; "Glimpses of a Woman's Work"; SLF, "An Indian's View of 'The Lonesome Trail,'" *New York Times*, June 15, 1907.

35. SLF, Diary, December 21, 1910, LFP-NSHS.

36. "May Build an Indian Hospital," *Hartford Courant*, February 19, 1908, Scrapbook 1, Box 3, STK-CSL; "Indian Association," *Litchfield Enquirer*, October 15, 1908, Scrapbook 1, Box 3, STK-CSL; "Hartford Branch of Indian Association," *Hartford Courant*, November 6, 1908, Scrapbook 1, Box 3, STK-CSL; "Executive and Mission Committees of the Connecticut Indian Association," June 4, 1909, "28th Annual Meeting,"

December 3, 1909, "29th Annual Meeting," November 15, 1910, Minute Book no. 5, 1900–1923, Box 3, STK-CSL; "Christmas Dinner for Old Indians," *Waterbury American*, November 16, 1910, Scrapbook 1, Box 3, STK-CSL.

37. Pascoe, *Relations of Rescue*, 139–43; for an overview of "sisterhood" in U.S. history, see Hewitt, "Beyond the Search for Sisterhood," 1–19.

38. Putney, "Fighting the Scourge," 79; CIA, *AR*, 1910, 10; CIA, *AR*, 1911, 5–6.

39. SLF, "From the Omahas," *The Word Carrier* 39 (July/August 1910): 16.

40. SLF, Diary, December 5, 21, 1910, January 6, 11, 1911, LFP-NSHS.

41. Susan Pingry to Marguerite La Flesche Diddock, October 3, 1917, LFP-NSHS; Board of Home Missions of the Presbyterian Church in the U.S.A., "Minutes of Regular Meetings of the Board of Home Missions of the Presbyterian Church in the U.S.A.," September 14, 1911, 143, October 12, 1911, 172, November 16, 1911, 198, PHS; "Contract for the New Hospital is Signed," *WT*, January 12, 1912.

42. "Plans for the New Hospital are Completed," *WT*, October 6, 1911; "Contract for the New Hospital is Signed."

43. "Presbyterian Hospital Opened with Appropriate Services," *WT*, January 10, 1913.

44. Ibid.

45. *C.W.A. West*, 1912, clipping, SAF-HUA; *WT*, September 27, 1912; "Presbyterian Hospital Opened with Appropriate Services."

46. "Presbyterian Hospital Opened with Appropriate Services."

47. Ibid.; Elizabeth Shaffer to Marguerite La Flesche Diddock, April 30, 1914, LFP-NSHS.

48. *WT*, February 7, 1913; "Annual Report, Omaha School, 1914," *SNSR*; *Indian News*, January 13, clipping, SAF-HUA; *SW*, April, 1913, SAF-HUA; Tyler, *History of Medicine in Nebraska*, 28–29.

49. "Dr. Picotte Passes Away," *Peace Pipe*, September 1915, clipping, SAF-HUA; *WT*, March 5, 1915; *WT*, March 26, 1915; *WT*, September 3, 1915.

50. *WT*, May 28, 1915; *WT*, September 17, 1915.

51. "Funeral of Dr. Picotte Marked by Simplicity," *WT*, September 24, 1915.

52. "Dr. Picotte: An Appreciation," *WT*, September 24, 1915; "Dr. Picotte Passes Away"; "Susan La Flesche Picotte," *SW*, November 1915, clipping, SAF-HUA; see also "Daughter of Indian Chief, Well Known as Author, Dies in Nebraska Home," *Washington Post*, September 19, 1915,

clipping, SAF-HUA; *Indian Leader*, November, 1915, clipping, SAF-HUA; "Noted Indian Woman Dies," *New York Sun*, clipping, SAF-HUA.

53. Alice C. Fletcher to Marguerite La Flesche Diddock, September 25, 1915, LFP-NSHS; Harry L. Keefe, "The Mystery of Her Genius," *WT*, September 24, 1915; Josephine E. Richards to Marguerite La Flesche Diddock, October 4, 1915, LFP-NSHS.

54. SLF, "My Childhood," 78.

55. Thomas Dublin, ed., *Becoming American, Becoming Ethnic: College Students Explore Their Roots* (Philadelphia: Temple University Press, 1996), 231.

56. Fletcher and La Flesche, *Omaha Tribe*, 326.

57. Szasz, "Conclusion," 297.

58. *Indian Leader*, November, 1915, clipping, SAF-HUA.

59. *Heritage of Bancroft, Nebraska, 1884–1954* (n.p.: The Heritage Book Committee, 1984), 243; Orr, *Selected Pages from the History of Medicine in Nebraska*, 12.

60. Green, *Iron Eye's Family*, 160; "Ex-Hospital May Honor Indian Woman," *Omaha World-Herald*, October 6, 1988; "Picotte Hospital Put in Historic Register," *Omaha World-Herald*, March 12, 1989, 3B; Exhibition program book, Susan La Flesche Picotte Center, September 16, 1989, SAF-HUA.

61. *Congressional Record*, August 3, 1989, v. 135, no. 108, H 4952–53.

62. Dedication program, Susan L. Picotte School, May 16, 1993, SAF-HUA.

63. Theodore Finks, ed., "The First Indian Woman Physician," *Home Mission Monthly* 38 (February 1924): 87.

Bibliography

PRIMARY SOURCES

Published Letters and Writings of Susan La Flesche

La Flesche, Susan. "Another Appeal." *The Indian's Friend* 12 (March 1900): 8–9.

————."Dr. Picotte Discusses the New Policy." *WT*, December 31, 1909.

————. "Dr. Picotte's Appeal." *WT*, March 4, 1910.

————. "From Dr. Susan La Flesche." In *The Hampton Normal and Agricultural Institute and Its Work for the Education of the Indian*, clipping, SAF-HUA.

————. "From the Omahas." *The Word Carrier* 39 (July/August 1910): 16.

————. "Health Department." In *Nebraska Federation of Women's Clubs Yearbook, 1910–1911*, 36–37. Lincoln: n.p., 1911.

————. "The Home Life of the Indian." *The Indian's Friend* 4 (June 1892): 39–40.

————. "An Indian Mud Lodge: A Peculiar Home." *The Indian Helper*, June 17, 1892, 1, 4.

————. "An Indian on Home Building." *The Indian's Friend* 1 (July 1889): 1.

————. "An Indian's View of 'The Lonesome Trail.'" *New York Times*, June 15, 1907.

————. Letter, December 19, 1887. In *Hampton Institute, Ten Years' Work for Indians at Hampton, Virginia, Record of Negro and Indian Graduates and Ex-Students*. Hampton: Normal School Press, 1893.

_____. Letter, probably spring 1893. Reprinted in "From Dr. Susan La Flesche." *The Indian's Friend* 5 (June 1893): 3.

_____. Letter, undated. Reprinted in "From Dr. La Flesche." *The Indian's Friend* 3 (February 1891): 3.

_____. Letter, undated. Reprinted in *IB* 10 (March 1896): 1.

_____. Letter, undated. Reprinted in *The Indian's Friend* 6 (November 1890): 2.

_____. "My Childhood and Womanhood." *SW* (15 July 1886): 78–79.

_____. "My Work as Physician among My People." *SW* 21 (August 1892): 133.

_____. "Omaha-Winnebago Merger." *WT*, January 7, 1910.

_____. "The Omahas and Citizenship." *SW* 20 (April 1891): 177.

_____. "The Origin of the Corn." *WT*, March 8, 1912.

_____. *Report of Susan La Flesche, M.D., Medical Missionary of the Women's National Indian Association Among the Omaha Indians.* Women's National Indian Association, October 24, 1891, Sophia Smith Collection, Smith College, Northampton, Massachusetts.

_____. "Report of Physician for Omahas." In U.S. Commissioner of Indian Affairs, *Annual Report of the Commissioner of Indian Affairs to the Secretary of the Interior*, 1893, 197.

_____. "The Varied Work of an Indian Missionary." *Home Mission Monthly* 22 (August 1908): 246–47.

_____ to Dear Friends, probably April 1894. Reprinted in "Letter from Dr. Susan La Flesche." *IB* 8 (May 1894): 3.

_____ to Members of the Connecticut Indian Association, January 13, 1890. Reprinted in "Some Interesting Letters," The Bulletin 1 (April 1890): 3.

_____ to Miss Burbanks, November 6, 1891. Reprinted in "A Letter from Dr. La Flesche," *IB* 3 (December 1891): 4.

_____ to Mrs. Kinney, November 14, 1896. Reprinted in "News from Dr. Picotte," *IB* 11 (February 1897): 2.

_____ to Mrs. Quinton, undated. Reprinted in "From Dr. Susan La Flesche," *The Indian's Friend* 2 (December 1889): 2.

_____ to Sara Thomson Kinney, April 2, 1888. Reprinted in *The Bulletin* 1 (April 1888): 1.

Archival Materials

American Indian Correspondence, PHS.

Board of Home Missions of the Presbyterian Church in the U.S.A., "Minutes of Regular Meetings of the Board of Home Missions of the Presbyterian Church in the U.S.A.", PHS.

Bodley, Rachel L. Papers, Archives and Special Collections on Women in Medicine, The Medical College of Pennsylvania and Hospital, Philadelphia, Pennsylvania.

Cuming County, "Nebraska Marriages, Book V, 1894–1898," NSHS.

Fletcher–La Flesche Papers, National Anthropological Archives, Smithsonian Institution, Washington, D.C.

Furnas, Robert W. Papers, NSHS.

Gilmore, Melvin R. Papers, NSHS.

Indian Rights Association Papers, 1868–1968, 136 microfilm reels. Glen Rock, N.J.: Microfilming Corporation of America, 1974.

Kinney, Sara Thomson. Papers, Connecticut State Library, Hartford, Connecticut.

La Flesche Family Papers, NSHS.

La Flesche, Susan. Alumni File, HUA.

Picotte, Susan La Flesche. Alumna File, Archives and Special Collections on Women in Medicine, The Medical College of Pennsylvania and Hospital, Philadelphia.

Presbyterian Church in the U.S.A., "Niobrara Presbytery, Minutes, 1885–1950," 4 vols., PHS.

"Presbyterian Missionary Letters Relating to the American Indians in Nebraska Country," PHS.

Waldron, Martha M. Papers, HUA.

Government Documents and Publications

Central Consolidated Files, 1907–1939. Record Group 75, Bureau of Indian Affairs, National Archives and Records Service, Washington, D.C.

Dorsey, James Owen. *Omaha and Ponka Letters.* Bureau of American Ethnology Bulletin 11. Smithsonian Institution. Washington, D.C.: Government Printing Office, 1891.

———. *Omaha Sociology.* Bureau of American Ethnology Third Annual Report. Washington, D.C.: Government Printing Office, 1884.

Federal Indian Law. Washington, D.C.: Government Printing Office, 1958. Reprint, New York: Association on American Indian Affairs, 1966.

Fletcher, Alice C., and Francis La Flesche. *The Omaha Tribe.* Bureau of American Ethnology Twenty-Seventh Annual Report, 1905–1906. Washington, D.C.: Government Printing Office, 1911.

Hailmann, William N. *Circular Letter of Instruction.* Washington, D.C.: Government Printing Office, 1895.

Hrdlicka, Ales. *Tuberculosis among Certain Indian Tribes of the United States*. Washington, D.C.: Government Printing Office, 1909.

Kappler, Charles J. *Indian Affairs: Laws and Treaties*. 2 vols. Washington, D.C.: Government Printing Office, 1904.

Letters Received by the Indian Office, 1881–1907. RG 75, BIA, NA.

Letters Received by the Indian Office, 1824–1881. Nebraska Agencies, 1876–1880. RG 75, BIA, M234, reel 524, NA.

Letters Received by the Indian Office, 1824–1881. Omaha Agency, 1824–1870. RG 75, BIA, M234, reel 605, NA.

In The Matter of Heff. 25 Sup. Ct. 605 (1905).

Reports of Inspection of the Field Jurisdictions of the Office of Indian Affairs, 1873–1900. RG 75, BIA, M1016, reel 32, NA.

Smith, G. Hubert. *Omaha Indians: Ethnohistorical Report on the Omaha People*. Indian Claims Commission docket no. 225A. Washington, D.C.: Government Printing Office, 1957. Reprint, New York: Garland Publishing, 1974.

Superintendents' Annual Narrative and Statistical Reports from Field Jurisdictions of the Bureau of Indian Affairs, 1907–1938. RG 75, BIA, M1011, reel 169, NA.

U.S. Commissioner of Indian Affairs. *Annual Report of the Commissioner of Indian Affairs to the Secretary of the Interior*, 1845, 1855–1857, 1861–1915.

U.S. Congress. *Congressional Record*.

_____. Senate. *Memorial of the Members of the Omaha Tribe of Indians for a Grant of Land in Severalty*. S. Misc. Doc. 31, 47th Cong., 1st sess., 1882, serial 1993.

_____. *Notes on the Returned Indian Students of the Normal and Agricultural Institute*. S. Rept. Exec. Doc. 31, 52d Cong., 1st sess., 1892, serial 2892.

_____. *Sale of Intoxicating Liquors to Indians*. S. Rept. Doc. 1294, 54th Cong., 2d sess., 1897, serial 3474.

U.S. Statutes at Large 27 (1892), 29 (1897).

Articles

Armstrong, Samuel Chapman. "Education of the Indian." *The Journal of Proceedings and Addresses of the National Education Association* (1884): 177.

Dougherty, John. "A Description of the Fur Trade in 1831 by John Dougherty." Edited by Richard E. Jensen. *Nebraska History* 56 (Spring 1975): 109–20.

Eastman, Charles. "The Indian's Health Problem." *American Indian Magazine* 4 (April/June 1916):139–45.

Fletcher, Alice C. "Glimpses of Child-Life Among the Omaha Tribe of Indians." *Journal of American Folklore* 1 (July/September 1888): 115–23.

———. "Glimpses of Indian Child Life." *The Outlook*, May 16, 1896, 891–92.

———. "The Indian Woman and Her Problems." *SW* 28 (May 1899): 172–76.

———. "Lands in Severalty to Indians: Illustrated by Experiences with the Omaha Tribe." *Proceedings of the American Association for the Advancement of Science* 33 (1884): 654–65.

———. "Obituary Notice." *Journal of American Folklore* 2 (January/March 1889): 11.

———. "Preparation of Indians for Citizenship." *SW* 34 (August 1905): 425–28.

———. "The Preparation of the Indian for Citizenship." *Lend a Hand* 9 (September 1892): 190–98.

"Glimpses of a Woman's Work among the Omahas," *Omaha World-Herald*, March 22, 1908.

Hrdlicka, Ales. "Contribution to the Knowledge of Tuberculosis." *SW* 5 (November 1908): 626–34.

"An Indian Chief's Crusade for Temperance," *The Indian School Journal* 9 (March 1909): 35.

"Joseph La Flesche." *SW* 17 (December 1888): 127.

Kearns, W. H. "The New Presbyterian Hospital for the Omaha Indians." In *American Indian Missions, Reprint of Assembly Herald Articles, 1913*, 5. N.p., n.d.

Kinney, Sara T. "Indian Home Building." *The Indian's Friend* 2 (April 1889): 3.

La Flesche, Francis. "An Indian Allotment." *The Independent* 52 (November 8, 1900): 2686–88.

———. "Protection of Indian Lands." In *Report of the Annual Lake Mohonk Conference on the Indian and Other Dependent Peoples*, 70–72. Mohonk Lake, N.Y.: The Conference, 1914–1916.

La Flesche, Marguerite. "Some Indian Customs: Commencement Address of Marguerite La Flesche." *SW* 16 (August 1887): 88–89.

La Flesche, Susette. "Nedawi." *St. Nicholas Magazine* 8 (January 1881): 225–30.

"Letterbox." *St. Nicholas Magazine* 7 (September 1880): 918.

MacKay, James. "Journal." In *Before Lewis and Clark: Documents Illustrating the History of the Missouri, 1783–1804*, edited by Abraham P. Nasatir, 1:354–64. 2 vols. St Louis: St. Louis Historical Documents Foundation, 1952.

Murphy, Joseph A. "Health Problems of the Indians." *Annals of the American Academy of Political and Social Science* 37 (March 1911): 347–53.

"Omahas Drinking," *The Word Carrier* 21 (August 1892): 21.

Philbrick, Inez C. "Health Committee." In *Nebraska Federation of Women's Clubs Yearbook, 1909–1910*, 28–29. Lincoln: n.p., 1910.

"Pioneer Medical Women: Dr. Susan La Flesche Picotte." *The Medical Woman's Journal* 37 (1930): 19–20.

"Quaker Report on Indian Agencies in Nebraska, 1869." *Nebraska History* 54 (Summer 1973): 151–220.

Roddy, Thomas R., "The Winnebago Mescal-Eaters," in *The Indian Tribes of the Upper Mississippi Valley and Region of the Great Lakes*, edited by Emma Helen Blair, 281–83. 2 vols. Cleveland: Arthur H. Clark, 1912.

Sellers, James L., ed. "Diary of Dr. Joseph A. Paxson, Physician to the Winnebago Indians, 1869–1870." *Nebraska History* 27 (July/September 1946): 143–204.

"State Indian Associations." *Lend a Hand* 4 (December 1889): 863–82.

Waldron, Martha M. "The Indian Health Question." *Lend a Hand* 5 (November 1890): 766–74.

Books and Pamphlets

Annual Report of the Women's National Indian Association, December 1892. Philadelphia: n.p., 1892.

Armstrong, Samuel Chapman. *Annual Report of the Principal to the Board of Trustees, 1891*. Hampton, Va.: Hampton Institute Press, 1891.

_____. *The Ideas on Education Expressed by Samuel C. Armstrong*. Hampton, Va.: For the Armstrong League of Hampton Workers by the Hampton Institute Press, 1909.

_____. *Indian Education in the East: At Hampton, Va. and Carlisle, Penn.* Hampton, Va.: Normal School Steam Press, 1980.

_____. *The Indian Question*. Hampton, Va.: Normal School Steam Press, 1883.

Board of Foreign Missions of the Presbyterian Church in the U.S.A. *Thirty-Third Annual Report of the Board of Foreign Missions of the Presbyterian Church in the United States of America.* New York: Board of Foreign Missions, 1870.

Bradbury, John. *Travels in the Interior of America, in the Years 1809, 1810, and 1811.* London: Sherwood, Neely, & Jones, 1817. Reprint, Ann Arbor: University Microfilms, 1966.

The City of Elizabeth, New Jersey Illustrated. Elizabeth, N.J.: Elizabeth Daily Journal, 1889.

De Smet, Pierre-Jean. *Life, Letters, and Travels of Father Pierre-Jean De Smet, S.J., 1801–1873.* 4 vols. Edited by Hiram M. Chittenden and Alfred Talbot Richardson. New York: Francis P. Harper, 1905. Reprint, New York: Arno Press, 1969.

Fortieth Annual Announcement of the Woman's Medical College of Pennsylvania. Philadelphia: n.p., 1889.

Giffen, Fannie Reed. *Oo-Ma-Ha-Ta-Wa-Tha (Omaha City).* Lincoln: n.p., 1898.

Hampton Institute. *Concerning Indians.* Hampton, Va.: Normal School Steam Press, 1883.

_____. *The Hampton Normal and Agricultural Institute and its Work for Negro and Indian Youth.* Hampton, Va.: n.p., 1894.

_____. *Ten Years' Work for Indians at Hampton, Virginia, 1878–1888.* Hampton, Va.: Hampton Institute Press, 1888.

_____. *Twenty-Two Years' Work of the Hampton Normal and Agricultural Institute at Hampton, Virginia, Record of Negro and Indian Graduates and Ex-Students.* Hampton, Va.: Normal School Press, 1893.

Hensel, Lawrence M. *Report of Our Omaha Mission.* N.p.: 1888.

Historical Sketch of the Missions. Philadelphia: Women's Board of Home Missions, 1891.

James, Edwin. *Account of an Expedition from Pittsburgh to the Rocky Mountains.* 2 vols. Philadelphia: H. C. Carey & I. Lea, 1823. Reprint, Ann Arbor: University Microfilms, 1966.

Johnson, Ellen Terry. *Historical Sketch of the Connecticut Indian Association from 1881 to 1888.* Hartford: Fowler & Miller, 1888.

Kurz, Rudolph Friederich. *Journal of Rudolph Friederich Kurz.* Edited by J. N. B. Hewitt. Bureau of American Ethnology, Bulletin 115. Washington, D.C.: Government Printing Office, 1937. Reprint, Lincoln: University of Nebraska Press, 1970.

Lake Mohonk Conference of Friends of the Indian and Other Dependent Peoples. *Annual Report of Proceedings,* 1889–1894, 1900, 1906.

Ludlow, Helen W. Hampton *Normal and Agricultural Institute: Its Work for Indians.* Springfield, Mass.: n.p., n.d.

Marshall, Clara. *The Woman's Medical College of Pennsylvania: An Historical Outline* Philadelphia: P. Blakiston, Son, 1897.

Maximilian, Prince of Wied-Neuwied. *Travels in the Interior of North America, 1832–1834.* Edited by Reuben Gold Thwaites. 3 vols. Cleveland: Arthur H. Clark, 1906.

Moulton, Gary E., ed. *The Journals of the Lewis and Clark Expedition.* 8 vols. Lincoln: University of Nebraska Press, 1983–.

Nasatir, Abraham P., ed. *Before Lewis and Clark: Documents Illustrating the History of the Missouri, 1783–1804,* 2 vols. St. Louis: St. Louis Historical Documents Foundation, 1952.

Nebraska Federation of Women's Clubs Yearbook, 1909–10. Lincoln: n.p., 1910.

Nebraska Federation of Women's Clubs Yearbook, 1911–1912. Lincoln: n.p., 1912.

Nebraska State Medical Society Proceedings. Lincoln: n.p., 1890–1899.

Neihardt, John G. *Patterns and Coincidences: A Sequel to All is But a Beginning.* Columbia: University of Missouri Press, 1978.

Nichols, Roger L., ed. *The Missouri Expedition, 1818–1820: The Journal of Surgeon John Gale with Related Documents.* Norman: University Of Oklahoma Press, 1969.

Olson, Paul A., ed. *The Book of the Omaha: Literature of the Omaha People.* Lincoln: Nebraska Curriculum Development Center, 1979.

Osler, William. *Principles and Practice of Medicine.* 2d ed. New York: Appleton, 1895.

Paul Wilhelm, Duke of Wurttemberg. *Travels in North America, 1822–1824.* Edited by Savoie Lottinville. Norman: University of Oklahoma Press, 1973.

Pratt, Richard H. *Battlefield and Classroom: Four Decades with the American Indian, 1867–1904.* Edited by Robert M. Utley. New Haven, Conn.: Yale University Press, 1964.

Quinton, Amelia Stone. *Missionary Work of the Women's National Indian Association.* N.p., 1885?

Scharf, John Thomas, and Thompson Westcott. *History of Philadelphia, 1609–1884.* 3 vols. Philadelphia: L. H. Everts, 1884.

Schmeckebier, Laurence F. *The Office of Indian Affairs: Its History, Activities and Organization.* Baltimore: Johns Hopkins Press, 1927.

Schwarz, Julius F. *History of the Presbyterian Church in Nebraska.* N.p., 1924.

Thirty-Seventh Annual Announcement of the Woman's Medical College of Pennsylvania. Philadelphia: n.p., 1886.

Thirty-Eighth Annual Announcement of the Woman's Medical College of Pennsylvania. Philadelphia: n.p., 1887.

Thirty-Ninth Annual Announcement of the Woman's Medical College of Pennsylvania. Philadelphia: n.p., 1888.

Thwaites, Reuben Gold, ed. *Original Journals of the Lewis and Clark Expedition, 1804–1806.* 8 vols. New York: Dodd, Mead, 1904–1905. Reprint, New York: Arno Press, 1969.

Tibbles, Thomas H. *Buckskin and Blanket Days: Memoirs of a Friend of the Indians.* Edited by Theodora Bates Cogswell. Garden City, N.Y.: Doubleday, 1957.

Welsch, Roger L. *Omaha Tribal Myths and Trickster Tales.* Athens, Ohio: Sage/Swallow Press Books, 1981.

Women's National Indian Association. *Sketches of Delightful Work.* N.p., 1893.

Wood, Mary I. *The History of the General Federation of Women's Clubs.* New York: The History Department, General Federation of Women's Clubs, n.d.

Newspapers and Periodicals

Bancroft Blade, 1899–1908.
The Bulletin, 1888–1890.
Hartford Courant, 1886–1891.
The Indian Bulletin, 1889–1898.
The Indian's Friend, 1888–1915.
Lend a Hand, 1889–1890.
Omaha World-Herald, 1908–1910, 1988–1989.
Southern Workman, 1882–1895.
Talks and Thoughts, 1889–1893.
Walthill Times, 1907–1912, 1909–1915.

SECONDARY SOURCES
Dissertations and Theses

Adams, David Wallace. "The Federal Indian Boarding School: A Study of Environment and Response." Ph.D. diss., Indiana University, 1975.

BIBLIOGRAPHY

Boughter, Judith A. "Betraying Their Trust: The Dispossession of the Omaha Nation, 1790–1916." Master's thesis, University of Nebraska at Omaha, 1995.

Drachman, Virginia G. "Women Doctors and the Women's Medical Movement: Feminism and Medicine, 1850–1895." Ph.D. diss., State University of New York at Buffalo, 1976.

Evers, Lawrence J. "The Literature of the Omahas." Ph.D. diss., University of Nebraska, Lincoln, 1972.

Marsh, Barbara R. "Intertribal Conflicts of the Omaha Indians: Traditional and Contemporary Accounts, 1673–1837." Master's thesis, Wichita State University, 1956.

Putney, Diane Theresa. "Fighting the Scourge: American Indian Morbidity and Federal Policy, 1897–1928." Ph.D. diss., Marquette University, 1980.

Schnier, Donald. "A History of Bancroft, Nebraska." Master's thesis, University of Nebraska at Omaha, 1967.

Thorne, Janis Chapman. "People of the River: Mixed Blood Families on the Lower Missouri." Ph.D. diss., University of California, Los Angeles, 1987.

Tingey, Joseph Willard. "Blacks and Indians Together: An Experiment in Biracial Education at Hampton Institute (1878–1923)." Ph.D. diss., Columbia Teachers' College, 1978.

Wanken, Helen M. "Woman's Sphere and Indian Reform: The Women's National Indian Association, 1875–1901." Ph.D. diss., Marquette University, 1981.

Welch, Rebecca Hancock. "Alice Cunningham Fletcher, Anthropologist and Indian Rights Reformer." Ph.D. diss., George Washington University, 1980.

Articles

Abram, Ruth J. "Give Her Knowledge: The Class of 1879 in Training." In *"Send Us a Lady Physician": Women Doctors in America, 1835–1920*, edited by Ruth J. Abram, 139–52. New York: W. W. Norton, 1985.

———. "Private Practice: Taking Every Case to Heart." In *"Send Us a Lady Physician": Women Doctors in America, 1835–1920*, edited by Ruth J. Abram, 153–62. New York: W. W. Norton, 1985.

———. "Soon the Baby Died: Medical Training in Nineteenth-Century America." In *"Send Us a Lady Physician": Women Doctors in America, 1835–1920*, edited by Ruth J. Abram, 17–20. New York: W. W. Norton, 1985.

_____. "Will There Be a Monument?: Six Pioneer Women Doctors Tell Their Own Stories." In *"Send Us a Lady Physician": Women Doctors in America, 1835–1920*, edited by Ruth J. Abram, 71–106. New York: W. W. Norton, 1985.

Albers, Patricia C. "Autonomy and Dependency in the Lives of Dakota Women: A Study in Historical Change." *Review of Radical Political Economics* 17, no. 3 (1985): 109–34.

_____. "From Illusion to Illumination: Anthropological Studies of American Indian Women." In *Gender and Anthropology: Critical Reviews for Research and Teaching*, edited by Sandra Morgan, 137–70. Washington, D.C.: American Anthropological Association, 1989.

Allen, Virginia R. "Agency Physicians to the Southern Plains Indians, 1868–1900." *Bulletin of the History of Medicine* 49 (Fall 1975):318–30.

Anson, Bert. "Variations of the Indian Conflict: The Effects of the Emigrant Indian Removal Policy, 1830–1854." *Missouri Historical Review* 59 (October 1964): 64–89.

Arth, Malcolm J. "A Functional View of Peyotism in Omaha Culture." *Plains Anthropologist* 2 (October 1956): 25–29.

Attneave, Carolyn L., and Agnes Dill. "Indian Boarding Schools and Indian Women: Blessing or Curse?" In *Proceedings of the Conference on the Educational and Occupational Needs of American Indian Women*, 211–30. Washington, D.C.: Government Printing Office, 1976.

Baker, Paula. "The Domestication of Politics: Women and American Political Society, 1780–1920." In *Unequal Sisters: A Multicultural Reader in U.S. Women's History*, 2d ed., edited by Vicki L. Ruiz and Ellen Carol Dubois, 85–110. New York: Routledge, 1994.

Bangs, S. D. "History of Sarpy County." In *Transactions and Reports of the Nebraska State Historical Society*, vol. 2, 293–308. Lincoln: State Journal, 1887.

Barnes, R. H. "A Legacy of Misperception and Invention: The Omaha Indians in Anthropology." In *The Invented Indian: Cultural Fictions and Government Policies*, edited by James A. Clifton, 211–22. New Brunswick: Transaction Publishers, 1990.

Barry, Kathleen. "The New Historical Syntheses: Women's Biography." *Journal of Women's History* 1 (Spring 1989): 74–105.

Clifton, James A. "Alternate Identities and Cultural Frontiers." In *Being and Becoming Indian: Biographical Studies of North American Frontiers*, edited by James A. Clifton, 1–37. Chicago: Dorsey Press, 1989.

Coleman, Michael C. "American Indian School Pupils as Cultural Brokers: Cherokee Girls at Brainerd Mission, 1828–1829." In *Between Indian and*

White Worlds: The Cultural Broker, edited by Margaret Connell Szasz, 122–36. Norman: University of Oklahoma Press, 1994.

————. "The Mission Education of Francis La Flesche: An American Indian Response to the Presbyterian Boarding School in the 1860s," *American Studies in Scandinavia*, 18 (1986): 67–82.

————. "Not Race but Grace: Presbyterian Missionaries and American Indians, 1837–1893." *Journal of American History* 67 (June 1980): 41–60.

Darder, Antonio. "The Politics of Biculturalism: Culture and Difference in the Formation of Warriors for *Gringostroika* and The New Mestizas." In *Culture and Difference: Critical Perspectives on the Bicultural Experience in the United States*, edited by Antonio Darder, 1–20. Westport, Conn.: Bergin & Garvey, 1995.

Davies, Phillips G. "Davis Jones and Gwen Davies, Missionaries in Nebraska Territory, 1853–1860." *Nebraska History* 60 (Spring 1979): 77–91.

Diffendel, Anne P. "The La Flesche Sisters: Susette, Rosalie, Marguerite, Lucy, Susan." In *Perspectives: Women in Nebraska History,* edited by Susan Pierce, 215–25. Lincoln: Nebraska Department of Education and the Nebraska State Council for the Social Studies, 1984.

Dozier, E. P. "Problem Drinking Among American Indians: The Role of Sociocultural Deprivation." *Quarterly Journal of Studies on Alcohol* 27, no. 1 (1966): 77–87.

Duffin, Lorna. "The Conspicuous Consumptive: Woman as an Invalid." In *The Nineteenth-Century Woman: Her Cultural and Physical World*, edited by Sara Delamont and Lorna Duffin, 26–56. New York: Barnes & Nobles Books, 1978.

Duffy, John. "School Buildings and the Health of American School Children in the Nineteenth Century." In *Healing and History: Essays for George Rosen*, edited by Charles E. Rosenberg, 161–78. New York: Science History Publications, 1979.

Dye, Nancy S. "Introduction." *In Gender, Class, Race, and Reform in the Progressive Era*, edited by Noralee Frankel and Nancy S. Dye, 1–9. Lexington: University Press of Kentucky, 1991.

Emmerich, Lisa E. "Marguerite La Flesche Diddock: Office of Indian Affairs Field Matron." *Great Plains Quarterly* 13 (Summer 1993): 162–71.

————. "'Right in the Midst of My Own People'": Native American Women and the Field Matron Program." *American Indian Quarterly* 15 (Spring 1991): 201–16.

Etienne, Mona, and Eleanor Leacock. "Introduction." In *Women and Colonization: Anthropological Perspectives*, edited by Mona Etienne and Eleanor Leacock, 1–24. New York: Praeger Publishers, 1980.

Ewers, John. "Intertribal Warfare as the Precursor of Indian-White Warfare on the Northern Great Plains." *Western Historical Quarterly* 6 (October 1975): 397–410. Reprinted in *Plains Indian History and Culture: Essays on Continuity and Change* (Norman: University of Oklahoma Press, 1997).

_____. "Mothers of Mixed Bloods: The Marginal Women in the History of the Upper Missouri." In *Probing the American West: Papers from the Santa Fe Conference*, edited by K. Ross Toole, 62–70. Santa Fe: Museum of New Mexico Press, 1962.

Farb, Robert C. "Robert C. Furnas as Omaha Indian Agent, 1864–1866." *Nebraska History* 32 (September 1951): 186–203.

Finks, Theodore, ed. "The First Indian Woman Physician." *Home Mission Monthly* 38 (February 1924): 86–87.

Fox, L. Webster. "Trachoma Problem among North American Indians." *Journal of the American Medical Association* 86 (February 1926): 404–406.

Freedman, Estelle. "Separatism as Strategy: Female Institution Building and American Feminism, 1870–1930." In *Women and Power in American History: A Reader, vol. II from 1870*, edited by Kathryn Kish Sklar and Thomas Dublin, 10–24. Englewood Cliffs, N.J.: Prentice Hall, 1991.

Gilmore, Melvin R. "First Prohibition Law in America." *Journal of American History* 4 (July/September 1910): 397.

Gleason, Philip. "American Identity and Americanization," in *Harvard Encyclopedia of American Ethnic Groups*, edited by Stephen Thernstrom, 31–58. Cambridge, Mass.: Belknap Press, 1980.

Gordon, Linda. "Putting Children First: Women, Maternalism, and Welfare in the Early Twentieth Century." In *U.S. History as Women's History: New Feminist Essays*, edited by Linda K. Kerber, Alice Kessler-Harris, and Kathryn Kish Sklar, 63–86. Chapel Hill: University of North Carolina Press, 1995.

Green, Norma Kidd. "Four Sisters: Daughters of Joseph La Flesche." *Nebraska History* 45 (June 1964): 165–76

_____. "The Make-Believe White Man's Village." *Nebraska History* 56 (Summer 1975): 242–47.

_____. "The Presbyterian Mission to the Omaha Indian Tribe." *Nebraska History* 48 (Autumn 1967): 267–88.

Green, Rayna. "The Pocahontas Perplex: The Image of the Indian Woman in American Culture," *Massachusetts Review* 16 (1975): 698–714.

Griswold, Robert L. "Anglo Women and Domestic Ideology in the American West in the Nineteenth and Early Twentieth Centuries." In *Western Women: Their Land, Their Lives*, edited by Lillian Schlissel, Vicki L.

Ruiz, and Janice Monk, 15–34. Albuquerque: University of New Mexico Press, 1988.

Hagan, William T. "Daniel M. Browning (1893–1897)." In *The Commissioners of Indian Affairs, 1824–1977*, edited by Robert M. Kvasnicka and Herman J. Viola, 205–10. Lincoln: University of Nebraska, 1979.

Hall, Stuart. "Cultural Identity and Diaspora." In *Identity: Community, Culture, Difference*, edited by Jonathan Rutherford, 222–37. London: Lawrence & Wishart, 1990.

————. "Ethnicity: Identity and Difference." *Radical America* 23, no. 4 (1989): 9–20.

Hauptman, Laurence M. "Medicine Woman: Susan La Flesche, 1865–1915." *New York State Journal of Medicine* 78 (September 1978): 1783–88.

Herzog, Kristin. "The La Flesche Family: Native American Spirituality, Calvinism, and Presbyterian Missions." *American Presbyterians* 65 (Fall 1987): 222–32.

Hewitt, Nancy A. "Beyond the Search for Sisterhood: American Women's History in the 1980s." In *Unequal Sisters: A Multicultural Reader in U.S. Women's History*, 2d ed., edited by Vicki L. Ruiz and Ellen Carol Dubois, 1–19. New York: Routledge, 1994.

Hill, Thomas W. "Peyotism and the Control of Heavy Drinking: The Nebraska Winnebago in the Early 1900s." *Human Organization* 49 (Fall 1990): 255–65.

Hinckley, Ted C. "Glimpses of Societal Change Among Nineteenth-Century Tlingit Women." *Journal of the West* 32 (July 1993): 12–24.

Holder, Preston. "The Fur Trade as Seen from the Indian Point of View." In *The Frontier Re-examined*, edited by John Francis McDermott, 129–39. Urbana: University of Illinois Press, 1967.

Howard, James H. "Omaha Peyotism." *Hobbies—The Magazine for Collectors* 56 (September 1951): 142.

"An Indian Chief's Crusade for Temperance." *The Indian School Journal* 9 (March 1909): 35.

Ingham, Alan G. "Games, Structures, and Agency: Historians on the American Play Movement." *Journal of Social History* 17 (Winter 1983): 285–302.

Jacobi, Mary Putnam. "Woman in Medicine," In *Woman's Work in America*, edited by Annie Nathan Meyer, 139–205. New York: Henry Holt, 1891.

Jameson, Elizabeth. "Women as Workers, Women as Civilizers: True Womanhood in the American West." In *The Women's West*, edited by Susan Armitage and Elizabeth Jameson, 145–64. Norman: University of Oklahoma Press, 1987.

Janiewski, Dolores. "Learning to Live 'Just Like White Folks': Gender, Ethnicity, and the State in the Inland Northwest." In *Gendered Domains: Rethinking Public and Private in Women's History*, edited by Dorothy O. Helly and Susan M. Reverby, 167–82. Ithaca, N.Y.: Cornell University, 1992.

Kerber, Linda K. "Separate Spheres, Female Worlds, Woman's Place: The Rhetoric of Women's History." *Journal of American History* 75 (June 1988): 9–39.

King, James T. "A Better Way: General George Crook and the Ponca Indians." *Nebraska History* 50 (Fall 1969): 239–55.

Klein, Alan. "The Political-Economy of Gender: A 19th Century Plains Indian Case Study." In *The Hidden Half: Studies of Plains Indian Women*, edited by Patricia Albers and Beatrice Medicine, 143–65. Washington, D.C.: University Press of America, 1983.

Klein, Laura F. "'She's One of Us, You Know,' The Public Life of Tlingit Women: Traditional, Historical, and Contemporary Perspectives." *The Western Canadian Journal of Anthropology* 6, no. 3 (1976): 164–83.

_____., and Lillian A. Ackerman. "Introduction." In *Women and Power in Native North America*, edited by Laura F. Klein and Lillian A. Ackerman, 3–16. Norman: University Of Oklahoma Press, 1995.

La Barre, Weston. "Twenty Years of Peyote Studies," *Current Anthropology* 1 (January 1960): 45.

Liberty, Margot. "Hell Came with Horses: Plains Indian Women in the Equestrian Era." *Montana, The Magazine of Western History* 32 (Summer 1982): 10–19.

Lomawaima, K. Tsianina. "Domesticity in the Federal Indian Schools: The Power of Authority over Mind and Body." *American Ethnologist* 20 (May 1993): 227–40.

Lurie, Nancy Oestreich. "The Lady from Boston and the Omaha Indians." *American West* 3 (Fall 1966): 31–33, 80–85.

_____. "The World's Oldest On-Going Protest Demonstration: North American Indian Drinking Patterns." *Pacific Historical Review* 40 (August 1971): 311–32.

McDonnell, Janet A. "Land Policy on the Omaha Reservation: Competency Commissions and Forced Fee Patents." *Nebraska History* 63 (Fall 1982): 399–412.

McFee, Malcolm. "The 150% Man, A Product of Blackfeet Acculturation." *American Anthropologist* 70 (1968): 1096–1103.

MacMurphy, J. A. "Some Frenchmen of Early Days on the Missouri River." In *Transactions and Reports of the Nebraska State Historical Society* 5 (1893): 43–63.

Mathes, Valerie Sherer. "Dr. Susan La Flesche Picotte: The Reformed and the Reformer." In *Indian Lives: Essays on Nineteenth and Twentieth-Century Native American Leaders*, edited by L. G. Moses and Raymond Wilson, 63–90. 2d ed. Albuquerque: University of New Mexico Press, 1993.

——. "Native American Women in Medicine and the Military." *American Indian Quarterly* 2, no. 2 (1975): 41–48.

——. "Nineteenth Century Women and Reform: The Women's National Indian Association." *American Indian Quarterly* 14 (Winter 1990): 1–18.

——. "Portrait for a Western Album." *American West* 16 (May/June 1979): 38–39.

——. "Susan La Flesche Picotte, M.D.: Nineteenth-century Physician and Reformer." *Great Plains Quarterly* 13 (Summer 1993): 172–96.

Matthews, Jean. "'Woman's Place' and the Search for Identity in Ante-Bellum America." *The Canadian Review of American Studies* 10 (Winter 1979): 288–304.

Mattison, Ray H. "The Indian Frontier on the Upper Missouri to 1865." *Nebraska History* 39 (September 1958): 241–66.

——. "Indian Missions and Missionaries on the Upper Missouri to 1900." *Nebraska History* 38 (June 1957): 127–54.

Morantz-Sanchez, Regina. "The Female Student Has Arrived: The Rise of the Women's Medical Movement." In *"Send Us a Lady Physician": Women Doctors in America, 1835–1920*, edited by Ruth J. Abram, 59–70. New York: W. W. Norton, 1985.

Moses, L. G., and Raymond Wilson, eds. "Introduction." In *Indian Lives: Essays on Nineteenth- and Twentieth-Century Native American Leaders*, 2d ed., 1–18. Albuquerque: University of New Mexico Press, 1993.

Murphy, Lucy Eldersveld. "Business Ladies: Midwestern Women and Enterprise, 1850–1880." *Journal of Women's History* 3 (Spring 1991): 65–89.

Nasatir, Abraham. "John Evans, Explorer and Surveyor." *Missouri Historical Review* 25 (April 1931): 432–60.

Ogbu, John. "Cultural Discontinuities and Schooling." *Anthropology and Education Quarterly* 8 (December 1982): 290–307.

O'Shea, John M., and John Ludwickson. "Omaha Chieftainship in the Nineteenth Century." *Ethnohistory* 39 (Summer 1992): 319–23.

Parker, Kay. "American Indian Women and Religion on the Southern Plains." In *Women and Religion in America: The Nineteenth Century*, vol. 1 of *Women and Religion in America*, edited by Rosemary Radford Ruether and Rosemary Skinner Keller, 48–79. San Francisco: Harper & Row, 1983.

Patterson, Victoria D. "Evolving Gender Roles in Pomo Society." In *Women and Power in Native North America*, edited by Laura F. Klein and Lillian A. Ackerman, 126–45. Norman: University Of Oklahoma Press, 1995.

Peterson, Jacqueline, and Mary Drake. "American Indian Women and Religion." In *Women and Religion in America: The Colonial and Revolutionary Periods*, vol. 2 of *Women and Religion in America*, edited by Rosemary Radford Ruether and Rosemary Skinner Keller, 1–11. San Francisco: Harper & Row, 1983.

Pool, Carolyn Garrett. "Reservation Policy and the Economic Position of Wichita Women." *Great Plains Quarterly* 8 (Summer 1988): 158–71.

Prucha, Francis Paul. "Thomas Jefferson Morgan (1889–93)." In *The Commissioners of Indian Affairs, 1824–1977*, edited by Robert M. Kvasnicka and Herman J. Viola, 193–203. Lincoln: University of Nebraska Press, 1979.

Reverby, Susan M., and Dorothy O. Helly. "Introduction: Converging on History." In *Gendered Domains: Rethinking Public and Private in Women's History*, edited by Dorothy O. Helly and Susan M. Reverby, 1–26. Ithaca, N.Y.: Cornell University Press, 1992.

Ridington, Robin. "Images of Cosmic Union: Omaha Ceremonies of Renewal." *History of Religions* 28 (November 1978): 135–50.

———. "Omaha Survival: A Vanishing Indian Tribe that would Not Vanish." *The American Indian Quarterly* 11 (Winter 1987): 37–51.

Riley, Glenda. "Some European (Mis)perceptions of American Indian Women," *New Mexico Historical Review* 59 (July 1984): 237–66.

Ritcher, Daniel K. "Cultural Brokers and Intercultural Politics: New York–Iroquois Relations, 1664–1701." *Journal of American History* 75 (June 1988): 40–67.

Rosenberg, Charles E. "American Medicine in 1879." In *"Send Us a Lady Physician": Women Doctors in America, 1835–1920*, edited by Ruth J. Abram, 21–34. New York: W. W. Norton, 1985.

Rowland, S. James, Jr.. "Susan La Flesche: Princess, Physician, Prairie Preacher." *A.D.* 4 (November 1975): 40.

Schliz, Thomas F., and Jodye L. D. Schliz. "Beads, Bangles, and Buffalo Robes: The Rise and Fall of the Indian Fur Trade Along the Missouri and Des Moines Rivers, 1720–1820." *Annals of Iowa* 49 (Summer/Fall 1987): 5–25.

Scott, Anne F. "On Seeing and Not Seeing: A Case of Historical Invisibility." *Journal of American History* 71 (June 1984): 7–21.

Sicherman, Barbara. "The Uses of a Diagnosis: Doctors, Patients, and Neurasthenia." *Journal of the History of Medicine* 32 (January 1977): 33–54.

Shoemaker, Nancy. "Introduction." In *Negotiators of Change: Historical Perspectives on Native American Women*, edited by Nancy Shoemaker, 1–25. New York: Routledge, 1995.

———. "Rise or Fall of Iroquois Women." *Journal of Women's History* 2 (Winter 1991): 39–57.

Smith, Ellen J. "Family and Community Life: Cordial Social Recognition." In *"Send Us a Lady Physician": Women Doctors in America, 1835–1920*, edited by Ruth J. Abram, 213–24. New York: W. W. Norton, 1985.

———. "Medical Societies: Lifted from the Ranks of Mere Pretenders." In *"Send Us a Lady Physician": Women Doctors in America, 1835–1920*, edited by Ruth J. Abram, 205–12. New York: W. W. Norton, 1985.

Smith, G. Hubert. "Notes on Omaha Ethnohistory, 1763–1820." *Plains Anthropologist* 18 (November 1973): 257–71.

Smits, David D. "'Squaw Men,' 'Half-Breeds,' and Amalgamators: Late Nineteenth Century Anglo-American Attitudes Toward Indian-White Race-Mixing." *American Indian Culture and Research Journal* 15, no. 3 (1991): 29–61.

Spindler, George D. "Psychocultural Adaption." In *The Study of Personality: An Interdisciplinary Appraisal*, edited by Edward Norbeck, Douglas Price-Williams, and William M. McCord, 337–43. New York: Holt, Rinehart, and Winston, 1968.

Stein, Gary C. "A Fearful Drunkenness: The Liquor Trade to the Western Indians as Seen by European Travelers in America, 1800–1860." *Red River Valley Historical Review* 1 (Summer 1974): 109–21.

Szasz, Margaret Connell. "Conclusion." In *Between Indian and White Worlds: The Cultural Broker*, edited by Margaret Connell Szasz, 294–300. Norman: University of Oklahoma Press, 1994.

———. "Introduction." In *Between Indian and White Worlds: The Cultural Broker*, edited by Margaret Connell Szasz, 3–20. Norman: University of Oklahoma Press, 1994.

———. "Native American Children." In *American Childhood: A Research Guide and Historical Handbook*, edited by Joseph M. Hawes and N. Ray Hiner, 11–42. Westport, Conn.: Greenwood Press, 1985.

Thomas, Robert K. "History of North American Indian Alcohol Use as a Community-Based Phenomenon." *Journal of Studies on Alcohol* 42, no. 9 (1981): 29–39.

Tsosie, Rebecca. "Changing Women: The Cross-Currents of American Indian Feminine Identity." *American Indian Culture and Research Journal* 12, no. 1 (1988): 1–37.

Trennert, Robert A. "Educating Indian Girls at Nonreservation Boarding Schools, 1878–1920." *Western Historical Quarterly* 13 (July 1982): 271–90.

Twin, Stephanie L. "Women and Sport." In *Sport in America: New Historical Perspectives*, edited by Donald Spivey, 193–218. Westport,Conn.: Greenwood Press, 1985.

Utley, Robert M. "The Celebrated Peace Policy of General Grant." *North Dakota History* 20 (1953): 121–42.

Van De Wetering, Maxine. "The Popular Concept of 'Home' in Nineteenth-Century America." *Journal of American Studies* 18 (April 1984): 5–28.

Welter, Barbara. "The Cult of True Womanhood, 1820–1860." *American Quarterly* 18 (Summer 1966): 151–74.

_____. "She Hath Done What She Could: Protestant Women's Missionary Careers in Nineteenth-Century America." *American Quarterly* 30 (Winter 1978): 624–38.

White, Richard. "The Winning of the West: The Expansion of the Western Sioux in the Eighteenth and Nineteenth Centuries." *Journal of American History* 65 (September 1978): 319–43.

Winkler, Allan M. "Drinking on the American Frontier." *Quarterly Journal of Studies on Alcohol* 29, no. 6 (1968): 413–45.

Wolcott, Harry F. "The Teacher as an Enemy." In *Education and Cultural Process: Toward an Anthropology of Education*, edited by George D. Spindler, 411–25. New York: Holt, Rinehart, and Winston, 1974.

Wood, W. Raymond. "Plains Trade in Prehistoric and Protohistorical Intertribal Relations." In *Anthropology on the Great Plains*, edited by W. Raymond Wood and Margot Liberty, 98–109. Lincoln: University of Nebraska Press, 1980.

Wright, Mary C. "Economic Development and Native American Women in the Early Nineteenth Century." *American Quarterly* 33 (Fall 1981): 525–536.

Books

Adams, David Wallace. *Education for Extinction: American Indians and the Boarding School Experience, 1875–1928*. Lawrence: University Press of Kansas, 1995.

Alsop, Gulielma Fell. *History of the Woman's Medical College, Philadelphia, Pennsylvania, 1850–1950*. Philadelphia: J. B. Lippincott, n.d.

Anderson, Karen. *Changing Woman: A History of Racial Ethnic Women in Modern America*. New York: Oxford University Press, 1996.

Bannan, Helen M. *"True Womanhood" on the Reservation: Field Matrons in the United States Indian Service*. Tucson: University of Arizona Southwest Institute for Research on Women, 1984.

Berg, Barbara J. *The Remembered Gate: Origins of American Feminism: The Woman and the City, 1800–1860*. New York: Oxford University Press, 1978.

Berkhofer, Robert F., Jr. *Salvation and Savage: An Analysis of Protestant Missions and American Indian Response, 1787–1862*. Lexington: University Press of Kentucky, 1965.

Blair, Karen J. *Clubwoman as Feminist: True Womanhood Redefined, 1868–1914*. New York: Holmes & Meier, 1980.

Blocker, Jack S., Jr. *American Temperance Movements: Cycles of Reform*. Boston: Twayne, 1989.

Bordin, Ruth. *Woman and Temperance: The Quest for Power and Liberty, 1873–1900*. Philadelphia: Temple University Press, 1981.

Cavallo, Dominick. *Muscles and Morals: Organized Playgrounds and Urban Reform, 1880–1920*. Philadelphia: University of Pennsylvania Press, 1981.

Chambers, John Whiteclay, II. *The Tyranny of Change: America in the Progressive Era, 1900–1917*. New York: St. Martin's Press, 1980.

Cogan, Frances B. *All-American Girl: The Ideal of Real Womanhood in Mid-Nineteenth-Century America*. Athens: University Of Georgia Press, 1989.

Coleman, Michael C. *Presbyterian Missionary Attitudes toward American Indians, 1837–1893*. Jackson: University Press of Mississippi, 1985.

Cott, Nancy. *The Bonds of Womanhood: "Woman's Sphere" in New England, 1780–1835*. New Haven: Yale University Press, 1987.

Crary, Margaret. *Susette La Flesche: Voice of the Omaha Indians*. New York: Hawthorn Books, 1973.

Cutter, Irving S. *Dr. John Gale, A Pioneer Army Surgeon*. Springfield, Ill.: Schnepp & Barnes, 1931.

DeJong, David H. *Promises of the Past: A History of Indian Education in the United States*. Golden, Colo.: North American Press, 1993.

Devens, Carol. *Countering Civilization: Native American Women and Great Lakes Missions, 1630–1900*. Berkeley: University of California Press, 1992.

Dippie, Brian W. *The Vanishing American: White Attitudes and U.S. Indian Policy*. Lawrence: University Press of Kansas, 1982.

Dublin, Thomas, ed. *Becoming American, Becoming Ethnic: College Students Explore Their Roots*. Philadelphia: Temple University Press, 1996.

Duffy, John. *From Humors to Medical Science: A History of American Medicine*. Urbana: University of Illinois Press, 1993.

Epstein, Barbara Leslie. *The Politics of Domesticity: Women, Evangelism, and Temperance in Nineteenth-Century America*. Middletown, Conn.: Wesleyan University Press, 1981.

Ferris, Jeri. *Native American Doctor: The Story of Susan La Flesche Picotte*. Minneapolis: Carolrhoda Books, 1991.

Fritz, Henry E. *The Movement for Indian Assimilation, 1860–1890*. Philadelphia: University of Pennsylvania Press, 1963.

Galishoff, Stuart. *Safeguarding the Public Health: Newark, 1895–1918*. Westport, Conn.: Greenwood Press, 1975.

Giele, Janet Zollinger. *Two Paths to Women's Equality: Temperance, Suffrage, and the Origins of Modern Feminism*. New York: Twayne Publishers, 1995.

Goodman, Cary. *Choosing Sides: Playground and Street Life on the Lower East Side*. New York: Schocken Books, 1979.

Green, Norma Kidd. *Iron Eye's Family: The Children of Joseph La Flesche*. Lincoln: Nebraska State Historical Society, 1969.

Guttmann, Allen. *Women's Sports: A History*. New York: Columbia University Press, 1991.

Hagan, William T. *Indian Police and Judges: Experiments in Acculturation and Control*. New Haven: Yale University Press, 1966.

Hailmann, William N. *Education of the Indian*. Monographs on Education in the U.S., no. 19. St. Louis: Division of Exhibits, Department of Education, Universal Exposition, 1904.

Harrison, Tinsley Randolph. *Principles of Internal Medicine*. 7th ed. New York: McGraw Hill, 1974.

Heritage of Bancroft, Nebraska, 1884–1954. N.p.: The Heritage Book Committee, 1984.

Hertzberg, Hazel W. *The Search for an American Identity: Modern Pan-Indian Movements*. Syracuse, N.Y.: Syracuse University Press, 1971.

Hofstadter, Richard. *Social Darwinism in American Thought*, rev. ed. New York: George Braziller, 1959.

Holder, Preston. *The Hoe and the Horse on the Plains: A Study of Cultural Development among North American Indians*. Lincoln: University of Nebraska Press, 1970.

Hoxie, Frederick E. *A Final Promise: The Campaign to Assimilate the Indians, 1880–1920*. Lincoln: University of Nebraska Press, 1984.

Hultkrantz, Ake. *Native Religions of North America: The Power of Visions and Fertility.* San Francisco: Harper & Row, 1987.

_____. *Shamanic Healing and Ritual Drama: Health and Medicine in Native American Religious Traditions.* New York: Crossroads Publishing, 1992.

Hyde, George E. *The Pawnee Indians.* Norman: University of Oklahoma Press, 1951.

Indian Voices: The First Convocation of American Indian Scholars San Francisco: Indian Historian Press, 1970.

Iverson, Peter. *Carlos Montezuma and the Changing World of American Indians.* Albuquerque: University of New Mexico Press, 1982.

Jablow, Joseph. *Ethnohistory of the Ponca.* New York: Garland Publishing, 1974.

Kaufman, Polly Welts. *National Parks and the Woman's Voice: A History.* Albuquerque: University of New Mexico Press, 1996.

Keller, Robert H., Jr. *American Protestantism and United States Indian Policy, 1869–82.* Lincoln: University of Nebraska Press, 1983.

Kerr, K. Austin. *Organized for Prohibition: A New History of the Anti-Saloon League.* New Haven, Conn.: Yale University Press, 1985.

Kessler-Harris, Alice. *Out to Work: A History of Wage-Earning Women in the United States.* New York: Oxford University Press, 1982.

La Barre, Weston. *The Peyote Cult.* 5th ed. Norman: University of Oklahoma Press, 1989.

Leach, William. *True Love and Perfect Union: The Feminist Reform of Sex and Society.* 2d ed. Middletown, Conn.: Wesleyan University Press, 1989.

Leavitt, Judith Walker. *The Healthiest City: Milwaukee and the Politics of Health Reform.* Princeton, N.J.: Princeton University Press, 1982.

Lindsey, Donal F. *Indians at Hampton Institute, 1877–1923.* Urbana: University of Illinois Press, 1995.

Lomawaima, K. Tsianina. *They Called it Prairie Light: The Story of Chilocco Indian School.* Lincoln: University of Nebraska Press, 1994.

Lopate, Carol. *Women in Medicine.* Baltimore: Johns Hopkins University Press, 1968.

McDonnell, Janet A. *The Dispossession of the American Indian, 1887–1934.* Bloomington: Indiana University Press, 1991.

Mark, Joan. *A Stranger in Her Native Land: Alice Fletcher and the American Indians.* Lincoln: University of Nebraska Press, 1984.

Marty, Martin E. *Righteous Empire: The Protestant Experience in America.* New York: Dial Press, 1970.

Matthews, Glenna. *"Just a Housewife": The Rise and Fall of Domesticity in America.* New York: Oxford University Press, 1987.

Milner, Clyde A., II. *With Good Intentions: Quaker Work among the Pawnees, Otos, and Omahas in the 1870s.* Lincoln: University of Nebraska Press, 1982.

Moldow, Gloria. *Women Doctors in Gilded-Age Washington: Race, Gender, and Professionalization.* Urbana: University of Illinois Press, 1987.

Morantz-Sanchez, Regina M. *Sympathy and Science: Women Physicians in American Medicine.* New York: Oxford University Press, 1985.

Nasatir, Abraham P., ed. *Before Lewis and Clark: Documents Illustrating the History of the Missouri, 1783–1804,* 2 vols. St. Louis: St. Louis Historical Documents Foundation, 1952.

Oates, Stephen B. *Biography as History.* Waco: Markham Press Fund, 1991.

————, ed. *Biography as High Adventure: Life-Writers Speak on Their Art.* Amherst: University of Massachusetts Press, 1986.

Orr, H. Winnett. *Selected Pages from the History of Medicine in Nebraska.* Lincoln: n.p., 1952.

O'Shea, John M., and John Ludwickson. *Archaeology and Ethnohistory of the Omaha Indians: The Big Village Site.* Lincoln: University of Nebraska Press, 1992.

Otis, Delos Socket. *The Dawes Act and the Allotment of Indian Lands.* Edited by Francis Paul Prucha. Norman: University of Oklahoma Press, 1973.

Painter, Orrin C. *William Painter and His Father, Dr. Edward Painter: Sketches and Reminiscences.* Baltimore: Arundel Press, 1914.

Pascoe, Peggy. *Relations of Rescue: The Search for Female Moral Authority in the American West, 1874–1939.* New York: Oxford University Press, 1990.

Peabody, Francis Greenwood. *Education for Life: The Story of Hampton Institute.* Garden City, N.Y.: Doubleday, 1919.

Peterson, Jacqueline, and Jennifer S. H. Brown, eds. *The New Peoples: Being and Becoming Métis in North America.* Lincoln: University of Nebraska Press, 1985.

Pioneer-Pacesetter-Innovator: The Story of the Medical College of Pennsylvania. New York: Newcomen Society in North America, 1971.

Powers, Marla N. Oglala *Women: Myth, Ritual, and Reality.* Chicago: University of Chicago Press, 1986.

Prucha, Francis Paul. *American Indian Policy in Crisis: Christian Reformers and the Indian, 1865–1900.* Norman: University of Oklahoma Press, 1976.

_____. *American Indian Policy in the Formative Years: The Indian Trade and Intercourse Acts, 1790–1834*. Cambridge: Harvard University Press, 1962.

_____. *The Great Father: The United States Government and the American Indians*. 2 vols. Lincoln: University of Nebraska Press, 1984.

Raup, Ruth M. *The Indian Health Program from 1800 to 1955*. Washington, D.C.: U.S. Public Health Service, Division of Indian Health, 1955.

Riley, Glenda. *The Female Frontier: A Comparative View of Women on the Prairie and the Plains*. Lawrence: University Press of Kansas, 1988.

Rosen, George A. *A History of Public Health*. New York: MD Publications, 1957.

_____. *Preventive Medicine in the United States, 1900–1975: Trends and Interpretations*. New York: Science History Publications, 1975.

Rosenberg, Rosalind. *Beyond Separate Spheres: Intellectual Roots of Modern Feminism*. New Haven: University of Yale Press, 1982.

Rumbarger, John J. *Profits, Power, and Prohibition: Alcohol Reform and the Industrializing of America, 1800–1930*. Albany: State University of New York Press, 1989.

Scott, Anne Firor. *Natural Allies: Women's Associations in American History*. Urbana: University of Illinois Press, 1991.

Sheldon, Addison E. *Land Systems and Land Policies in Nebraska*. Publications of the Nebraska State Historical Society, vol. 22. Lincoln: Nebraska State Historical Society, 1936.

Shyrock, Richard H. *Medicine in America: Historical Essays*. Baltimore: Johns Hopkins University Press, 1966.

Sixty Years of Nebraska Federation of Women's Clubs, Inc., 1894–1954. Lincoln: n.p., 1954.

Sklar, Kathryn Kish. *Catharine Beecher: A Study in American Domesticity*. New York: W. W. Norton, 1973.

Slotkin, J. S. *The Peyote Religion*. Glencoe, Ill.: Free Press, 1956.

Smith, Elias D. *The School Interests of Elizabeth, A City of New Jersey, U.S.A.* Elizabeth, N.J.: n.p., 1911.

Smith, Henry Nash. *Virgin Land: The American West as Symbol and Myth*. New York: Vintage Books, 1950.

Smith, Sherry L. *The View from Officers' Row*. Tucson: University of Arizona Press, 1990.

Soper, J. Christopher. *Evangelical Christianity in the United States and Great Britain: Religious Beliefs, Political Choices*. New York: New York University Press, 1994.

BIBLIOGRAPHY

Spector, Janet D. What *This Awl Means: Feminist Archaeology at a Wahpeton Dakota Village*. St. Paul: Minnesota Historical Society Press, 1993.

Stern, Theodore. *The Klamath Tribe: A People and Their Reservation*. Seattle: University of Washington Press, 1965.

Stewart, Omer C. *Peyote Religion: A History*. Norman: University of Oklahoma Press, 1987.

Szasz, Margaret Connell. *Education and the American Indian: The Road to Self-Determination since 1928*. Albuquerque: University of New Mexico Press, 1977.

Talbot, Edith Armstrong. *Samuel Chapman Armstrong: A Biographical Study*. New York: Doubleday, Page, 1904.

Timberlake, James H. *Prohibition and the Progressive Movement, 1900–1920*. Cambridge: Harvard University Press, 1963.

Trennert, Robert A., Jr. *Alternative to Extinction: Federal Indian Policy and the Beginnings of the Reservation System, 1846–51*. Philadelphia: Temple University Press, 1975.

Tyler, Albert F., ed. *History of Medicine in Nebraska*. Omaha: Magic City Printing, 1977.

Tyrell, Ian. *Woman's World, Woman's Empire: The Woman's Christian Temperance Union in International Perspective, 1880–1930*. Chapel Hill: University of North Carolina Press, 1991.

Verbrugge, Martha. *Able-Bodied Womanhood: Personal Health and Social Change in Nineteenth-Century Boston*. New York: Oxford University Press, 1988.

Walsh, Mary Roth. *"Doctors Wanted: No Women Need Apply": Sexual Barriers in the Medical Profession, 1835–1975*. New Haven: Yale University Press, 1977.

Washburn, Wilcomb E. *The Assault on Indian Tribalism: The General Allotment Law (Dawes Act) of 1887*. Edited by Harold H. Hyman. Philadelphia: Lippincott, 1975.

Weaver, John Ernest. *Native Vegetation of Nebraska*. Lincoln: University of Nebraska Press, 1965.

Wells, Mildred W. *Unity in Diversity: The History of the General Federation of Women's Clubs*. N.p.: General Federation of Women's Clubs, 1953.

White, Richard. *The Roots of Dependency: Subsistence, Environment, and Social Change among the Choctaws, Pawnees, and Navajos*. Lincoln: University of Nebraska Press, 1983.

Wilson, Raymond. *Ohiyesa: Charles Eastman, Santee Sioux*. Urbana: University of Illinois Press, 1983.

Wishart, David J. *The Fur Trade of the American West, 1807–1840: A Geographical Synthesis.* Lincoln: University of Nebraska Press, 1979.

_____. *An Unspeakable Sadness: The Dispossession of the Nebraska Indians.* Lincoln: University of Nebraska Press, 1994.

Young, T. Kue. *The Health of Native Americans: Toward a Biocultural Epidemiology.* New York: Oxford University Press, 1994.

Index

(La Flesche, Francis, *continued*)
employee, 48; as interpreter, 44;
Omaha dispossession and, 109–10
La Flesche, Joseph (Iron Eye/E-sta-
ma-za), 25, 78, 117; acculturation
and, 15, 17–18, 25; allotment and,
18, 42, 174–75; as cultural broker,
11, 13, 19; birthdate, 10;
chieftainship of, 13–14, 24; death
of, 81–82, 115; education and, 16;
farming and, 16, 22, 27; Mary Gale
and, 13; Omaha Indians' rights and,
18; parents' background, 9;
polygamy and, 18; prohibition and,
17–18, 117; Quaker day schools
and, 40; Susan La Flesche and, 15,
28, 31, 55, 191–92, 194;
temperance and, 17, 107, 117;
traditionalism and, 17–18
La Flesche, Joseph, Sr., 9
La Flesche, Lucy, 51, 121
La Flesche, Marguerite, 20, 41, 48,
77, 80, 82, 99, 101, 117, 189, 191,
194, 197
La Flesche, Noah, 51, 121, 157
La Flesche, Susan, 3, 7, 20, 75; Alice
C. Fletcher and, 43–44, 55, 60–62,
65, 103, 191; as agency physician,
86, 93–99; as assistant teacher,
43–44; as health inspector, 179–80;
as interpreter, 94, 153–55, 163; as
medical missionary, 123–26; as
missionary society president,
126–27; as school physician,
87–91, 99–100; assimilation and,
20, 53, 82; bicultural identity of,
51–53, 75, 82, 89, 101, 158, 186,
192; buffalo hunt and, 5; birthdate
of, 22; calisthenics and, 75; career
goals of, 64–66; childhood play of,
28–29; Christianity and, 34, 39, 52,
64–65, 75, 106–107; "civilization"
and, 64, 76, 99, 109, 124; coercive

anti-drinking methods and, 107,
111, 114–15, 121, 124, 127;
Connecticut Indian Association
and, 61, 65–67, 70, 83–85, 89, 92,
100, 102, 186–87; consolidation
plan and, 160–69, 197; cultural
brokerage and, 26, 44, 53, 56,
63–66, 82–83, 89, 94, 105, 113,
124, 153–56, 161, 163–64, 169,
188, 196; cultural mediation, *see*
cultural brokerage; death of, 190;
Elizabeth Institute for Young
Ladies and, 140–42;
entrepreneurship and, 149–53, 197;
Euro-American gender roles and,
64–65, 151, 162, 164; Euro-
American images of, 41, 85;
evangelism of, 34, 52, 75, 106,
123–26; family's health and,
77–78, 81–82; family lands and,
174–75; field matron program and,
122; funding for medical education
of, 57–58, 60–61, 65, 67, 70;
Gallagher Bill and, 174; Hampton
Institute education of, 49, 47, 52,
54–55; Henry Picotte and,
100–103, 121–22, 147; in defense
of Omaha Indians, 64, 88, 94, 109,
113, 115, 118, 166, 168–72; in
defense of Omaha Indians' rights,
64, 85, 88, 105, 153, 156–59,
161–63; in defense of
traditionalism, 53, 66, 80, 89, 99,
186, 197; land disputes and,
147–53, 174–75; legacy of,
197–99; "mark of honor" and, 25;
marriage and, 100–102; medical
college education of, 71–75;
medical college graduation of, 84;
Omaha Indians, western medicine
and, 81, 83, 91–92, 96; medical
internship of, 84–85; motherhood
and, 101–102; motivation for

medical education and, 55–57;
Nebraska Federation of Women's
Clubs and, 181–85; Office of
Indian Affairs (OIA) bureaucracy
and, 70, 93–96, 147–54, 165–66,
169–70, 174–75; OIA paternalism
and, 64, 158–61, 165–66, 169–71,
175, 195, 197; Omaha Indians'
alcoholism and, 106, 108, 110–11,
114–15, 118, 120, 122, 124–25,
132; Omaha language and, 51;
Omaha Tribal Council and, 104,
111, 115; Omaha Indians'
competency and, 147–48, 154,
159–61, 166, 169–70, 172, 174;
oratorical skills of, 65, 76, 120,
184; organized-play movement
and, 178; parents' influence on, 12,
15, 28; personal ambition of, 77,
101, 105, 123–24, 175, 180,
192–93; personal health of, 99,
102, 104–105, 123, 168, 189;
peyotism and, 129–31; physical
appearance of, 42; Presbyterian
education of, 31, 34–35; preventive
health and, 78, 90, 96–98, 177,
182; prohibition and, 106, 111,
113–16, 118–20, 122–23, 127, 132;
public health movement and,
177–78, 181; published writings of,
21–22, 26–31, 34, 38, 53, 63–65,
74, 87–88, 104, 112–14, 119,
124–25; Quaker education of,
37–38; Quakerism and, 39;
reservation hospital and, 76,
185–90; salutatorian address of,
162–65; self-employment and,
102–103; self-pride of, 77, 81, 105,
175–76, 180, 198; sons of, 102–13,
143, 148, 190, 197–98; temperance
and, 52, 75, 106, 125; Thomas
Ikinicapi and, 78–79, 100;
traditional education of, 26–27;

traditional gender roles
and, 6, 9, 26–27, 57, 91, 164;
traditional medicine and, 26; trival
factionalism and, 23, 38, 116–17,
123, 161, 164, 175, 195–97; tribal
leadership of, 161, 175, 194;
tributes for, 190–91; tuberculosis
and, 97–99, 182–85; "turning of the
child ceremony" and, 25;
upbringing of, 22, 26–27, 29–30;
Walthill health board and, 178–79.
See also American Indian women;
Connecticut Indian Association;
"Indian Princess"; Omaha Indians;
Omaha reservation
La Flesche, Rosalie, 20, 47, 52, 63,
68, 73, 76–77, 79, 100, 102–103,
117, 121
La Flesche, Susette ("Bright Eyes"/
Inshtatheamba), 21, 25, 28, 39,
194; and Eastern education, 40,
174, 197; political activism of,
40–41
Lake Mohonk, N.Y., 62
Latter-Day Saints (Mormons), 14
Lend-a-Hand Club, 52. *See also* La
Flesche, Susan, Christianity and
Leupp, Francis E., 124, 147–48,
150–52, 183, 187
Levering, Louis, 109, 172
Lewis, Meriwether, 7
Lincoln Institute, Philadelphia, Pa.,
76
Lockrey, Sarah, 75
Lonesome Trail, The, 186
Lyons, Nebr., 104

Macy, Nebr., 124, 126, 154, 165, 166
Maize ritual song, 4. *See also* Omaha
Indians, religiosity of
Manifest Destiny, 14–15, 23
"Manly detachment," 59
Marshall, Clara, 59, 73

Public health movement, 177–78, 181.
　See also La Flesche, Susan, public
　health movement and
"Quaker Policy." *See* United States,
　Peace Policy
Quakers. *See* Society of Friends
Quapaw Indians, 4
Quinton, Amelia S., 91

Ramona, 86
Read, Nettie C., 41
Reid, Jane, 74
Rolph, I. R., 33
Roosevelt, Theodore, 127, 160
Russell Sage Foundation, 182

Sac and Fox Indians, 20
Sacred bundles, 26
Sacred Legend, 3–4, 8, 30. *See also*
　Omaha Indians, religiosity of
Sacred Pole, 24. *See also* Omaha
　Indians, religiosity of
St. Louis, Mo., 11
St. Nicholas Magazine, 21
Sam (schoolmate), 52
Sand Creek Massacre, 35–36
Sarpy, Peter A., 9, 12
Sauk Indians, 7
Sioux Indians, 10, 13, 20, 30, 101,
　153
Sloan, Thomas, 109, 157–58
Smith, Harriet Whitehall, 107
Smith College, 48
Sniffen, Matthew K., 157
Social Darwinism, 20, 42, 45
Social Evolution, 45, 50, 64. *See also*
　Social Darwinism
Society of American Indians, 88
Society of Friends: American Indians
　and, 39; Hicksite Friends of, 37;
　Inner Light and, 39; and Omaha
　day schools, 37–38, 40

Southern Workman
Standing Bear (Ponca chief), 40
Standing Bear decision, 114
Sun Dance, 129
Susan La Flesche Picotte Center, 198
Szasz, Margaret Connell, 196

Ta–in–ne, 18
Taft, William Howard, 159
Talcott, Seth, 65, 68
Talks and Thoughts, 114
Taylor, R. J., 148–53
Temperance. *See* La Flesche, Susan,
　prohibition and; La Flesche, Susan,
　temperance and; Omaha Indians,
　prohibition among; Omaha
　reservation, prohibition on
Thurston County, 112, 159
Thurston County Medical Society,
　178
Tinker, Arthur M., 93
Trade and Intercourse Acts, 112
Treaty of Prairie de Chien, 13, 15, 31
Trennert, Robert, A. Jr., 14
Turner, Joel, 154
Two Crows (Omaha tribal policeman),
　17
Tyndall, Mary, 76

Uk'ite, 6, 8, 164
United States: Congress, 42; House of
　Representatives, 131; westward
　expansion of, 8–10, 14–15, 23–24.
　See also United States government
United States government,
　Americanization policy of, 21,
　44–45, 48, 54, 122, 131; army of,
　11; assimilation and, 20–21, 36, 54,
　174; "concentration" policy of, 15,
　23, 44; American Indians' higher
　education and, 57–58, 86; "Peace
　Policy" of, 35–36, 40; purchase of
　Lousiana by, 8

INDEX

Upshaw, Alexander, 70

"Upstream People," 3–4, 6–7, 10. *See also* Omaha Indians; Omaha reservation

Valentine, Robert G., 156, 158, 160, 164–65, 168, 171, 187

"Wa-han-the-shu-gae," 29
Wade, Margaret C., 44
Wajapa, 113
Wakon'da, 38, 25
Waldron, Martha W., 60, 62
Walker, James, 84
Walter (schoolmate), 47
Walthill, Nebr., 126–27, 155, 190, 196
Walthill Times, 178–79, 189–91
Waterbury, Conn., 84
Wathin'ethe, 13
Wa tun-na (Susan's grandmother), 9
Wa'wan, 6
Webster, Daniel, 168
Welsh, Herbert, 119
White Horse (Omaha leader), 171
White, Luke, 154
Wickersham, George W., 168
Willard, Francis, 107
Winnebago Indians, 18–19, 23, 166–67

Winona Lodge, 48–49
Winsted, Conn., 84
Wolf, Dan, 153–54
Wolf, James, 158
Woman's Hospital of Pennsylvania, 71, 84–85
Women, prescriptive ideology for, 5, 33–34, 37, 58–60, 66. *See also* "Cult of true womanhood"
Women's Clubs movement, 179
Women's Medical College of Pennyslvania, 44, 46, 55, 58–60, 67; curriculum of, 71–72; entrance requirements of, 71; physical description of, 69; mission of, 69. See also La Flesche, Susan, medical college education of
Women's National Indian Association, 61, 112–13, 115, 185–86; mission of, 61; and Omaha mission, 90–91. *See also* Connecticut Indian Association; La Flesche, Susan, Connecticut Indian Association and
Women physicians, opposition to, 58–59, 91; societal expectations for, 92; support for, 59–60

Young Elk (Omaha chief), 13–14
Yankton Sioux Indians, 4, 7, 101, 151, 153

— *285* —